AF478640

Progress in
AIDS Pathology

VOLUME I

Progress in
AIDS Pathology

VOLUME I

Edited by

Heidrun Rotterdam, M.D.
Associate Professor of Surgical Pathology
New York University Medical Center
New York, NY

Sheldon C. Sommers, M.D.
Clinical Professor of Pathology
Columbia University College of Physicians & Surgeons
New York, NY
Clinical Professor of Pathology
University of Southern California School of Medicine
Los Angeles, CA

with the assistance of
Paul Raćz, M.D.
Bernhard–Nocht–Institut
Hamburg, West Germany
Paul R. Meyer, M.D.
University of Southern California
Los Angeles, CA

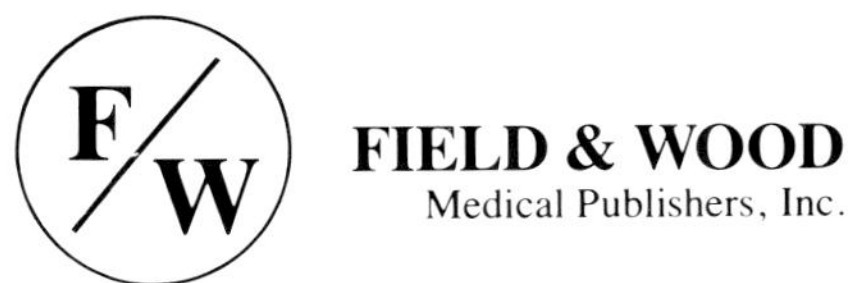

FIELD & WOOD
Medical Publishers, Inc.

Distributed by W. W. Norton & Company, Inc.

500 Fifth Avenue, New York, NY 10110

Distributed by:

W. W. Norton & Company, Inc.
500 Fifth Avenue
New York, New York 10110

ISBN 0-938607-21-9
ISSN 1042-363X

Printed in the United States of America

Printing: 1 2 3 4 5 6 7 8 9 10

Contents

Contributors

Slobodan N. Aleksic, M.D.
Department of Neurology
New York University–Bellevue Hospital Medical Center
New York, NY

Karl H. Anders, M.D.
Department of Pathology
Kaiser-Permanente Hospital
Woodland Hills, CA

Ann Avitabile, M.D.
Department of Pathology
Roosevelt Hospital–St. Luke's Medical Center
New York, NY

Jay H. Beckstead, M.D.
Department of Pathology
University of California School of Medicine
San Francisco, CA

Ira J. Bleiweiss, M.D.
Immunopathology Laboratory
Veterans Administration Medical Center
Bronx, NY
Department of Pathology
Mount Sinai School of Medicine
New York, NY

Gleb N. Budzilovich, M.D.
Department of Pathology
New York University–Bellevue Hospital Medical Center
New York, NY

Russell K. Byrnes, M.D.
Department of Pathology
University of Southern California
Los Angeles, CA

Barbara Chaitin, M.D.
Department of Pathology
Lenox Hill Hospital
New York, NY

Wing C. Chan, M.B., B.S.
Department of Pathology and Laboratory Medicine
Emory University School of Medicine
Atlanta, GA

Francis W. Chandler, M.D.
Experimental Pathology Branch
Division of Host Factors
Center for Infectious Diseases
Centers for Disease Control
Atlanta, GA

Eun-Sook Cho, M.D.
Department of Pathology
UMD–New Jersey Medical School
Newark, NJ

Manfred Dietrich, M.D.
Department of Medicine
Bernhard-Nocht-Institut
für Schiffs- und Tropenkrankheiten
Hamburg, West Germany

Edwin P. Ewing, Jr., M.D.
Experimental Pathology Branch
Divison of Host Factors
Center for Infectious Diseases
Centers for Disease Control
Atlanta, GA

Cheryl P. Frydman, M.D.
Immunopathology Laboratory
Veterans Administration Medical Center
Bronx, NY
Department of Pathology
Mount Sinai School of Medicine
New York, NY

Suzanne Gartner, M.D.
National Institutes of Health
National Cancer Institute
Bethesda, MD

Stephen A. Geller, M.D.
Department of Pathology and Laboratory Medicine
Cedars-Sinai Medical Center
Los Angeles, CA

Jean-Claude Gluckman, M.D.
Laboratoire d'Immunologie,
Nephrologie et Transplantation
UFR Pitie-Salpétriere
Paris, France

Miroslaw K. Gorny, M.D.
Department of Clinical Pathomorphology
Academy of Medicine
Poznan, Poland

Elliot Gross, M.D.
Former Chief Medical Examiner
of the City of New York, NY

Jaishree Jagidar, M.D.
Immunopathology Laboratory
Veterans Administration Medical Center
Bronx, NY
Department of Pathology
Mount Sinai School of Medicine
New York, NY

Joseph Jankovic, M.D.
Department of Neurology
Baylor College of Medicine
Houston, TX

Stephen C. Joseph, M.D., M.P.H.
Commissioner of Health
New York, NY

Vijay V. Joshi, M.D.
Department of Pathology
Children's Hospital for New Jersey
United Hospitals Medical Center
Newark, NJ

Edward C. Klatt, M.D.
Department of Pathology
University of Southern California
Los Angeles, CA

Ernest E. Lack, M.D.
Laboratory of Pathology
National Cancer Institute
National Institutes of Health
Bethesda, MD

Paul R. Meyer, M.D.
Department of Pathology
University of Southern California
Los Angeles, CA

Avindra Nath, M.D.
Department of Neurology
University of Texas Health Science Center
Houston, TX

George Niedt, M.D.
Department of Dermatopathology
New York Hospital
Cornell Medical Center
New York, NY

Frederick P. Ognibene, M.D.
Critical Care Medicine Department
National Institutes of Health
Bethesda, MD

Jan Marc Orenstein, M.D., Ph.D
Department of Pathology
George Washington University Medical Center
Washington, D.C.

Abraham Pinter, M.D.
New York City Department of Health
Public Health Research Institute
New York, NY

Mikulas Popovic, M.D.
Laboratory of Tumor Cell Biology
National Institutes of Health
National Cancer Institute
Bethesda, MD

Paul Raćz, M.D.
Department of Pathology & Körber
Laboratory for AIDS Research
Bernhard-Nocht-Institut für
Schiffs- und Tropenkrankheiten
Hamburg, West Germany

Julia Ramsauer, M.D.
Department of Pathology & Körber
Laboratory for AIDS Research
Bernhard-Nocht-Institut für
Schiffs- und Tropenkrankheiten
Hamburg, West Germany

Roy H. Rhodes, Ph.D, M.D.
Department of Pathology
University of Southern California
School of Medicine
Los Angeles, CA

Marc K. Rosenblum, M.D.
Department of Pathology
Memorial Sloan-Kettering Cancer Center
New York, NY

Roger Schinella, M.D.
Department of Pathology
New York University–Bellevue Hospital Medical Center
New York, NY

Richard S. Schulof, M.D., Ph.D.
Department of Medicine
George Washington University Medical Center
Washington, D.C.

Leroy R. Sharer, M.D.
Department of Pathology
UMD-New Jersey Medical School
Newark, NJ

James Shelhamer, M.D.
Critical Care Medicine Department
National Institutes of Health
Bethesda, MD

Anthony F. Suffredini, M.D.
Critical Care Medicine Department
National Institutes of Health
Bethesda, MD

Klara Tenner-Rácz, M.D.
Department of Hematology
Allgemeines Krankenhaus St. Georg
Hamburg, West Germany

Uwamie Tomiyasu, M.D.
Laboratory Services (Pathology)
Wadsworth Veterans Administration Hospital
Los Angeles, CA

William D. Travis, M.D.
Laboratory of Pathology
National Cancer Institute
National Institutes of Health
Bethesda, MD

Harry V. Vinters, M.D.
Department of Pathology (Neuropathology)
UCLA Medical Center
Los Angeles, CA

Jerrold M. Ward, D.V.M., Ph.D.
Tumor Pathology & Pathogenesis Section
Laboratory of Comparative Carcinogenesis
Division of Cancer Etiology
National Cancer Institute
Frederick, MD

Ok H. Yoo, M.D.
Department of Pulmonary Medicine
Veterans Administration Medical Center
Bronx, NY
Mount Sinai School of Medicine
New York, NY

Susan Zolla-Pazner, M.D.
Department of Pathology
Veterans Administration Medical Center
New York, NY

Preface

We have come to recognize, since the initial description of AIDS in July of
1981, that clinical symptoms are not reflected by specific morphologic
findings and that the complications, in particular the opportunistic infections, are more relevant to the diagnosis than morphologic changes in
lymphoid organs, as one would expect from the action of a lymphotropic
virus. Furthermore, the spectrum of complicating diseases, infections as
well as tumors, has undergone continuous change and has widened to
include hitherto poorly known or unknown conditions. Pathologists need
to keep abreast of new developments and be aware that an old, well known
condition may acquire a new appearance, in patients with AIDS.

Progress in AIDS offers a forum to diagnostic pathologists and researchers dealing with AIDS to discuss their findings and thoughts, thus
enabling the pathology community at large to keep up to date with the ever
changing manifestations of this protean disease. It is also hoped that the
greater the familiarity with the facts of the disease the more the hysteria
spreading in lay as well as medical communities will be kept under control.

There are overviews of the histopathology of AIDS in general, as well as
of single organ systems in specific. Much emphasis is placed on the nervous
system, which has evolved as one of the major target organs of the human
immunodeficiency virus (HIV). Various aspects of the HIV virus per se are
discussed, including tissue changes, immunologic parameters, and possible
applications of the latter in predicting disease outcome or determining
treatment. New techniques applicable to the diagnosis of certain infections
are shown to open new perspectives to their pathogenesis.

1

The Histopathology of HIV Infection: An Overview

Russell K. Brynes
Edwin P. Ewing, Jr.
Vijay V. Joshi
Wing C. Chan

MANY HISTOLOGIC ALTERATIONS are associated with symptomatic human immunodeficiency virus (HIV) infections. Some are related directly to the virus, such as changes in lymph nodes, blood, and bone marrow. Others are strictly secondary to immune deficiency, and include certain neoplasms and opportunistic infections that are particularly characteristic of the acquired immune deficiency syndrome (AIDS). A few changes are, as yet, of uncertain classification. None of these tissue changes are diagnostic of AIDS by themselves, but together with an appropriate clinical history and/or a positive serologic test for HIV infection, they can help establish a diagnosis of AIDS or AIDS-related complex (ARC). Histopathologic findings also correlate well with laboratory tests of immunologic function and are useful in the assessment of disease progression. Finally, early histologic detection of secondary diseases permits institution of appropriate therapy.

PRIMARY HISTOPATHOLOGY

Lymph Nodes

For many individuals a syndrome of persistent generalized lymphadenopathy (PGL) represents an early, often mild manifestation of HIV infection. The lymph node is a focus of interest in PGL because of its conspicuous enlargement, its relatively easy surgical access, and the likelihood that it represents a major anatomic site of T-helper cell destruction by HIV.

Lymph node histology in PGL and in AIDS extends across a wide spectrum of microscopic changes ranging from florid lymphoid hyperplasia to marked lymphoid depletion. These changes occur serially, and serve as morphologic evidence of progressive damage to the immune system.[1] Three histologic patterns are recognized, and have been arbitrarily designated Type I, Type II

1

and Type III.[2,3] Type I and Type II patterns may be associated with PGL or AIDS, while Type III is characteristic of fatal AIDS.

In Type I morphology (Fig. 1), the normal architecture is altered by a profound hyperplasia of mitotically active germinal centers that expand the cortical zone, and often appear in deeper parts of the lymph node as well. Because germinal centers can vary in size and shape, they may sometimes appear confluent. Interfollicular tissue, however, is always demonstrable. The mantle zones are often attenuated. In many cases, disruption of the follicles is evident. This feature is characterized by invagination of the small lymphocytes of the mantle zone into germinal centers, with resultant geographic compartmentalization of germinal center cells and dendritic reticulum cells. Small hemorrhages are seen in some cases.[4] When stained with monoclonal antibodies directed against dendritic reticulum cells (DRC), the normal meshwork of DRC cytoplasmic processes is seen to be disrupted by aggregates of invaginated mantle zone cells.[5]

The DRC express CD4 antigen, the membrane receptor for HIV. Recent immunocytochemical and ultrastructural studies have shown that DRC bear HIV antigens and are associated with retroviral particles.[6-8] Degenerative changes have also been noted in these cells by electron microscopy.[8] Infection and subsequent damage to this antigen processing cell are likely to play a significant role in producing the morphologic changes seen in PGL lymph node germinal centers.

The paracortex in Type I cases is irregularly expanded by nodular and/or diffuse hyperplasia. In the former, scattered histiocytes dispersed among small lymphocytes often confer a "starry sky" pattern. In the diffuse form, there are fewer histiocytes, but scattered immunoblasts and mitotic figures are present. Small lymphocytes with pyknotic nuclei may also be seen. There are numerous postcapillary venules lined by plump endothelium, usually with abundant intramural small lymphocytes. Intramural neutrophils are also seen occasionally. In some cases, the venules show a moderately

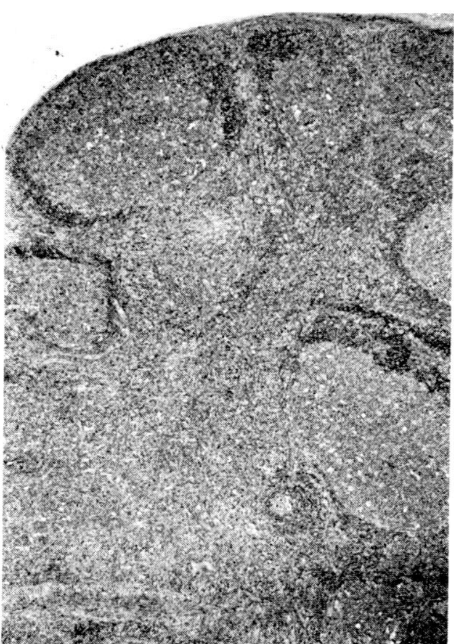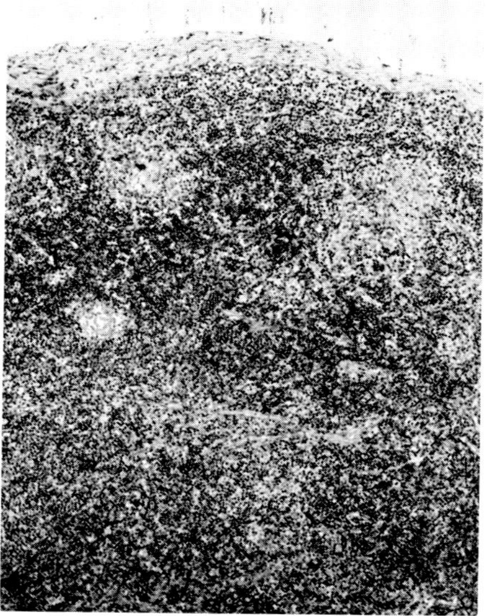

Figure 1. Left: Lymph node section with Type I morphology shows prominent follicular and paracortical hyperplasia. Right: Lymph node section from a patient with Type II morphology demonstrates partial effacement of nodal architecture. Two burnt-out appearing germinal centers are seen beneath the capsule (H&E, original magnification ×25). (From Brynes RK, et al: JAMA 1983: 50:1313–1317)

thickened adventitia. Small parenchymal hemorrhages are occasionally present in this region of the lymph node also.

The medulla in lymph nodes with the Type I pattern contains small indistinct cords. Subcapsular and medullary sinuses are occasionally prominent, and usually contain histiocytes, neutrophils, lymphocytes, and red cells. Hemophagocytosis by histiocytes is a subtle feature in about half of the cases with Type I morphology, and phagocytosis of both erythrocytes and neutrophils may be seen. Trabecular sinuses and adjacent interfollicular tissues sometimes contain an infiltrate of monocytoid B cells. These cells are characterized by medium-sized round to oval nuclei and copious pale to clear cytoplasm.[9] They are also commonly found in toxoplasmic lymphadenitis.[10] Their significance is unknown.

In half of the cases, multinucleated giant cells that resemble the Warthin-Finkeldey giant cells of measles are identified.[2,3] These cells have sparse cytoplasm and their nuclei contain finely stippled chromatin, and inconspicuous nucleoli. They may be found in any region of the lymph node, including germinal centers. In in vitro studies of HIV-infected CD4-positive cell lines, multinucleated lymphoid giant cells are formed through cell-to-cell fusion. This process involves binding of cell surface viral gp120 protein to the CD4 receptor on adjacent cells. As a result, uninfected cells fuse to infected cells to form giant cells.[11]

In situ quantitation of T lymphocyte subsets in the germinal centers of PGL specimens exhibiting a Type I pattern demonstrates an increase in CD8+ lymphocytes that is due to increased numbers of T-suppressor cells associated with a decrease in T-cytotoxic cells and T-helper cells.[12] The germinal center cells and mantle zone lymphocytes have a polyclonal staining pattern for immunoglobulin.[13]

Enumeration of paracortical T-lymphocyte subsets by immunohistochemical methods (Fig. 2) demonstrates a relative loss of T-helper cells as manifested by a reduction in the T-helper to T-suppressor ratio to 1.5 or less.[14-16] In contrast, the T-helper to T-suppressor ratio of hyperplastic lymph nodes from individuals not known to be at risk for AIDS is usually greater than 2.0.[14]

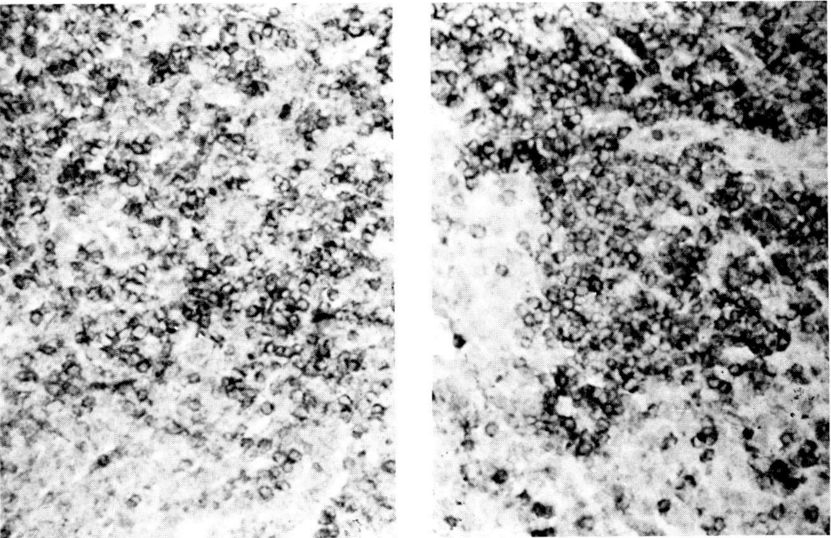

Figure 2. Paracortical region of lymph node with Type I morphology shows approximately equal numbers of T-helper (left), and T-suppressor cells (right). The morphometrically determined T helper/suppressor ratio was 1.05 (peroxidase-antiperoxidase, original magnification ×250).

The distribution of T-cell subsets is not uniform. Hyperplastic paracortical nodules that normally consist of helper cells retain this composition. In some cases, Leu 7-positive natural killer cells and histiocytes are increased.[17]

Study of serial biopsies from individuals with the Type I pattern demonstrates evidence of gradual germinal center loss through follicular involution. This change occurs in 50–66% of patients over a period of 1–2 years or more, and progresses to the Type II pattern.[1,3,18] Specimens from patients with this histology show partial effacement of nodal architecture by a polymorphic population of lymphoid cells and an irregularly distributed proliferation of small blood vessels. The lymph node capsules are often thickened. Germinal centers are either absent, small and inactive, or completely involuted with a burnt-out appearance (Fig. 1, 3, upper inset). The cellular composition of the paracortex varies somewhat in this group, and within individual lymph nodes. Generally, it consists of normal to moderately reduced numbers of small lymphocytes, moderate numbers of mature plasma cells, and variable numbers of large transformed lymphocytes with either clear or pyroninophilic cytoplasm, and scattered histiocytes. Numerous branching vessels of the size of postcapillary venules are observed, and they may show a mild hyaline fibrosis of the adventitia and many intramural lymphocytes. This picture superficially resembles angioimmunoblastic lymphadenopathy with dysproteinemia, but differs from the latter in that immunoblasts are not particularly numerous, and characteristic deposits of PAS-positive interstitial material are absent (Fig. 3). Warthin-Finkeldey-like multinucleated lymphoid cells are seen in this group of patients also (Fig. 3, lower inset). Limited available immunohistochemical data from lymph nodes with the Type II histologic pattern demonstrate the anticipated marked reduction of the T-helper cell to T-suppressor cell ratio (Fig. 4).[12–14]

The prognosis of individuals with the Type I pattern is not entirely clear. Kaposi's

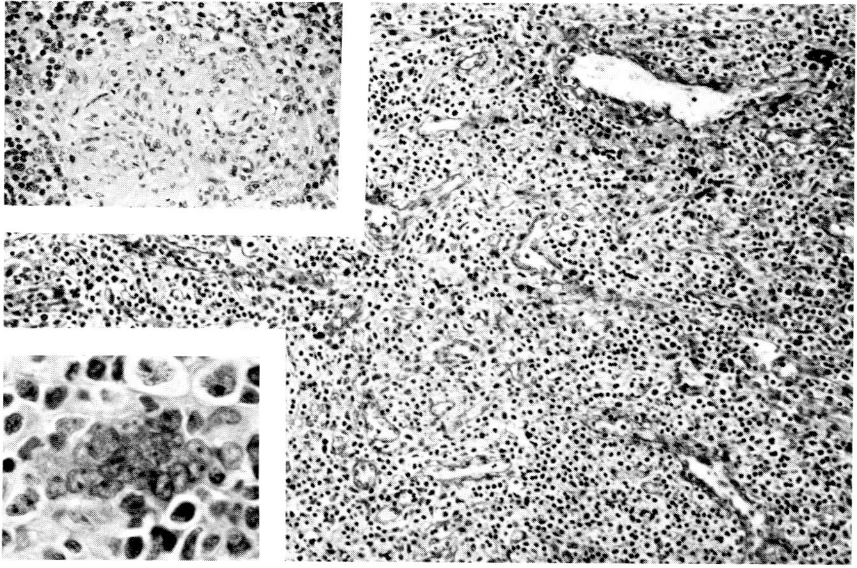

Figure 3. Lymph node section with Type II morphology shows extensive proliferation of postcapillary venules in paracortex (PAS, original magnification ×75). Burnt-out appearing germinal center (upper inset) (H&E, original magnification ×125), and multinucleated lymphoid giant cell (lower inset) (H&E, original magnification ×300) were also seen. (From Brynes RK, et al: JAMA 1983; 250:1313–1317)

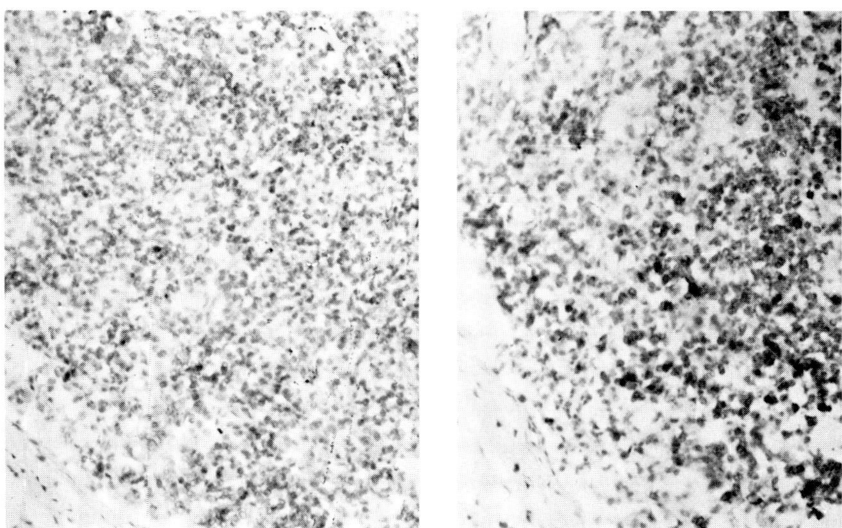

Figure 4. Paracortical region of lymph node with Type II morphology shows virtually no T-helper cells in this field (left), and only small numbers of T-suppressor cells (right). The morphometrically determined T-helper/suppressor ratio was 0.5 (peroxidase-antiperoxidase, original magnification ×200).

sarcoma has been found in the lymph nodes of some patients with this pattern, and some patients have subsequently developed opportunistic infections or lymphoma and died.[19-20] Most patients with this histologic pattern have periods of stable followup for 1 or 2 years,[1,2,18] but appear to have a cumulative 5-year progression to AIDS of 30%.[21]

The Type II pattern is strongly associated with the imminent development of AIDS.[2,18] Just as Kaposi's sarcoma occasionally develops at or shortly after the time that lymph nodes with Type I morphology are biopsied, secondary diseases indicative of AIDS may already be present when lymph nodes with the Type II pattern are biopsied.

Type I and Type II patterns show hyperplasia, whereas the outstanding feature of the Type III pattern is lymphocyte depletion.[3,22] A corresponding reduction in the size of lymph nodes has been observed. Lymph nodes in patients with AIDS are generally enlarged only when involved by secondary diseases such as Kaposi's sarcoma, lymphoma, or mycobacteriosis. Uninvolved small lymph nodes with the un-

complicated Type III pattern are unlikely to be biopsied and are commonly encountered only at autopsy.[3,22]

The Type III lymph node is little more than a reticuloendothelial skeleton populated by variable numbers of stromal cells and plasma cells. It is markedly depleted of lymphocytes, and germinal centers are absent or vestigial. Postcapillary venules are lined by a flattened endothelium, and intramural lymphocytes are sparse or absent. The sinuses are dilated and usually contain abundant histiocytes. Erythrophagocytosis is usually seen, and may appear quite brisk.

The histopathologic patterns of lymphadenopathy found in children infected by HIV are similar to those seen in adults, although prominent follicular hyperplasia may coexist with paracortical depletion.[23]

Peripheral Blood and Bone Marrow

In addition to lymphopenia, cytopenia in one or more additional cell lines is common in AIDS.[24] Occasionally, pancytopenia is present. Mild to moderate normochromic normocytic anemia is thought to be due to a hypoproliferative mechanism, since reticulocyte production is usually low.[25] In AIDS and its prodromes, immune platelet destruction is associated with increased platelet-associated IgG, nonspecific coating of platelets by complement and circulating immune complexes.[26] A paradoxical impairment of reticuloendothelial Fc receptor-mediated antibody-coated cell clearance is seen in some patients.[27]

Bone marrow trephine and aspiration biopsies are normocellular to moderately hypercellular with normal percentages of myeloid and erythroid precursors (Fig. 5). Megakaryocytes are normal in number except in cases of ITP, where their number is increased. A mild plasmacytosis is common, and a delicate reticulin fibrosis is nearly always seen with a reticulin stain.[24] In a substantial number of AIDS patients, subtle myelodysplastic changes are seen in developing erythroid, myeloid, and megakaryocytic elements. These include megaloblas-toid maturation in all three lines, plus occasional binucleation or bizarre-shaped nuclei in red cell precursors; hypogranulation and pseudo-Pelger-Huet changes in the myeloid series; and small or hypolobated megakaryocytes.[28] Circulating dyspoietic neutrophils, which may be found by careful examination of peripheral blood smears, contain greater than normal amounts of myeloperoxidase and appear to be associated with advanced disease.[29] As in lymph nodes, hemophagocytosis is seen in some marrow specimens, and may reflect parts of the spectrum of the virus-associated hemophagocytic syndrome.[25] Nonparatrabecular lymphoid aggregates are found in more than one third of patients with AIDS.[25,30] Typically, these infiltrates are variable in both size and shape, and are composed of an admixture of small lymphocytes with slightly irregular nuclei, and scattered benign epithelioid histiocytes. In some cases, the aggregates contain one or two small venules lined by hypertrophic endothelium. Fre-

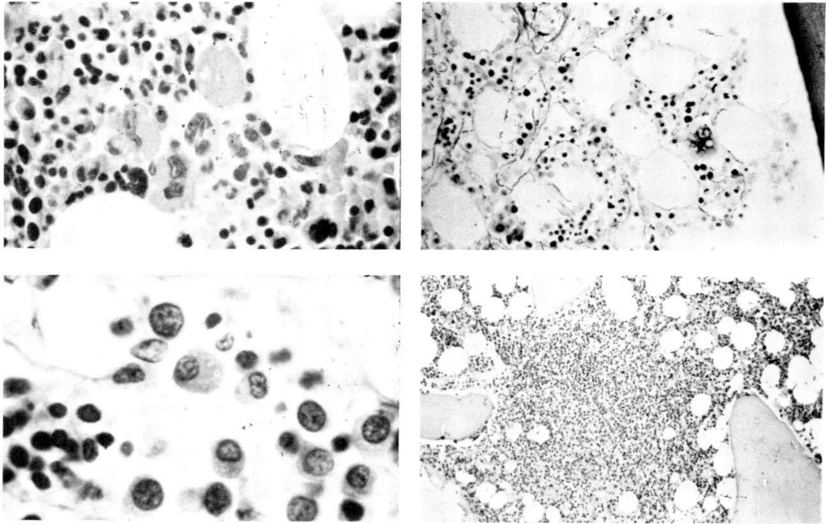

Figure 5. Normocellular bone marrow section from an AIDS patient with ITP shows increased numbers of megakaryocytes (upper left) (H&E, original magnification ×250). Delicate reticulin fibrosis (upper right) (Snooks reticulin, original magnification ×125), and mild plasmacytosis (lower left) (H&E, original magnification ×300) are commonly seen in marrow sections. Large ill-defined lymphoid aggregates such as this resemble those seen in angioimmunoblastic lymphadenopathy and peripheral T-cell lymphoma (lower right) (H&E, original magnification ×40).

quently surrounding the aggregates is an irregular collection of eosinophils and plasma cells. Morphologically, these lymphoid aggregates are similar to those seen in bone marrow involvement by angioimmunoblastic lymphadenopathy with dysproteinemia and peripheral T-cell lymphoma. Care must be taken not to misinterpret the large aggregates as lymphoma.[30]

In patients with AIDS, careful examination of marrow sections occasionally shows granulomas composed of small clusters of histiocytes and lymphocytes. These structures may be limited to only one or two levels of the tissue. Acid-fast stains often disclose *Mycobacterium avium-intracellulare*, although *Mycobacterium tuberculosis* may also be encountered.[31] A Gomori methenamine silver stain may reveal yeasts of *Crytococcus neoformans* or *Histoplasma capsulatum*.[32,33] Mycobacterial and fungal cultures should be routinely performed at the time of bone marrow biopsy in HIV seropositive individuals or patients with AIDS.

Spleen

The histopathology of the spleen in patients with PGL and early AIDS is not well characterized, since specimens are not available for study unless splenectomy is performed for ITP. In this condition, periarteriolar T-lymphocytes are variable in number, and active germinal centers may be seen. At autopsy, the spleen is often enlarged due to congestion and there is marked atrophy of the B-cell zone as well as the T-cell zone. Hemophagocytosis and deposition of hemosiderin are commonly seen. Foci of extramedullary hematopoiesis are noted in some cases.[22]

Thymus

When inspected at autopsy, the thymus is greatly atrophied, with loss of both lympho-

cytes and thymic epithelium (Fig. 6). A mild plasma cell infiltration is often found, and vascular changes including adventitial fibrosis and onion-skinning may be noted. Hassall's corpuscles are reduced numerically and are calcified, a finding that appears characteristic of AIDS.[34,35] In children, examination of the thymus is useful in presumptively differentiating AIDS from other immunodeficiency syndromes.[34] The gland is reduced in size and weight; however, the reduction appears to be less severe than in congenital immunodeficiency. Furthermore, the thymus is found in the normal anterior mediastinal location and has a normal configuration with the normal size and number of blood vessels. These features are in contrast to those in congenital immune deficiency states such as severe combined immune deficiency syndrome (i.e., Nezelof's syndrome, etc.), where the thymus is markedly reduced in size and weight and tends to be located high in the mediastinum or in the neck and has decreased numbers of blood vessels. In partial DiGeorge's syndrome, the thymus has an abnormal configuration.

Histopathologic study of thymus biopsies has revealed thymitis as well as precocious involution, and involution mimicking thymic dysplasia.[36] Thymitis is characterized by the presence of medullary lymphoid follicles with germinal centers, multinucleated giant cells, or a lymphohistiocytic infiltrate. In cases in which both biopsy and autopsy specimens of the thymus are available, progression from thymitis to involution or the simultaneous occurrence of the two lesions in the autopsy specimen is seen. This suggests that thymitis may represent an earlier active stage of thymic injury in pediatric AIDS.

It should be noted that marked reduction of Hassall's corpuscles has also been reported in certain other acquired diseases such as severe protein calorie malnutrition, graft-versus-host disease, and congenital (intrauterine) infections (i.e., rubella and neonatal hepatitis). While in the majority of

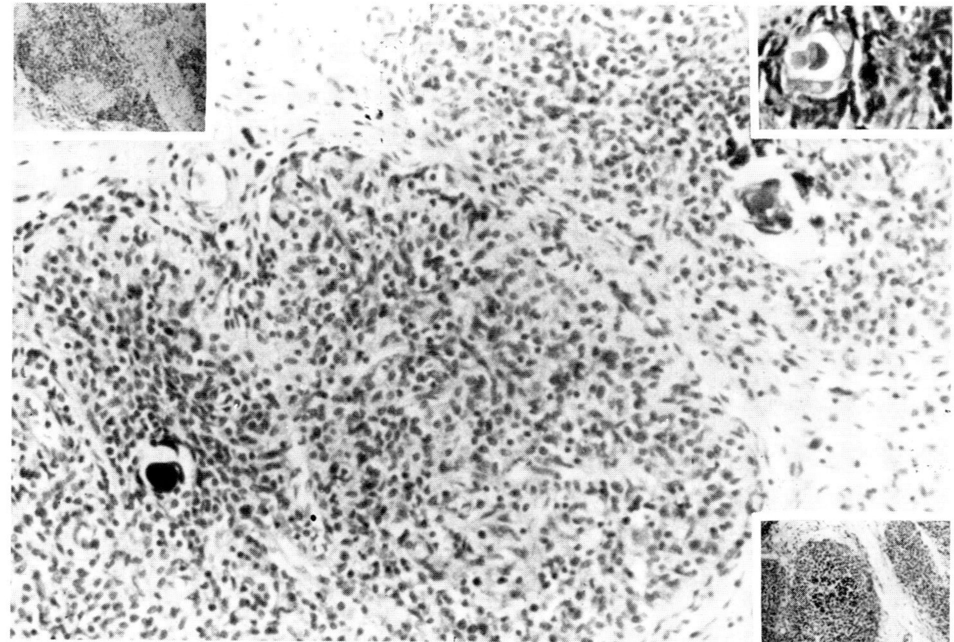

Figure 6. Lobules from the thymus of a 3-month-old child with AIDS are nearly devoid of lymphocytes, and contain calcified Hassall's corpuscles (H&E, original magnification ×250). Focal lobular hyalinization (upper left) (H&E, original magnification ×40); microcystic dilatation of Hassall's corpuscles (upper right) (H&E, original magnification ×250); and focal nodules of residual lymphocytes (lower right) (H&E, original magnification ×40) are also commonly found in the thymus of AIDS patients. (From Joshi VV, et al: Arch Pathol Lab Med 1985; 109:142–146)

children with AIDS the changes in Hassall's corpuscles mimic thymic dysplasia of congenital immune deficiency syndromes, the reduction of Hassall's corpuscles and the other features described above favor the interpretation of an acquired lesion.

SECONDARY HISTOPATHOLOGY

Opportunistic Infections

It is not surprising that risk factors for the transmission of HIV also apply to a number of other infectious agents, such as cytomegalovirus, *Entamoeba histolytica, Giardia lamblia,* hepatitis A and B, *Neisseria gonorrhoeae,* and *Treponema pallidum.* Thus members of risk groups for AIDS often present with infectious diseases not related

to AIDS. There is, however, a limited set of secondary infectious agents that is particularly characteristic of AIDS. The presence of any of these agents, especially in the appropriate clinicopathologic setting, suggests that AIDS should be considered as the underlying disease.

Cytomegalovirus

Cytomegalovirus (CMV) is a species-specific DNA virus of the family Herpesviridae that is endemic throughout the world. It is acquired through close contact including sexual activity.[37] Infection is asymptomatic in a majority of cases, and the virus persists in a latent state while the immune system is competent. In AIDS, CMV emerges to become a common and important cause of opportunistic disease.

As this virus infects a host cell, it transiently stimulates the cell's own protein synthesis, and the unique result is a megalic cell to which the virus owes its name. The nucleus of the infected cell develops a large round to cigar-shaped inclusion separated from the nuclear membrane by a clear halo, and the presence of multiple intracytoplasmic inclusions completes the diagnostic triad.

CMV can infect a variety of cells, but in AIDS the cells most often involved are pneumocytes, vascular endothelial cells, and secretory cells of exocrine and endocrine glands. Since one or more of these cell types exist in every organ of the body, evidence of CMV infection may appear in any type of tissue specimen. However, CMV infection is especially common and/or significant in certain organs described below, namely lung, alimentary tract, adrenal, eye, and brain.

Lung. CMV infection of the lung is frequently seen in autopsy specimens, usually accompanied by one or more additional opportunistic diseases. In cases where no other pulmonary pathogens are detected, damage to the lung may appear to be minimal. Attached and desquamated inclusion-bearing pneumocytes are seen, sometimes in large numbers. A mild diffuse lymphocytic infiltrate may be present in the interstitium. Since CMV infection is usually disseminated in patients with AIDS, detection of CMV-infected cells by bronchoalveolar lavage or biopsy makes it even more likely that significant involvement of other organs is present. Detection of CMV by bronchoalveolar lavage may be enhanced by direct immunofluorescence[38] or in situ hybridization techniques.[39]

Alimentary tract. Involvement of the alimentary tract by CMV can lead to diarrhea,[40] ulcers,[40] and perforations.[41] Infected mucosal epithelial cells are occasionally seen,[40] but inclusions are most often seen in capillary endothelial cells of the lamina propria. Ulcerations tend to be limited to the mucosa, but reactive changes including sub-mucosal granulation tissue, nonspecific inflammatory cell infiltrates, and thickening of the muscularis may be seen. Direct involvement of the muscularis with CMV infection of smooth muscle cells and focal necrosis is associated with perforation. The terminal ileum and proximal colon seem especially prone to this complication.

Adrenal. Necrotizing lesions due to CMV commonly affect both cortex and medulla of the adrenal glands, leading in some cases to adrenal insufficiency.[42] Foci of necrosis, often hemorrhagic, are accompanied by viral inclusions and variable numbers of neutrophils.[43]

Eye. CMV retinitis can lead to blurring or loss of vision; cotton wool spots are seen clinically.[44] There is focal necrosis of the retina, and inclusion-bearing cells are present. The underlying choroid may be thickened and infiltrated by lymphocytes.[45]

Brain. CMV can produce severe focal or diffuse encephalopathy, but in AIDS it is always accompanied in the brain by another neurotropic pathogen, HIV. Thus, the relative contribution of CMV versus HIV to brain pathology can be difficult to assess. There is, however, evidence that CMV infects neurons, astrocytes, oligodendroglial cells, ependymal cells, and brain capillary endothelial cells.[46] In CMV infections, microglial nodules are consistently present and tend to be located in subcortical gray matter.[46] Occasionally, CMV-infected cells are observed in such nodules. Isolated inclusion-bearing cells may be seen elsewhere.[46] In severe infections, focal demyelination and necrosis[46] are seen.

Herpes Simplex Virus

Herpes simplex virus (HSV), like CMV, is a member of the family Herpesviridae, and is found worldwide.[47] Man is the only reservoir, although a variety of nonhuman cell lines and laboratory animals can be productively infected experimentally. HSV is acquired by direct, often sexual, person-to-person contact. There are two closely related variants of HSV called HSV-1 and HSV-2. They are considered together here because they cause similar clinical disease, resemble each other biologically, and are indistinguishable from each other in their histopathologic effects. Primary infections show marked variation in intensity of symptoms,[47] and can occur anywhere on the skin or mucous membranes. From lesions established on these surfaces, the virus quickly enters sensory nerves and travels back along them to establish a latent infection in sensory ganglion neurons.[48] By poorly understood mechanisms, the virus can be reactivated to produce recurrent, but normally temporary, skin or mucosal lesions. In the profound immunodeficiency of AIDS, however, lesions may persist for months.

Early in HSV infection of a host cell, the nucleus develops a ground-glass appearance. Subsequently, the chromatin marginates and the nuclear membrane takes on a thick, deeply basophilic appearance. A rounded, finely granular, lightly eosinophilic intranuclear inclusion forms and then develops a more distinct margin, more pronounced eosinophilia, and a clear halo separating it from the nuclear membrane. Infected cells vary somewhat in size and appearance, but cytomegaly and intracytoplasmic inclusions are not seen. Multinucleated cells, formed by fusion of adjacent cells, are characteristically present. Cells at various stages of infection, with one or multiple nuclei, are seen concurrently.

HSV has a distinct tropism for squamous epithelial cells, and the sites most often affected reflect its propensity to be sexually transmitted. The chronic lesions seen in AIDS are often anal,[49] genital, and oral. Esophageal[50] and pulmonary lesions are also seen in some cases.

On skin and mucosal surfaces, the characteristic lesion is an ulcer flanked by a narrow zone of altered, inclusion-bearing epithelial cells. In the lung, lesions consist of foci of necrosis with associated viral inclu-

sions. The presence of HSV antigen can be confirmed by immunoperoxidase staining.

Epstein-Barr Virus

The Epstein-Barr virus (EBV) is another DNA virus of the family Herpesviridae, with worldwide distribution in man. EBV is transmitted from person to person; efficient transmission is achieved by intimate oral-oral contact. Infection by EBV can be manifested clinically in a variety of ways in healthy persons, after which the virus persists in a latent state. In AIDS, EBV cooperates with a papillomavirus of the family Papovaviridae to produce a distinctive oral lesion called hairy leukoplakia (HL).[51]

HL presents as a white, slightly raised, poorly demarcated epithelial lesion involving the lateral borders of the tongue almost exclusively. It has not been found in the anus or rectum, or in other extra-oral sites. The presence of HL indicates AIDS or likely progression to AIDS.[52] Microscopic features of HL include fine keratin projections, parakeratosis, koilocytosis of prickle cells, acanthosis, and little or no subjacent inflammatory cell infiltrate (Fig. 7).[51,53] *Candida* organisms are often associated with the surface of the lesion.[53] Diagnosis of HL largely depends on biopsy.

EBV may also be involved in the etiology of various lymphoid neoplasms and lymphoid infiltrates seen in AIDS. These are discussed elsewhere.

JC Virus

JC virus (JCV) derives its name from the initials of the patient from whom it was first isolated. This neurotropic DNA virus is a polyomavirus of the family Papovaviridae; it is known to exist only in man, and is found in most populations throughout the world. It is asymptomatically acquired in childhood by an unknown route, and like the herpes viruses, establishes a persistent, latent infection.

Upon activation by profound immunode-

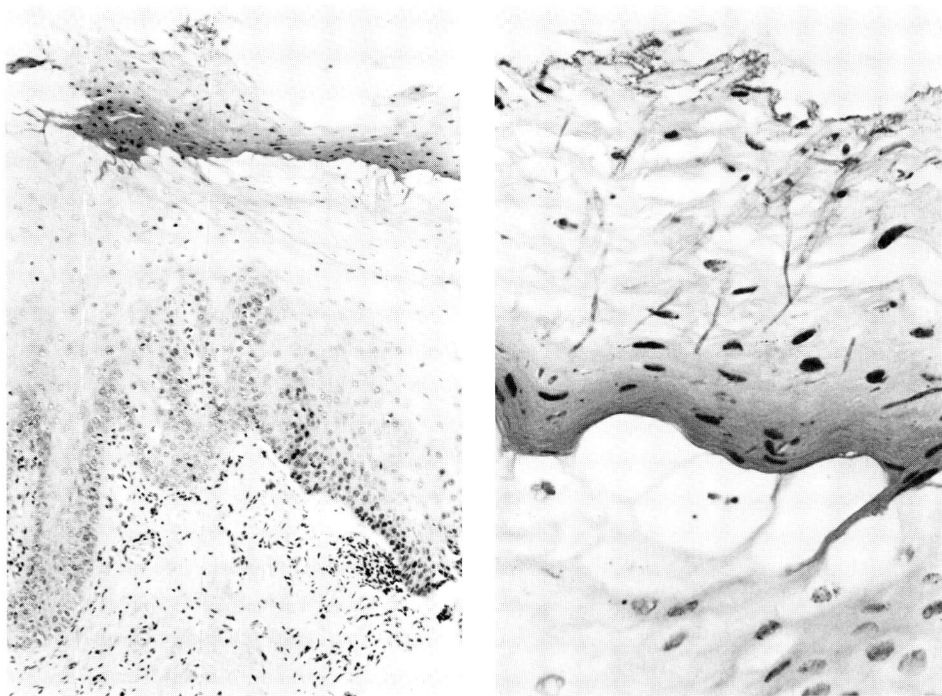

Figure 7. Section of tongue biopsy with hairy leukoplakia showing parakeratosis and koilocytosis (left) (H&E, original magnification ×20). Koilocytotic prickle cells are seen beneath the parakeratotic layer. Note presence of *Candida* hyphae within the epithelium (right) (H&E, original magnification ×85). (Section courtesy of R. J. Melrose, DDS, University of Southern California School of Dentistry, Los Angeles)

ficiency, JCV replicates mainly in oligodendrocytes, which develop large, hyperchromatic nuclei containing one to several poorly defined amphophilic intranuclear inclusions without halos. The inclusions represent crystalline arrays of JC virions that can be identified by electron microscopy,[54] immunoperoxidase technique[55] or in situ hybridization.[56] Destruction of oligodendrocytes, which normally produce and maintain the myelin sheaths, leads to progressive, multifocal, demyelinating lesions of the brain—hence the name of the resultant disease: progressive multifocal leukoencephalopathy (PML). PML is much more common in AIDS than in other immunodeficiency diseases,[55] but it is still seen in only a small fraction of persons with AIDS. The multifocal nature of the disease results in a varied constellation of symptoms such as

hemiparesis, blindness, intellectual deficits, and cerebellar and brain stem signs. Grossly, multiple discrete foci of myelin destruction are seen, usually starting near the gray-white matter margin. These tend to expand and coalesce with deeper involvement of the white matter. Microscopically, there are areas of demyelination that may progress to necrosis. At the periphery of these areas are oligodendrocytes that are altered as described above. Another distinct feature, especially in later lesions, is the presence of large, bizarre astrocytes that may show multiple or multilobed nuclei and atypical mitotic figures (Fig. 8). Some of these astrocytes can be shown to contain JCV.[56] Lesions may contain numerous foamy histiocytes, but there is a remarkable absence of neutrophils, lymphocytes, and plasma cells.

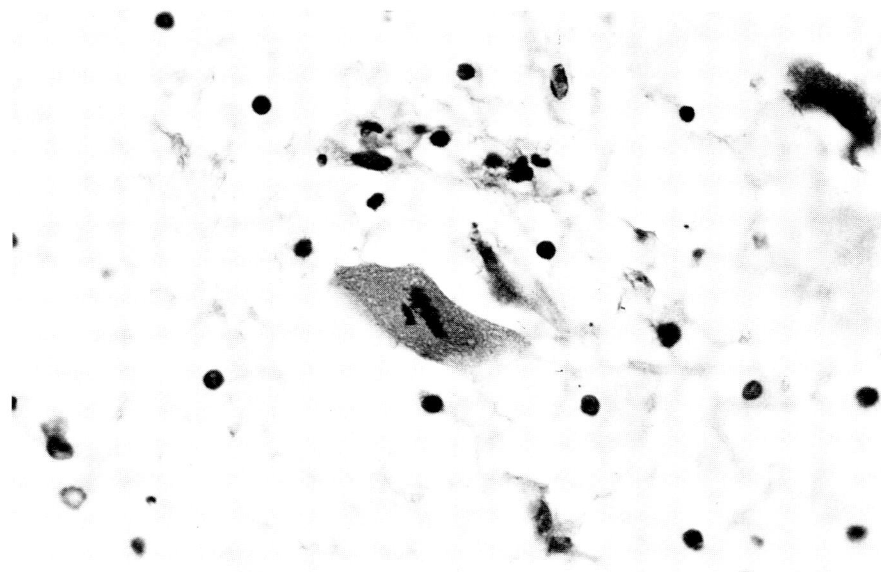

Figure 8. Section of brain with progressive multifocal leukoencephalopathy; an infection due to JC virus. The large, bizarre astrocyte contains a mitotic figure and is surrounded by a focus of necrosis. This lesion is usually seen late in PML (H&E, original magnification ×300).

Mycobacterium Avium-Intracellulare

Mycobacterium avium-intracellulare (MAI) is an acid-fast bacillus that owes its double species name to the fact that it actually represents a number of very similar strains.[57] In tissue, it is not only strongly acid-fast with a Ziehl-Neelsen stain, but is also strongly periodic acid-Schiff-positive. It is moderately positive with Gomori's methenamine silver stain, and weakly gram-positive with a Brown and Brenn stain. MAI is acquired directly from the environment, where it is ubiquitous. Infections occur naturally in man as well as in a variety of animals and birds. Despite universal human exposure to MAI, infections in immunocompetent individuals are uncommon and usually involve cervical lymph nodes of young children[58] or pneumoconiotic lungs of adult males.[57] In such persons, MAI elicits caseating granulomas, and disseminated infection is rare. In AIDS, however, MAI is the preeminent agent of disseminated bacterial infection.[59] It shows a predilection for lymphoreticular and hematopoietic tissues, although it occasionally appears elsewhere, e.g., in lung or adrenal. Signs and symptoms are often nonspecific, and include fever, night sweats, weakness, and diarrhea.[60] Mycobacteremia is often demonstrable,[61] as expected in disseminated infection.

The route of infection is not known, but MAI probably enters the body by ingestion or inhalation. Histiocytes take up the bacilli but are unable to kill them because of the immune deficit. Consequently, the organisms proliferate intracellularly until they completely fill the cells. Because of the deficiency of T-helper lymphocytes, histiocytes form granulomas poorly or not at all. Caseating necrosis is usually not a feature. Below, some typical organ involvement is described.

Lymph node. Any lymph node in the body may be infected, and progressive enlargement of a previously small or shrinking lymph node in an AIDS patient is a clue to possible MAI infection. Usually, multiple lymph nodes are involved. Histiocytic infiltration begins in the superficial paracortex and then extends to involve the entire parenchyma (Fig. 9). The architecture is effaced and the entire node becomes occupied by sheets of bland, round, or polygonal histiocytes. Granuloma formation and necrosis are usually absent, but an acid-fast stain may reveal tremendous numbers of acid-fast bacilli filling virtually every histiocyte.

Spleen. Collections of histiocytes in follicles and other areas are seen, and some of the collections may take the form of large, poorly formed granulomas. Some necrosis may be present. An acid-fast stain reveals numerous intracellular acid-fast bacilli.

Liver. Acid-fast organisms may be seen in portal collections of histiocytes, individual Kupffer cells, and in loose, poorly formed granulomas.

Bone marrow. Bone marrow trephine and aspiration biopsies are easily and safely done, and are likely to contain MAI when disseminated infection is present. Although poorly formed granulomas may be present, often they are not. Scattered histiocytes may contain large numbers of bacilli that would be unsuspected from the histology on hematoxylin and eosin staining. Therefore, an acid-fast stain should be routine on bone marrow specimens from patients with AIDS.

Alimentary tract. MAI infection of the small and large intestine is one of the causes of diarrhea in AIDS,[61] and may be encountered in intestinal biopsies. Microscopically, the lamina propria contains small to great numbers of histiocytes laden with acid-fast bacilli. The lesion may somewhat resemble that of Whipple's disease, but differs from the latter in that mycobacteria are acid-fast while the Whipple bacillus is not.[62] Mycobacteria are also several times larger than

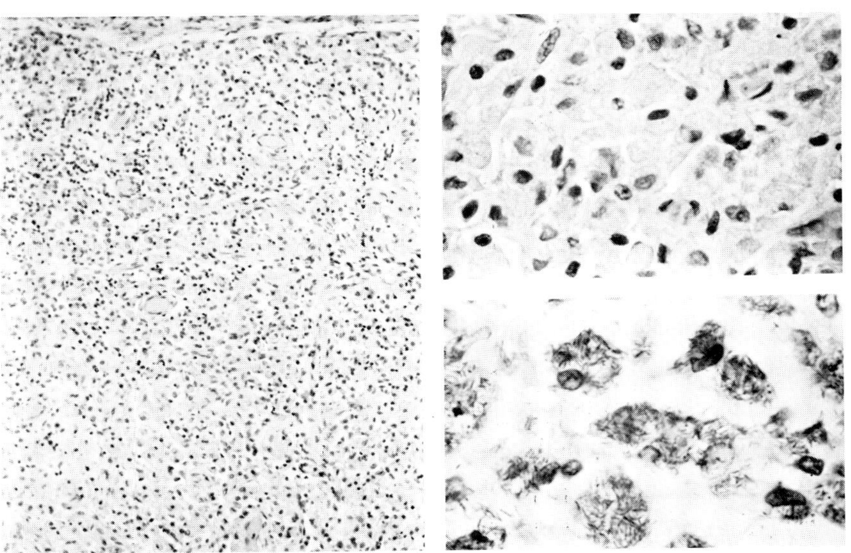

Figure 9. Lymph node section totally replaced by loosely coherent histiocytes (left and upper right) (H&E, original magnification ×80; ×250). Acid-fast stain demonstrates numerous positively stained bacilli in each cell (lower right) (Ziehl-Neelsen, original magnification ×300). A culture of this specimen grew *Mycobacterium avium-intracellulare.*

the Whipple bacillus. MAI has been reported to produce a clinical and radiologic picture resembling that of Crohn's disease in a patient with AIDS; histopathologic examination of resected bowel revealed noncaseating granulomas with numerous intracellular acid-fast bacilli.[63] MAI can be demonstrated by Ziehl-Neelsen staining and by culture of fecal specimens from many patients with AIDS,[61] even in the absence of known dissemination. It is possible that the intestine is a source of disseminated MAI infection.

Lung. Small numbers of histiocytes containing acid-fast bacilli may be observed in the interstitium, but significant pulmonary pathology is an uncharacteristic result of MAI infection in AIDS. Interestingly, respiratory secretions are culture positive in a majority of AIDS patients with disseminated MAI infection.[61]

Mycobacterium Tuberculosis

Mycobacterium tuberculosis (MTB), unlike MAI, is a virulent bacterium that is transmitted from person to person by aerosol and often causes disease in normal persons. Like MAI, it elicits caseating granulomas in such persons, after which it may remain as a latent infection for many years. Though much less common overall than MAI infections, MTB infections are nevertheless important complications of HIV infection in populations having a high prevalence of tuberculosis. Associations between MTB infection and HIV infection have been reported in intravenous drug abusers and Haitians in the United States,[64] and an association between these two infections has also been observed in Zaire.[65] In most cases, tuberculosis associated with HIV infection probably represents reactivation of an old MTB infection.[66] Unlike more strictly opportunistic infectious agents, MTB can emerge to cause clinical disease before the onset of AIDS as well as later.[67]

HIV-associated tuberculosis often in-volves one or more extrapulmonary sites such as lymph node, bone marrow, and brain.[64] Depending on the degree of immunodeficiency at the time, lesions may contain caseating granulomas, noncaseating granulomas, or no granulomas.[64]

Candida species

Certain members of the genus *Candida* are included in the normal flora of the oral cavity, throat, and vagina, as well as the skin. With Gomori's methenamine silver stain, the organisms appear as branching septate hyphae, pseudohyphae, and $3-5\,\mu$m round to oval blastoconidia. This combination of fungal structures is diagnostic for *Candida. Candida albicans* is the species most commonly observed in oral and vaginal candidiasis.

Superficial oral mucosal candidiasis is the most common fungal infection in patients with ARC or AIDS[68]; it is often, though not always, associated with esophageal candidiasis.[69] Biopsy shows the organisms superficially invading a somewhat hyperplastic stratified squamous epithelium. The subjacent stroma may contain a diffuse infiltrate of neutrophils, lymphocytes, and plasma cells. Vaginal candidiasis may occur in women with ARC or AIDS. Disseminated candidiasis is uncommon in ARC and AIDS.[70]

Cryptococcus Neoformans

Cryptococcus neoformans in tissue is a strikingly pleomorphic yeast that measures $2-20\,\mu$m in diameter and exhibits narrow-based budding. Its morphology is shown well by Gomori's methenamine silver stain. A thick mucopolysaccharide capsule that stains bright red with a mucicarmine stain is often present. The characteristic morphology of the yeast and the presence of a mucicarmine-positive capsule are usually sufficient to establish the identity of the organisms as cryptococci. A third stain, the Fontana-Masson silver stain, reacts with melanin-like substances in the cell wall to color it brown or black, and may be useful in identifying the organisms in the occasional cases when they are capsule-deficient.[71] Even in such cases, at least a few yeasts with mucicarmine capsules are likely to be present and should be sought, since the Fontana-Masson silver stain can also give a positive reaction in *Cryptococcus laurentii, Sporothrix schenckii,* and the immature spherules of *Coccidioides immitis.*[72]

C. neoformans exists in soil throughout the world, and is especially associated with areas where pigeons defecate. It is acquired from the environment by inhalation, and can infect both man and a variety of animals. Person to person or animal to person spread has not been described. Cryptococcosis is a frequent complication in AIDS, and severe, disseminated disease is common.

In the lung, yeasts are likely to be observed in the interstitium, where some histiocytes but no granulomas or other inflammatory cells are associated with them; in occasional cases, alveolar spaces are also invaded and filled with organisms, desquamated pneumocytes, and debris (Fig. 10).[73] The lung is regarded as the usual source of dissemination to the rest of the body, and there is evidence that this occurs via both blood vessels and lymphatics.[73] Meningitis with tremendous numbers of yeasts and little or no inflammatory cell reaction is a major manifestation of cryptococcosis in AIDS; it presents with headache and sometimes with nausea, vomiting, and photophobia.[74] In addition to lung and meninges, any organ of the body can be involved. Lesions consistently show lucent areas representing masses of organisms that are largely unstained by hematoxylin and eosin because of their large volume of capsular polysaccharide. Inflammatory cells are notably absent. Lesions due to *C. neoformans* can be subtle, especially in the lung. Gomori's methenamine silver stain should therefore be routinely employed to screen for this organism in lung specimens and in suspicious lesions elsewhere.

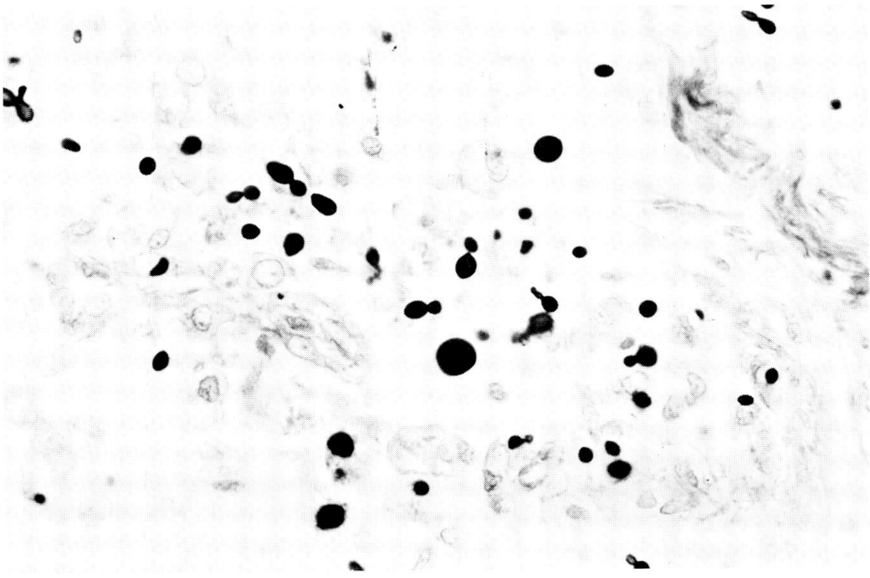

Figure 10. *Cryptococcus neoformans* in section of lung. The yeasts are characterized by narrow-based budding and marked variation in size and shape (Gomori methenamine silver, original magnification ×300).

Pneumocystis Carinii

Pneumocystis carinii is an extracellular protozoan parasite of the lung of man and many animals.[75] Proliferating organisms alternate between cyst and trophozoite forms, so demonstration of one form in lesions is sufficient for diagnosis. Cysts stain well with the Gomori's methenamine silver technique, for which rapid modifications are now available.[76] Cysts can be demonstrated in histologic sections, and appear as 4–6 μm round to oval structures with focal cyst wall thickening.[77] Some of the cysts are collapsed and cup-shaped. They are also readily demonstrated in lung biopsy imprints, and in bronchoalveolar lavage cell blocks and smears.[78]

This protozoan is universally acquired in early childhood, probably by aerosol spread from person to person. Infection is normally asymptomatic and latent for the lifetime of the host. Symptomatic infections are almost exclusively seen in persons who have some form of immune suppression. Once an uncommon disease, *P. carinii* pneumonia occurs in 80–85% of patients with AIDS.[79]

Sections of lung from patients with pulmonary pneumocystosis usually show alveolar spaces containing eosinophilic exudates that typically have a frothy or honeycombed appearance on hematoxylin and eosin staining. Exudates may appear retracted from alveolar walls, and they contain few intact host cells. The interstitium contains a mild diffuse infiltrate of lymphocytes, and may be thickened and fibrotic if the infection has been chronic. Plasma cells are also present in some cases. A Gomori's methanamine silver stain reveals the characteristic cysts embedded in the exudate. In some cases, the typical histopathology is not well developed or is partially obscured by concurrent opportunistic diseases; the hallmark exudates may be virtually absent. In addition, clinical and roentgenographic presentations of pulmonary pneumocystosis are notoriously subtle and protean. For these reasons and because of the very high incidence of pneumocystosis in AIDS,

screening of all lung specimens with the Gomori's methenamine silver stain from HIV-infected persons is essential.

There have been several reports of dissemination of *P. carinii* to one or more extrapulmonary sites.[80–82] Frothy eosinophilic exudates containing numerous cysts are the consistent histopathologic finding. Focal necrosis may be seen, but there is usually little or no inflammatory cell response.

Toxoplasma Gondii

Toxoplasma gondii is an intracellular protozoan parasite of man and of many animals. In active infections, trophozoites proliferate within membrane-bound vacuoles of host cells. The rapidly multiplying trophozoites are called tachyzoites, and collections of tachyzoites in host cell vacuoles are called pseudocysts. In hematoxylin and eosin stained sections, tachyzoites appear as 2–6 μm round to oval structures with single basophilic nuclei. The lack of a kinetoplast distinguishes them from members of the *Leishmania* and *Trypanosoma* genera. The thinner the section, the better the morphology of individual organisms can be appreciated. A good hematoxylin and eosin stain is often all that is needed to detect the organisms, but immunoperoxidase staining may also be of value in some cases.[83–85]

T. gondii is acquired by ingestion of oocysts from the feces of cats, the definitive host, or from consumption of inadequately cooked meat containing *T. gondii* cysts. This parasite is found throughout the world, and infection is especially prevalent in warm, humid climates. In the immunocompetent human host, infection is usually inapparent and followed by encystation of organisms in multiple sites, where they remain in a dormant state. In immunosuppressed patients such as those with AIDS, latent *T. gondii* becomes activated to produce symptomatic toxoplasmosis.[86] The most commonly involved organs are brain, heart, and lung,[87] though lesions may also be found in a variety of other organs. Some characteristic lesions of toxoplasmosis in AIDS are presented below.

Brain. Multiple focal lesions occur anywhere in the brain, but are most common in the cortex of the cerebrum and cerebellum.[85] The microscopic hallmarks of these lesions are necrosis,[85-87] a mixed infiltrate of neutrophils, lymphocytes, plasma cells, histiocytes,[85] and characteristic tachyzoites found both free and within pseudocysts (Fig. 11)[84]. Tachyzoites are usually found in the periphery of the lesions.[85] True *Toxoplasma* cysts—large, round structures packed with numerous bradyzoites and limited by a definite cyst wall—are seldom seen in AIDS.[84-85] It should be noted that multiple foci of necrosis occur in both toxoplasmosis and PML, but inflammatory infiltrates are usually present in toxoplasmosis and usually absent in PML.

Heart. The myocardium contains multiple ill-defined foci of inflammation containing neutrophils, lymphocytes, plasma cells, and histiocytes. Myocardial fibers in these areas are separated by edema, and show pallor, degeneration with dense cross-banding, and individual fiber necrosis. Pseudocysts within and conforming to the shape of myocardial fibers contain small to large numbers of tachyzoites, and may be seen both within inflammatory foci and elsewhere (Fig. 12). Where there is necrosis, scattered extracellular trophozoites may be seen (Fig. 13).

Lung. There are foci of necrosis with variable numbers of neutrophils, lymphocytes, plasma cells, and histiocytes. Pseudocysts are seen within pneumocytes, and free tachyzoites may be abundant.

Other organs. Focal involvement of any organ may be seen on occasion, not infrequently in the presence of lesions of one or more additional opportunistic infections.

Cryptosporidium

Cryptosporidium is a protozoan parasite of man and many animals[88] that does not yet possess the distinction of a species name.

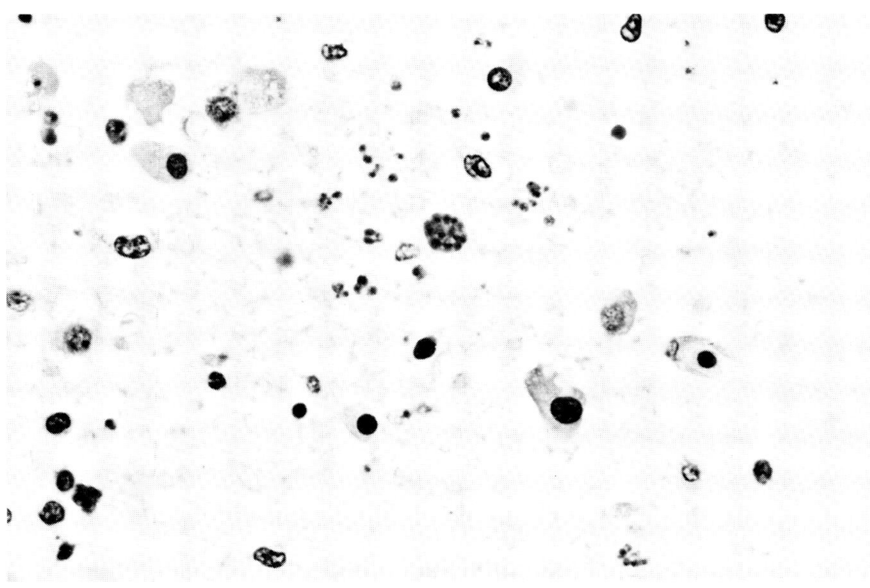

Figure 11. Necrotic area of brain containing *toxoplasma* tachyzoites in a small pseudocyst. Free tachyzoites are scattered around the pseudocyst (H&E, original magnification ×300).

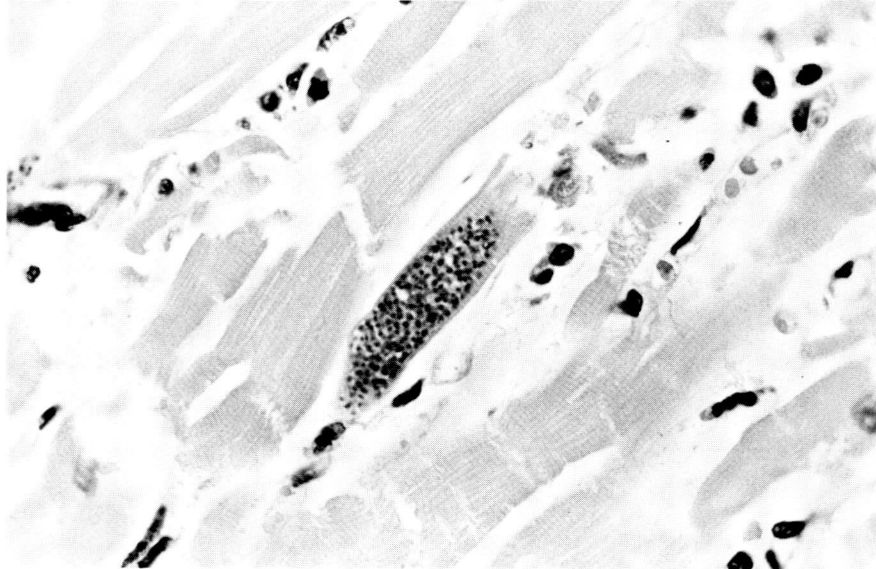

Figure 12.   Large myocardial pseudocyst of *Toxoplasma gondii* packed with tachyzoites (H&E, original magnification ×300).

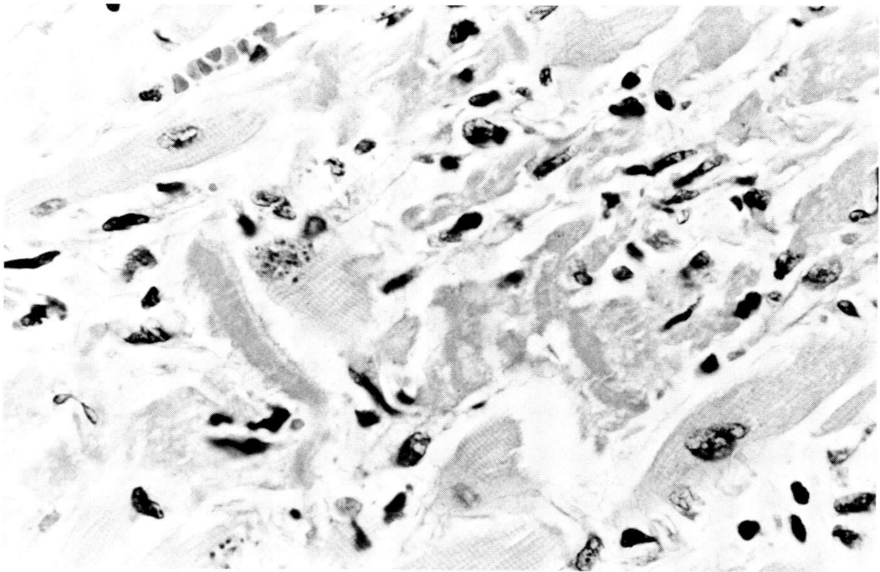

Figure 13.   Focus of myocardial necrosis with dense crossbanding demonstrates a small group of intracellular tachyzoites of *Toxoplasma gondii* (H&E, original magnification ×300).

This pathogen has a somewhat complicated life cycle detailed in recent reviews.[88] By light microscopy, the 1.5–6.0 μm, roughly spherical organisms appear to be attached individually to the luminal surfaces of epithelial cells. By electron microscopy, it is clear that the organisms are covered by a tight-fitting, blister-like evagination of the host cell's plasma membrane.[88-90] This superficial location in host cells differentiates *Cryptosporidium* from *Isospora belli* and microsporidians, which are rare but additionally known causes of diarrhea in AIDS patients.[90] Cryptosporidia are lightly basophilic and easily seen with a hematoxylin and eosin stain, despite their small size. As in the case of *T. gondii,* organisms are best seen in the thinnest sections. Special stains provide no advantage over hematoxylin and eosin.

Cryptosporidium is acquired by ingestion of oocysts shed in feces of infected humans or animals. Once regarded as extremely rare in humans, cryptosporidiosis is now recognized as an occasional cause of a diarrheal illness in normal children and adults that is self-limited.[91] In AIDS, however, cryptosporidiosis results in a chronic and debilitating diarrhea.

The chief target in cryptosporidiosis is the alimentary tract, which in AIDS patients may be involved at all levels, including the esophagus. Villous atrophy may be observed in the small intestine,[89-90] but inflammatory responses are generally minimal. Diagnosis therefore depends on close scrutiny of all epithelial surfaces, including those in the lumina of intestinal glands, for the characteristic organisms (Fig. 14). When cryptosporidia are present, they are usually abundant. Unlike mucin droplets, with which they might rarely be confused, they are mucicarmine-negative. Fusion of sexual stages ultimately results in the formation of the 4.5–6.0 μm thick-walled oocyst. The oocyst is passed in feces and is the infective form for the next host. It is positive by acid-fast staining and can be detected in smears prepared from feces or other specimens.[92] However, acid-fast stains are of no value in ordinary histologic sections because the solvents used in routine tissue processing abolish their acid-fastness.

Cryptosporidium has been observed in

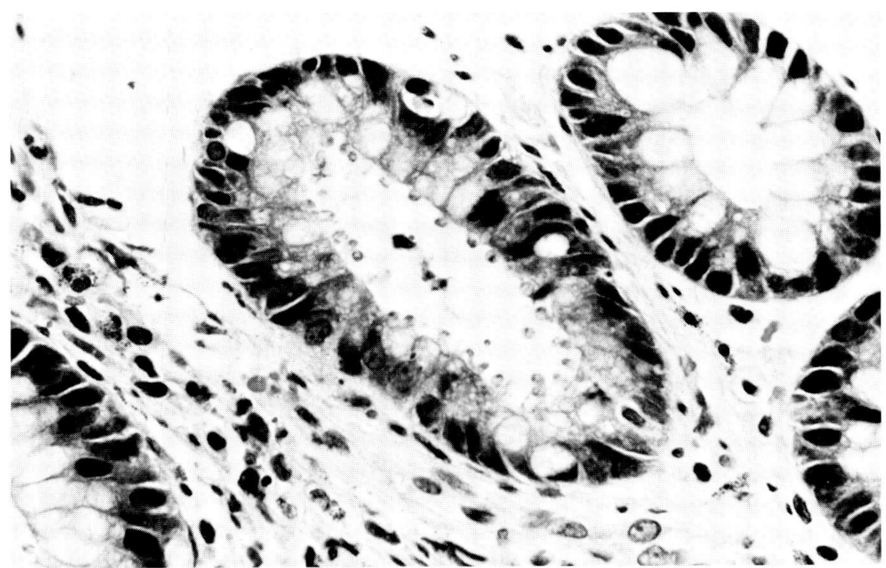

Figure 14. Numerous cryptosporidia project into the lumen of this colonic gland (H&E, original magnification ×300).

additional sites in AIDS patients, including gallbladder,[93] bronchus, and lung.[94] As in the alimentary tract, minimal inflammatory changes may be the only tissue reaction, and the cryptosporidia are easily missed unless epithelial surfaces are examined carefully.

Neoplasms

The close association between immunodeficiency states and an increased incidence of Kaposi's sarcoma and non-Hodgkin's lymphoma is well known. Organ transplant recipients and patients with lymphoreticular neoplasms have an increased incidence of Kaposi's sarcoma. Non-Hodgkin's lymphomas have been reported to arise in abnormal immune states associated with autoimmune disease, organ transplantation, and congenital immune deficiency states.[95-98] In view of the severe degree of immunodeficiency found in AIDS, it is not surprising to encounter these neoplasms.

Kaposi's Sarcoma

About one fourth of patients with AIDS have Kaposi's sarcoma. The lesion is typically multifocal and painless and can precede any other signs or symptoms. In AIDS, lesions are commonly found in skin, mucous membranes, and lymph nodes, but may be seen almost anywhere in the body.[22,99]

While the histologic features of Kaposi's sarcoma in well developed nodular lesions are readily recognizable, changes in the small patches and plaques that appear in the skin can be subtle.[100] Lesions are confined mainly to the upper half of the dermis and contain dilated, irregularly shaped, thin-walled, jagged vessels lined by a flattened endothelium. The vessels tend to be contiguous to pre-existing blood vessels and are typically accompanied by a sparse lymphoid infiltrate, often containing plasma cells. A few extravasated erythrocytes and hemosiderin granules may be seen at this early stage.

Plaque lesions of Kaposi's sarcoma tend to involve the entire dermis and may extend into the subcutaneous fat. Plaques contain increased numbers of spindle cells around the abnormal vessels and between collagen bundles in the dermis. These cells display little or no atypia and enclose irregular blood-filled clefts. As the number of spindle cells increases, raised nodules are produced. These have the characteristic histologic features of well developed Kaposi's sarcoma, which include interweaving fascicles of spindle cells, marked extravasation of erythrocytes, occasional cells containing intracytoplasmic eosinophilic globules, and deposition of hemosiderin. Plasma cells and lymphocytes are numerous at the margins of the tumor. Recent evidence suggests that the proliferating cell originates from lymphatic endothelial cells.[101] The striking predilection of Kaposi's sarcoma for the dermis of the skin, submucosa of the gastrointestinal tract, capsule of lymph node, and fibrovascular septa of various organs is not inconsistent with such an origin (Fig. 15). Interestingly, Kaposi's sarcoma rarely involves the brain, which lacks lymphatics.

Malignant Lymphoma

The lymphomas arising in immunodeficiency states differ from those developing in immunocompetent hosts. Follicular lymphomas comprise nearly half the lymphomas in otherwise healthy adults but are rare in immunodeficient individuals.[102] Lymphomas of the central nervous system, which ordinarily account for only 1–2% of non-Hodgkin's lymphomas, are found in nearly half of the lymphomas arising in renal transplant recipients. The majority of lymphomas described in patients with autoimmune disease and other non-AIDS related immunodeficiencies have been classified as large cell lymphomas, immunoblastic lymphoma or Burkitt-like lymphoma.[102,103]

The histopathology of lymphomas associated with AIDS parallels that seen in other

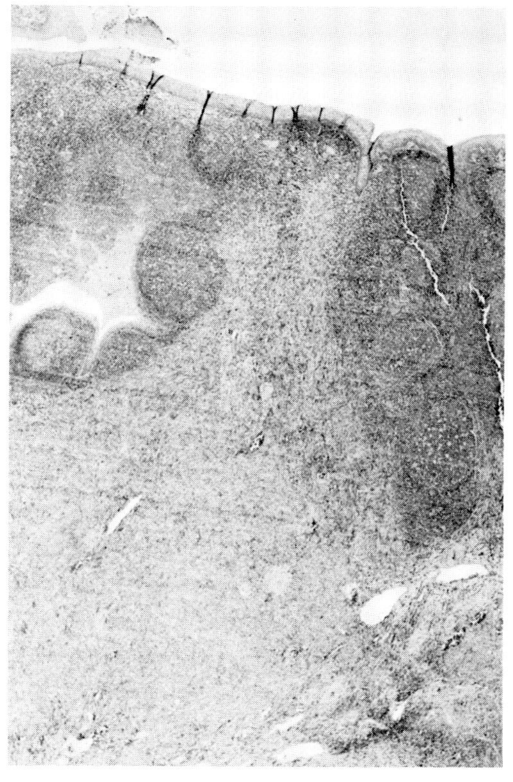

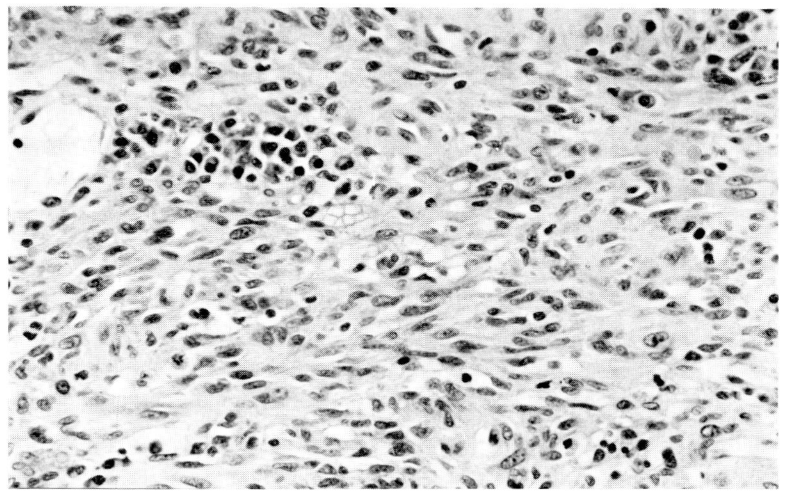

Figure 15. Kaposi's sarcoma involving tonsil. The medulla is diffusely infiltrated by tumor (top) (H&E, original magnification ×25). At a higher power there are typical interlacing tumor cells and slit-like vascular spaces. A cluster of plasma cells is also present (bottom) (H&E, original magnification ×250).

immune deficiency states.[104] Nearly all belong to the more aggressive histologic categories. Burkitt-like lymphoma, immunoblastic lymphoma with plasmacytoid features, and large cell lymphoma (histiocytic lymphoma) predominate. As in other immunosuppressed individuals, these tumors often arise in the central nervous system (Fig. 16) or gastrointestinal tract. The ileocecal region is a common site within this latter group. Most cases studied have demonstrated a B-cell phenotype, and evidence of Epstein-Barr virus infection has been reported in cases of Burkitt-like tumors in patients with AIDS as well as in cases of immunoblastic lymphoma associated with renal transplantation.[105,106]

Small numbers of cases of Hodgkin's disease have been reported in individuals with AIDS-related complex.[107-109] Much like non-Hodgkin's lymphoma in AIDS, Hodgkin's disease presents as an extensive disease that responds poorly to therapy and is associated with short survival intervals.[107-109] It has been suggested by some that the development of Hodgkin's disease in AIDS-related complex occurs at an increased incidence, but this has not been confirmed.[107-109]

UNCLASSIFIED LESIONS

A wide variety of pathologic lesions, not directly attributable to HIV infection, have been reported in AIDS-related complex and AIDS. It is unclear if they occur with increased frequency in HIV-infected individuals or are unrelated epiphenomena.

Lung

Five major lesions have been described in the respiratory system: opportunistic infections; diffuse alveolar damage associated with infections and/or oxygen therapy; Kaposi's sarcoma; pulmonary lymphoid hyperplasia/lymphoid interstitial pneumonitis complex (PLH/LIP complex); and desquamative interstitial pneumonitis (DIP).[110-113] Of these, the last two lesions are primarily diseases of children, but may be seen in adults as well.[110,111] Initially, PLH and LIP

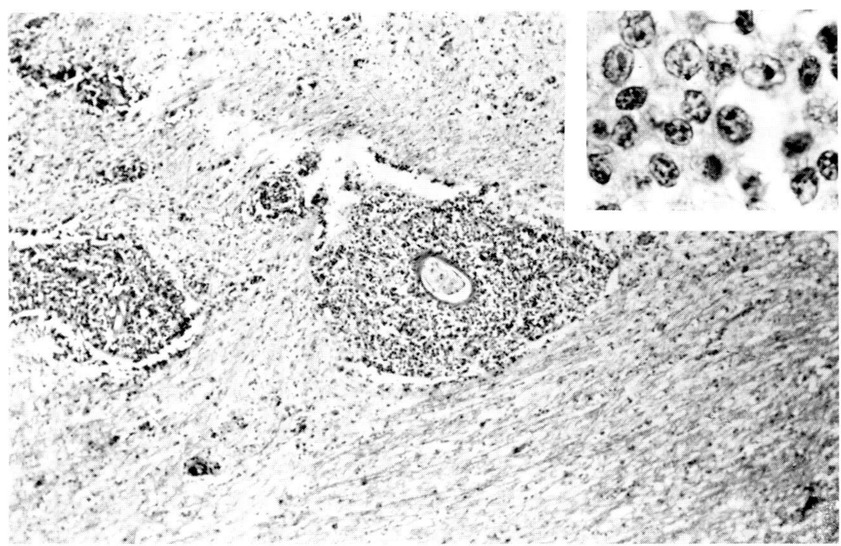

Figure 16. Large cell lymphoma of brain showing perivascular distribution (H&E, original magnification ×80). Inset demonstrates large noncleaved cell cytology (H&E, original magnification ×300).

appeared to be distinct lesions; however, now they appear to be part of the spectrum of the same lesion.[111] Similarly, DIP, which is considered to be a distinctive type of interstitial pneumonitis, appears to represent a reaction in association with other lesions of the lungs, particularly PLH/LIP complex.[111]

Pulmonary lymphoid hyperplasia is characterized by peribronchiolar aggregates of small lymphocytes that occasionally contain germinal centers. LIP consists of a diffuse infiltration of alveolar walls and peribronchiolar regions by small lymphocytes, plasma cells, plasmacytoid lymphocytes, and immunoblasts (Fig. 17). Lymphoid aggregates, occasionally demonstrating germinal centers, are seen in some cases.

In some cases of PLH/LIP complex, progression to a polyclonal polymorphic B-cell lymphoproliferative disorder (PBLD) may be seen.[114] PBLD is characterized by predominantly extranodal, systemic and prominent pulmonary involvement. The lymphoid nodules found in various organs consist of lymphocytes, plasma cells, plasmacytoid lymphocytes, and a few immunoblasts. Vessel wall infiltration or irregular infiltrative borders may be seen in these lesions but necrosis, cellular atypia, or prominent mitotic activity are not present. The pathogenesis of the PLH/LIP complex and PBLD is not clear, but there is evidence to suggest that these lesions may be related to Epstein-Barr virus.[113]

Heart

Cardiomyopathy with or without congestive heart failure has been described in AIDS.[115-116] Pathologic features consist of cardiomegaly with dilatation of ventricles, hypertrophy, and vacuolation of the myocardium, interstitial edema and microscopic foci of necrosis with a sparse inflammatory infiltrate, myocardial fibrosis, and endocardial thickening. The pathogenesis may be related to multiple factors including infec-

tion (undetermined etiology) and nutritional deficiencies.

Arteries

Lesions of small and medium-sized arteries have been described in children.[117] Two types of vascular lesions occur: vascular inflammation seen only in the brain, and fibrocalcific lesions associated with degeneration of elastic tissue of the media of arteries of the heart, lungs, thymus, lymph nodes, spleen, kidneys, and mesentery. A variable degree of luminal narrowing occurs. Very rarely, aneurysm formation can be seen in the coronary arteries. The pathogenesis of the arteriopathy may be related to increased exposure of the arterial wall to endogenous and exogenous elastases associated with opportunistic and other infections.

Kidney

A rapidly progressive nephrotic syndrome has developed in some patients with AIDS.[118-119] It is histologically characterized by focal and segmental glomerulosclerosis and segmental deposition of IgM and C3 in glomeruli. Focal loss of foot processes, shrinkage of glomerular tufts and rare mesangial dense deposits have been noted on ultrastructural examination. Less commonly, immune complex glomerulonephritis may be seen.[118] This lesion is characterized by an increase in glomerular mesangial matrix, extensive interstitial infiltration by lymphocytes and plasma cells, and loss of tubules. Deposition of IgM and C3 in the mesangium is seen when these specimens are immunostained.

The histologic picture found in AIDS-associated nephropathy is not specific, and similar changes have been reported in heroin-associated nephropathy, as well as in up to 10% of children and adults with idiopathic nephrotic syndrome.[118] AIDS patients both with and without a history of IV

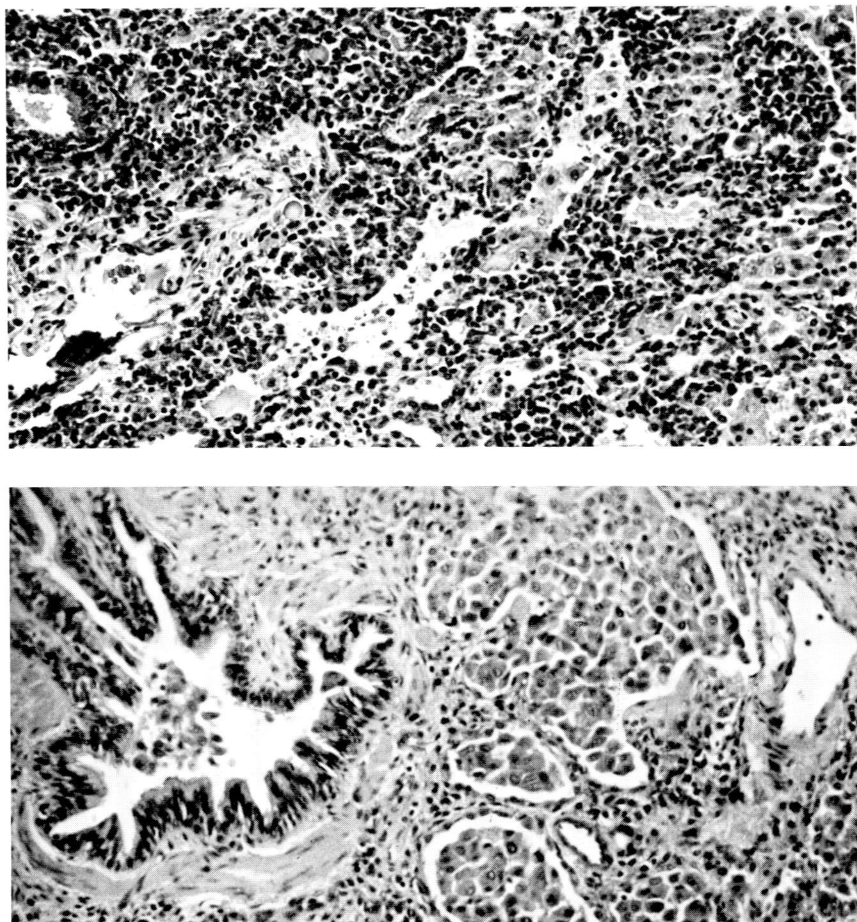

Figure 17. Lung biopsy section showing lymphoid interstitial pneumonitis (upper). A dense infiltration of alveolar septa by lymphoid cells is evident (H&E, original magnification ×150). Desquamative interstitial pneumonitis-like reaction in lung biopsy section is characterized by large clusters of hypertrophic pneumonocytes in alveolar spaces and cuboidal metaplasia of the alveolar lining epithelium (H&E, original magnification ×150). (From Joshi VV, et al: Hum Pathol 1985; 16:241–246)

drug abuse appear to be at risk to develop this lesion. Although the underlying cause is obscure, it appears that focal and segmental glomerulosclerosis is associated with AIDS.[118–119]

CONCLUSION

Careful correlation of clinical information with histopathologic observations is necessary to correctly diagnose the various infections, neoplasms, and lymphoid reactions present in patients infected by the human immunodeficiency virus. Serial sections may be required to demonstrate focal lesions of Kaposi's sarcoma, and compulsive use of cultures and special stains for infectious agents is often essential to detect opportunistic infections such as *Mycobacterium avium-intracellulare* or *cryptococcus* in the absence of a classical inflammatory reaction.

Our knowledge of the histopathology of

AIDS, only recently limited to a chronicle of opportunistic infections, malignancies, and unclassified reactions, is now developing into a detailed understanding of the direct effects of HIV on the host. Yet to come are the descriptions of new opportunistic agents, and morphologic reactions to new drugs. Through careful examination of biopsy and autopsy tissue specimens from patients infected with HIV, pathologists will continue to gain knowledge that is both valuable for individual patient care and for furthering our understanding of the consequences of this devastating infection.

REFERENCES

1. Turner RR, Levine AM, Gill PS, et al: Progressive histologic abnormalities in the persistent generalized lymphadenopathy syndrome. Am J Surg Pathol 1987; 11:625–632
2. Brynes RK, Chan WC, Spira TJ, et al: Value of lymph node biopsy in unexplained lymphadenopathy in homosexual men. JAMA 1983; 250:1313–1317
3. Ewing EP Jr, Chandler FW, Spira TJ, et al: Primary lymph node pathology in AIDS and AIDS-related lymphadenopathy. Arch Pathol Lab Med 1985; 109:977–981
4. Burns BF, Wood GS, Dorfman RF: The varied histopathology of lymphadenopathy in the homosexual male. Am J Surg Pathol 1985; 9:287–297
5. Wood GS, Garcia CF, Dorfman RF, Warnke RA: The immunohistology of follicle lysis in lymph node biopsies from homosexual men. Blood 1985; 66:1092–1097
6. Tenner-Racz K, Racz P, Dietrich M, Kern P: Altered follicular dendritic cells and virus-like particles in AIDS and AIDS-related lymphadenopathy. Lancet 1985; 1:105–106
7. Tenner-Racz K, Racz P, Bofill M, et al: HTLV-III viral antigens in lymph nodes of homosexual men with persistent generalized lymphadenopathy and AIDS. Am J Pathol 1986; 123:9–15
8. Piris MA, Rivas C, Morente M, et al: Persistent and generalized lymphadenopathy: a lesion of follicular dendritic cells. Am J Clin Pathol 1987; 87:716–724
9. Sohn CC, Sheibani K, Winberg CD, Rappaport H: Monocytoid B lymphocytes: Their relation to the patterns of the acquired immunodeficiency syndrome (AIDS) and AIDS-related lymphadenopathy. Hum Pathol 1985; 16:979–985
10. Dorfman RF, Warnke R: Lymphadenopathy simulating the malignant lymphomas. Hum Pathol 1974; 5:519–550
11. Lifson JD, Reyes GR, McGrath MS, et al: AIDS retrovirus induced cytopathology: giant cell formation and involvement of CD4 antigen. Science 1987; 232:1123–1127
12. Wood GS, Burns BF, Dorfman RF, Warnke RA: In situ quantitation of lymph node helper, suppressor, and cytotoxic T cell subsets in AIDS. Blood 1986; 67:596–603
13. Turner RR, Meyer PR, Taylor CR, et al: Immunohistology of persistent generalized lymphadenopathy: evidence for progressive lymph node abnormalities in some patients. Am J Clin Pathol 1987; 88:10–19
14. Chan WC, Brynes RK, Spira TJ, et al: Lymphocyte subsets in lymph nodes of homosexual men. Correlation of morphology and blood changes. Arch Pathol Lab Med 1985; 109:133–137
15. Raphael M, Puletty P, Cavaille-Coll M, et al: Lymphadenopathy in patients at risk for acquired immunodeficiency syndrome. Arch Pathol Lab Med 1985; 109:128–132
16. Garcia CF, Lifson JD, Engleman EG, et al: The immunohistology of the persistent generalized lymphadenopathy syndrome. Am J Clin Pathol 1986; 86:706–715
17. Wood GS, Burns BF, Dorfman RF, Warnke RA: The immunohistology of non-T cells in the acquired immunodeficiency syndrome. Am J Pathol 1985; 120:371–379
18. Chadburn A, Metroka C, Mouradian J: Progressive histopathology and prognostic value of sequential lymph node biopsies in acquired immunodeficiency syndrome in AIDS-related complex. Lab Invest 1987; 54:11A
19. Mathur-Waugh U, Spigland I, Sacks HS: Longitudinal study of persistent generalized lymphadenopathy in homosexual men: relation to acquired immunodeficiency syndrome. Lancet 1984; 2:1033–1038
20. Fishbein DB, Kaplan JE, Spira TJ, et al: Unexplained lymphadenopathy in homosexual men: a longitudinal study. JAMA 1985; 254:930–935
21. Kaplan JE, Spira TJ, Fishbein DB, et al: Lymphadenopathy syndrome in homosexual men: evidence for continuing risk of developing the acquired immunodeficiency syndrome. JAMA 1987; 257:335–337
22. Reichert CM, O'Leary TJ, Levins DL, et al: Autopsy pathology in the acquired immune deficiency syndrome. Am J Pathol 1983; 11:357–382
23. Joshi VV, Oleske JM, Minnefor AB, et al: Pathology of suspected acquired immune deficiency syndrome in children: a study of eight cases. Pediatr Pathol 1984; 2:71–87
24. Abrams DI, Chinn EK, Lewis BJ, et al: Hematologic manifestations in homosexual men with Kaposi's sarcoma. Am J Clin Pathol 1984; 81:13–18
25. Spivak JL, Bender BS, Quinn TC: Hematologic abnormalities in the acquired immunodeficiency syndrome. Am J Med 1984; 77:24–28
26. Walsh CM, Nardi MA, Karpatkin S: On the mechanism of thrombocytopenic purpura in sexually active homosexual men. N Engl J Med 1984; 311:635–639
27. Bender BS, Quinn TC, Spivak JL: Homosexual men with thrombocytopenia have impaired reticuloendothelial system Fc receptor-specific clearance. Blood 1987; 70:392–395

28. Schneider DR, Picker LJ: Myelodysplasia in the acquired immunodeficiency syndrome. Am J Clin Pathol 1985; 84:144–152

29. D'Onofrio G, Mancini S, Tamburrini E, et al: Giant neutrophils with increased peroxidase activity: another evidence of dysgranulopoiesis in AIDS. Am J Clin Pathol 1987; 87:584–591

30. Osborne BM, Guarda LA, Butler JJ: Bone marrow biopsies in patients with the acquired immunodeficiency syndrome. Hum Pathol 1984; 15:1048–1053

31. Fahri DC, Mason UG, Horsburgh CR. The bone marrow in disseminated *Mycobacterium avium-intracellulare* infection. Am J Clin Pathol 1985; 83:463–468

32. Witt D, Mckay D, Schwam L, et al: Acquired immune deficiency syndrome presenting as bone marrow and mediastinal cryptococcosis. Am J Med 1987; 82:149–150

33. Mandell W, Goldberg DM, Neu HC: Histoplasmosis in patients with the acquired immunodeficiency syndrome. Am J Med 1986; 81:974–978

34. Joshi VV, Oleske JM: Pathologic appraisal of the thymus in acquired immunodeficiency syndrome in children: a study of four cases and a review of the literature. Arch Pathol Lab Med 1985; 109:142–146

35. Grody WW, Fligiel S, Naeim F: Thymus involution in the acquired immunodeficiency syndrome. Am J Clin Pathol 1985; 85:85–95

36. Joshi VV, Oleske JM, Saad S, et al: Thymus biopsy in children with acquired immunodeficiency syndrome. Arch Pathol Lab Med 1986; 110:837–842

37. Drew WL, Mintz L, Miner RC, et al: Prevalence of cytomegalovirus infection in homosexual men. J Infect Dis 1981; 143:188–192

38. Emanuel D, Peppard J, Stover D, et al: Rapid immunodiagnosis of cytomegalovirus pneumonia by bronchoalveolar lavage using human and murine monoclonal antibodies. Ann Intern Med 1986; 104:476–481

39. Hilborne L, Nieberg R, Cheng L, et al: Direct in situ DNA hybridization for rapid detection of cytomegalovirus in bronchoalveolar lavage. Lab Invest 1986; 54:26A

40. Hinnant KL, Rotterdam HZ, Bell ET, et al: Cytomegalovirus infection of the alimentary tract: a clinicopathological correlation. Am J Gastroenterol 1986; 881:994–950

41. Frank D, Raicht RF: Intestinal perforation associated with cytomegalovirus infection in patients with acquired immune deficiency syndrome. Am J Gastroenterol 1984; 79:201–205

42. Greene LW, Cole W, Greene JB, et al: Adrenal insufficiency as a complication of the acquired immunodeficiency syndrome. Ann Intern Med 1984; 101:497–498

43. Tapper ML, Rotterdam HZ, Lerner CW, et al: Adrenal necrosis in the acquired immunodeficiency syndrome. Ann Intern Med 1984; 100:239–241

44. Kennedy PG, Newsome DA, Hess J, et al: Cytomegalovirus but not human T lymphotropic virus type III/lymphadenopathy associated virus detected by in situ hybridization in retinal lesions in patients with the acquired immune deficiency syndrome. Br Med J 1986; 293:162–164

45. Jenson OA, Gerstoft J, Thomsen HK, et al: Cytomegalovirus retinitis in the acquired immunodeficiency syndrome (AIDS). Light microscopical, ultrastructural and immunohistochemical examination of a case. Acta Ophthalmologia 1984; 62:1–9

46. Morgello S, Cho E-S, Nielsen S, et al: Cytomegalovirus encephalitis in patients with acquired immunodeficiency syndrome: an autopsy study of 30 cases and a review of the literature. Hum Pathol 1987; 18:289–297

47. Corey L, Spear PG: Infections with herpes simplex viruses. N Eng J Med 1986; 314:686–691; 740–757

48. Klein RJ. The pathogenesis of acute, latent and recurrent herpes simplex virus infections. Brief review. Arch Virol 1982; 72:143–168

49. Siegel FP, Lopez C, Hammer GS, et al: Severe acquired immunodeficiency in male homosexuals, manifested by chronic perianal ulcerative herpes simplex lesions. N Engl J Med 1981; 305:1439–1444

50. Matsumoto J, Sumiyoshi A: Herpes simplex esophagitis—a study in autopsy series. Am J Clin Pathol 1985; 84:96–99

51. Greenspan JS, Greenspan D, Lennette ET, et al: Oral viral leukoplakia—a new AIDS associated condition. Adv Exp Med Biol 1985; 187:123–128

52. Greenspan D, Greenspan JS, Hearst NG, et al: Relation of oral hairy leukoplakia to infection with human immunodeficiency virus and the risk of developing AIDS. J Infect Dis 1987; 155:475–481

53. Greenspan D, Greenspan JS, Conant M, et al: Oral "hairy leukoplakia" in male homosexuals: evidence of association with both papillomavirus and a herpes-group virus. Lancet 1984; 8:831–834

54. Bedri J, Weinstein W, DeGregorio P, et al: Progressive multifocal leukoencephalopathy in acquired immunodeficiency syndrome. N Engl J Med 1983; 309:492–493

55. Stoner GL, Ryschkewitsch CF, Walker DL, et al: JC papovavirus large tumor (T)-antigen expression in brain tissue of acquired immune deficiency syndrome (AIDS) and non-AIDS patients with progressive multifocal leukoencephalopathy. Proc Natl Acad Sci USA 1986; 83:2271–2275

56. Aksamit AJ, Mourrain P, Sever JL, et al: Progressive multifocal leukoencephalopathy: investigation of three cases using in situ hybridization with JC virus biotinylated DNA probe. Ann Neurol 1985; 18:490–496

57. Wolinsky E: Nontuberculous mycobacteria and associated diseases. Am Rev Resp Dis 1979; 119:107–159

58. Benjamin DR: Granulomatous lymphadenitis in children. Arch Pathol Lab Med 1987; 111:750–753

59. Greene JB, Sidhu GS, Lewin S, et al: *Mycobacterium avium-intracellulare:* a cause of disseminated life-threatening infection in homosexuals and drug abusers. Ann Intern Med 1982; 97:539–546

60. Young LS, Inderlied CB, Berlin OG, et al: Myco-bacterial infections in AIDS patients, with an emphasis on the *Mycobacterium avium* complex. Rev Infect Dis 1986; 8:1024–1033

61. Hawkins CC, Gold JWM, Whimbey E, et al: *Mycobacterium avium* complex infections in patients with the acquired immunodeficiency syndrome. Ann Intern Med 1986; 105:184–188

62. Roth RI, Owen RL, Keren DF: AIDS with *Mycobacterium avium-intracellulare* lesions resembling those of Whipple's disease. N Engl J Med 1983; 309:1324–1325

63. Schneebaum CW, Novick DM, Chabon AB, et al: Terminal ileitis associated with *Mycobacterium avium-intracellulare* infection in a homosexual man with acquired immune deficiency syndrome. Gastroenterology 1987; 93:1127–1132

64. Sunderam G, McDonald RJ, Maniatis T, et al: Tuberculosis as a manifestation of the acquired immunodeficiency syndrome (AIDS). JAMA 1986; 256:362–366

65. Mann J, Snider De Jr, Francis H, et al: Association between HTLV-III/LAV infection and tuberculosis in Zaire. JAMA 1986; 256:346

66. Centers for Disease Control: Tuberculosis and acquired immunodeficiency syndrome—Florida. MMWR 1986; 35:587–590

67. Louie E, Rice LB, Holzman RS: Tuberculosis in non-Haitian patients with acquired immunodeficiency syndrome. Chest 1986: 90:542–545

68. Holmberg K, Meyer RD: Fungal infections in patients with AIDS and AIDS-related complex. Scand J Infect Dis 1986; 18:179–192

69. Gelwan JS, Gold BM, Shih HJ, et al: Oral candidiasis and AIDS. NY State J Med 1987; 87:303–304

70. Rodgers VD, Kagnoff MF: Gastrointestinal manifestations of the acquired immunodeficiency syndrome. West J Med 1987; 146:57–67

71. Ro JY, Lee SS, Ayala AG: Advantage of Fontana-Masson stain in capsule-deficiency cryptococcal infection. Arch Pathol Lab Med 1987; 111:53–57

72. Watts JC, Chandler FW: Infection by capsule-deficient *Cryptococci.* Arch Pathol Lab Med 1987; 111:688

73. Gal AA, Koss MN, Hawkins J, et al: The pathology of pulmonary cryptococcal infections in the acquired immunodeficiency syndrome. Arch Pathol Lab Med 1986; 110:502–507

74. Kovacs JA, Kovacs AA, Polis M, et al: Cryptococcosis in the acquired immunodeficiency syndrome. Ann Intern Med 1985; 103:533–538

75. Chandler FW, McClure HM, Campbell WG Jr, et al: Pulmonary pneumocystosis in nonhuman primates. Arch Pathol Lab Med 1976; 100:163–167

76. Shimono LH, Hartman B: A simple and reliable rapid methenamine silver stain for *Pneumocystis carinii* and fungi. Arch Pathol Lab Med 1986; 110:855–856

77. Watts JC, Chandler FW: *Pneumocystis carinii* pneumonitis. The nature and diagnostic significance of the methenamine silver-positive "intracystic bodies". Am J Surg Pathol 1985; 9:744–751

78. Gal AA, Klatt EC, Koss MN, et al: The effectiveness of bronchoscopy in the diagnosis of *Pneumocystis carinii* and cytomegalovirus pulmonary infections in acquired immunodeficiency syndrome. JAMA 1987; 111:238–241

79. Mills J: *Pneumocystis carinii* and *Toxoplasma gondii* infections in patients with AIDS. Rev Infect Dis 1986; 8:1001–1011

80. Grimes MM, LaPook JD, Bar MH, et al: Disseminated *Pneumocystis carinii* infection in a patient with acquired immunodeficiency syndrome. Hum Pathol 1987; 18:307–308

81. Heyman MR, Rasmussen P. *Pneumocystis carinii* involvement of the bone marrow in acquired immunodeficiency syndrome. Am J Clin Pathol 1987; 87:780–783

82. Pilon VA, Echols RM, Celo JS, et al: Disseminated *Pneumocystis carinii* infection in AIDS. N Engl J Med 1987; 316:1410–1411

83. Luft BJ, Brooks RG, Conley FK, et al: Toxoplasmic encephalitis in patients with acquired immune deficiency syndrome. JAMA 1984; 252:913–917

84. Moskowitz LB, Hensley GT, Chan JC, et al: Brain biopsies in patients with acquired immune deficiency syndrome. Arch Pathol Lab Med 1984; 108:368–371

85. Navia BA, Petito CK, Gold JWM, et al: Cerebral toxoplasmosis complicating the acquired immune deficiency syndrome: clinical and neuropathological findings in 27 patients. Ann Neurol 1986; 19:224–238

86. Wong B, Gold JWM, Brown AE, et al: Central nervous system toxoplasmosis in homosexual men and parenteral drug abusers. Ann Intern Med 1984; 100:36–42

87. Yermakov V, Rashid RK, Vuletin JC, et al: Disseminated toxoplasmosis. Case report and review of the literature. Arch Pathol Lab Med 1982; 106:524–528

88. Casemore DP, Sands RL, Curry A: Cryptosporidium species—a "new" human pathogen. J Clin Pathol 1985; 38:1321–1336

89. Lefkowitch JH, Krumholz S, Feng-Chen K-C, et al: Cryptosporidiosis of the human small intestine: a light and electron microscopic study. Hum Pathol 1984; 15:746–752

90. Modigliani R, Bories C, Le Charpentier Y, et al: Diarrhea and malabsorption in acquired immune deficiency syndrome: a study of four cases with special emphasis on opportunistic protozoan infestations. Gut 1985; 26:179–187

91. Wolfson JS, Richter JM, Waldron MA, et al: Cryptosporidiosis in immunocompetent patients. N Engl J Med 1985; 312:1278–1282

92. Casemore DP, Armstrong M, Sands RL: Laboratory diagnosis of cryptosporidiosis. J Clin Pathol 1985; 38:1337–1341

93. Guarda LA, Stein SA, Cleary KA, et al: Human cryptosporidiosis in the acquired immune deficiency syndrome. Arch Pathol Lab Med 1983; 107:562–566

94. Ma P, Villanueva TG, Kaufman D, et al: Respiratory cryptosporidiosis in the acquired immune deficiency syndrome. Use of modified cold Kinyoun and hemacolor stains for rapid diagnosis. JAMA 1984; 252:1298–1301

95. Penn I: Kaposi's sarcoma in organ transplant recipients: report of 20 cases. Transplantation 1979; 27:8–11
96. Penn I, Hammond A, Brett-Schneider L, Starzl TE: Malignant lymphomas in transplantation patients. Transpl Proc 1969; 1:106
97. Ulbright TM, Santa Cruz J: Kaposi's sarcoma: its relationship with hematologic lymphoid and thymic neoplasia. Cancer 1981; 47:963–973
98. Gatti RA, Goud RA: Occurrence of malignancy in immunodeficiency diseases: a literature review. Cancer 1971; 28:89–98
99. Hymes KB, Cheung T, Greene JB, et al: Kaposi's sarcoma—a report of eight cases. Lancet 1981; 2:598–600
100. Gottlieb GJ, Ackerman AB: Kaposi's sarcoma: an extensively disseminated form in young homosexual men. Hum Pathol 1982; 13:882–892
101. Beckstead JH, Wood GH, Fletcher V: Evidence for the origin of Kaposi's sarcoma from lymphatic endothelium. Am J Pathol 1985; 119:294–300
102. Frizzera G, Rosai J, Dehner LP, et al: Lymphoreticular disorders in primary immunodeficiencies: new findings based on an up-to-date histologic classification of 35 cases. Cancer 1980; 46:692–699
103. Krikorian JG, Burke JS, Rosenberg SA, Kaplan HS: Occurrence of non-Hodgkin's lymphoma after therapy for Hodgkin's disease. N Engl J Med 1979; 300:452–458
104. Ziegler JL, Beckstead JA, Volberding PA, et al: Non-Hodgkin's lymphoma in 90 homosexual men: relation to generalized lymphadenopathy and the acquired immunodeficiency syndrome. N Engl J Med 1984; 311:565–570
105. Ziegler JL, Drew WL, Miner RL, et al: Outbreak of Burkitt's-like lymphoma in homosexual men. Lancet 1982; 2:631–633
106. Hanto D, Frizzera G, Purtillo DT: Clinical spectrum of lymphoproliferative disorders in renal transplant recipients and evidence for the role of Epstein-Barr virus. Cancer Res 1981; 41:4253–4261
107. Shoeppel SL, Hoppe RT, Dorfman RF, et al: Hodgkin's disease in homosexual men with generalized lymphadenopathy. Ann Intern Med 1985; 102:68–70
108. Unger PD, Strauchen JA: Hodgkin's disease in AIDS-related complex patients. Report of four patients and tissue immunologic marker studies. Cancer 1986; 58:821–825
109. Temple JJ, Andes WA: AIDS and Hodgkin's disease, Lancet 1986; 1:454–455
110. Joshi VV, Oleske JM, Minnefor AB, et al: Pathologic pulmonary findings in children with the acquired immunodeficiency syndrome. Hum Pathol 1986; 17:241–246
111. Joshi VV, Oleske JM: Pulmonary lesions in children with the acquired immunodeficiency syndrome: A reappraisal based on data in additional cases and follow-up study of previously reported cases. Hum Pathol 1986; 17:641–642
112. Marchevsky A, Rosen MJ, Chrystal G, Kleinerman J: Pulmonary complications of the acquired immunodeficiency syndrome: A clinicopathic study of 70 cases. Hum Pathol 1985; 16: 659–670
113. Andiman VA, Eastman R, Kelsey M, et al: Opportunistic lymphoproliferations associated with Epstein-Barr viral DNA in infants and children with AIDS. Lancet 1985; 1:1390–1393
114. Joshi VV, Kaufman S, Oleske JM, et al: Polyclonal polymorphic B-cell lymphoproliferative disorder with prominent pulmonary involvement in children with AIDS. Cancer 1987; 59:1455–1462
115. Joshi VV, Gadol C, Connor E, et al: Dilated cardiomyopathy in children with AIDS. Hum Pathol 1988; 10:69–73
116. Cohen IS, Anderson DW, Virmani R, et al: Congestive cardiomegaly in association with the acquired immunodeficiency syndrome. N Engl J Med 1986; 315:628–630
117. Joshi VV, Pawel B, Conner E, et al: Arteriopathy in children with AIDS. Pediatr Pathol 1987; 7:261–275
118. Rao TKS, Filippone EJ, Nicastri AD, et al: Associated focal and segmented glomerulosclerosis in the acquired immunodeficiency syndrome. N Engl J Med 1984; 310:669–673
119. Rao TKS, Friedman EA, Nicastri AD: The types of renal disease in the acquired immunodeficiency syndrome. N Engl J Med 1987; 316:1062–1068

2

Ultrastructural Analysis of Germinal Centers in Lymph Nodes of Patients with HIV-1-Induced Persistent Generalized Lymphadenopathy: Evidence for Persistence of Infection

Klara Tenner-Rácz
Paul Rácz
Suzanne Gartner
Julia Ramsauer
Manfred Dietrich
Jean-Claude Gluckman
Mikulas Popovic

CURRENTLY AVAILABLE DATA indicate that persons who are infected with the human immunodeficiency virus Type 1 (HIV-1) should be considered as infectious for life because HIV-1 persists in these individuals. Viremia in HIV-1 infection is not known in the classical sense. In the circulating blood, the number of cells expressing viral RNA is extremely low.[1] It is conceivable, however, that cells of the mononuclear phagocyte system throughout the tissues serve as the major reservoir of the virus.[2-7]

An often overlooked fact is that germinal centers (GC) of lymph nodes from patients with persistent generalized lymphadenopathy (PGL) or AIDS harbor many free retrovirus particles. Cell-free virions may also contribute to the persistence of HIV-1. Evidence that GC in these patients contain retrovirus particles was first obtained by ultrastructural analysis.[8-10] This constant finding emphasizes the diagnostic value of electron microscopic examinations of lymph nodes from patients with PGL or AIDS.[8,11-13]

In describing the presence of retrovirus particles in the GC, Armstrong and Horne also observed budding profiles on follicular dendritic cells (FDC) and suggested that

Supported by grants from Bundesministerium für Jugend, Familie, Frauen und Gesundheit, Bonn; and Körber-Stiftung, Hamburg.

viral nonlymphoid cell tropism may be a significant factor in the pathogenesis of the disease.[8,9] In addition, we noted severe lytic degeneration of FDC in the vicinity of virions[10] and the association of gag proteins of HIV-1 using immunohistochemical double labeling on frozen sections.[14-16]

The authors suggested that GC might serve as a major virus reservoir in PGL.[14-17] The deposition of gag proteins in the GC, also demonstrated by Baroni et al.,[18] is a characteristic finding in HIV-1-induced lymphadenopathy, and gag proteins can be detected even in degenerated GC as long as FDC are still present.[15,16]

The importance of the GC in the pathogenesis of the disease has gained further support by the observation that GC of the spleen also harbor retrovirus particles* and by results of in situ hybridization showing that within the lymph nodes, the majority of cells expressing viral RNA are inside the GC.[17,19] Similarly, other retroviruses (e.g., Rauscher leukemia virus, feline leukemia virus) appear to possess an affinity for GC.[20,21]

The present study was undertaken: (1) to evaluate the ultrastructural changes within GC in HIV-1-induced follicular hyperplasia; (2) to gain information regarding the dynamics of the infection of GC by comparing the alterations of lymph nodes obtained shortly after seroconversion with those seen in longstanding lymphadenopathy; and (3) to demonstrate the presence of free virus particles and their localization relative to sites of virus replication in repeated biopsy specimens.

MATERIAL AND METHODS

Lymph nodes were selected from a large series of cases of HIV-1-induced lymphadenopathy, which had been previously analyzed with light microscopic and immunohistochemical methods.[16] Forty lymph nodes from 36 homosexual males with PGL were chosen. In all cases the lymph nodes showed an exuberant follicular hyperplasia. The lymph nodes were divided into 3 groups: (1) early cases when the biopsy was performed 2–6 weeks after seroconversion (4 lymph nodes); (2) longstanding lymphadenopathy when the lymph node swelling had been present for at least 6 months before the biopsy (28 lymph nodes); and (3) repeated biopsies obtained 11, 16, 20, or 25 months after the initial biopsy (8 lymph nodes from 4 patients). Ten lymph nodes with follicular hyperplasia not related to HIV served as controls.

Tissues were fixed in 5% glutaraldehyde in cacodylate buffer (pH 7.2), postfixed in OsO_4 (cacodylate buffer, pH 7.2), dehydrated in graded acetons, and embedded in Araldite. Semithin sections were stained with methylene blue-azure II stain and examined for the presence of GC with a light microscope. To standardize the field to be investigated ultrastructurally, areas at the boundary of densely and sparsely populated zones of GC were chosen. Ultrathin sections from 3 blocks of each case were cut with a diamond knife, stained with uranyl acetate and lead citrate and examined with a Philips 201 electron microscope.

RESULTS

Germinal centers represent a complex immunologic environment composed of B cells, mainly centroblasts and centrocytes, T cells that are almost exclusively CD4+ lymphocytes, macrophages with or without signs of extensive phagocytosis, and FDC. No alterations were seen in centroblasts, centrocytes, and tingible body macrophages following HIV-1 infection; however, pathologic changes of varying degrees of severity were observed in FDC.

---

*Diebold, personal communication.

ULTRASTRUCTURE OF FOLLICULAR DENDRITIC CELLS IN THE CONTROL NODES

Follicular dendritic cells are big cells with a large nucleus containing loosely arranged chromatin and a small nucleolus. Deep nuclear invaginations may be present. The cytoplasmic rim around the nucleus is narrow. It contains a few mitochondria, several profiles of rough endoplasmic reticulum, moderate amounts of ribosomes, and, on favorable sections, a well developed Golgi apparatus. No phagosomes can be found. The cytoplasm continues in long slender processes (Fig. 1), dendrites, covered by an electron dense material known to contain antigen-antibody complexes. The dendrites are connected to each other by desmosomes creating a network over the entire GC.

ULTRASTRUCTURAL CHANGES IN GERMINAL CENTERS IN THE EARLY PHASE OF HIV-1 INFECTION

The ultrastructural appearance of FDC is practically the same as in control lymph nodes. In some areas, however, the number of dendrites was slightly increased, but no degenerative changes could be observed (Fig. 2). After an extensive search, characteristic retrovirus particles with an average diameter of 100 nm were found. They were located in the interdendritic extracellular spaces and embedded in the electron dense material covering the surface of FDC (Fig. 2). Occasionally, polymorphonuclear leukocytes and extravasated erythrocytes were seen in these areas.

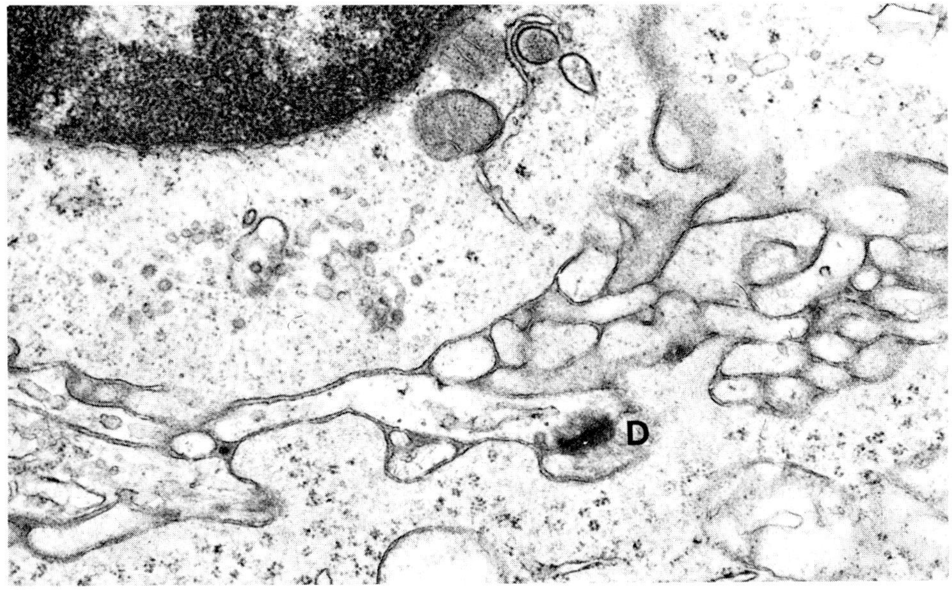

Figure 1. Cytoplasmic processes of FDC. The surface is covered by an electron dense material. D = desmosome. Control lymph node. Original magnification ×10,000.

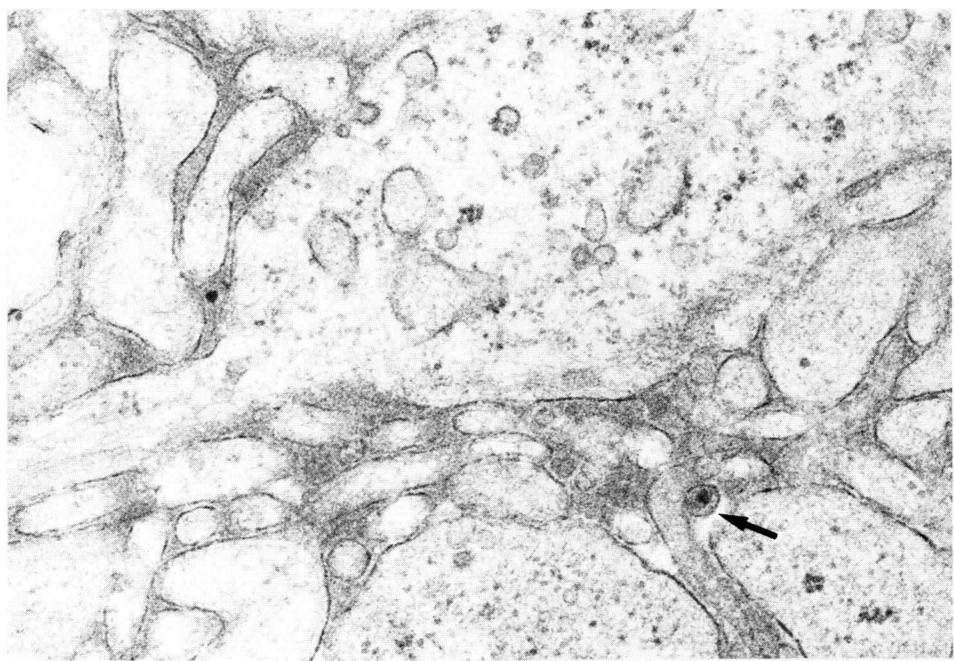

Figure 2. An extracellular retrovirus particle (arrow) in the infoldings of FDC. Slightly increased amount of electron dense material on the cell surface. No evidence of cell damage. Early phase of HIV-1 infection. Original magnification ×20,000.

ULTRASTRUCTURAL CHANGES IN GERMINAL CENTERS WITH LONGSTANDING HYPERPLASIA

In all lymph nodes, virus-associated hypertrophy of FDC was seen (Fig. 3). The hypertrophy was characterized by an increased number of organelles and dendrites, the latter often exhibiting swelling and fragmentation (Fig. 4). There was a considerable variation in the amount of electron dense material outside of the cells, some dendrites having lost this coat, while on others it was more prominent than in controls.

These lymph nodes harbor many free retrovirus particles within the extracellular compartment of the labyrinth formed by the abnormal dendrites (Fig. 4). Some virions possessed the characteristic cylindrical core, while in others it was round and located either centrally or eccentrically, depending on the plane of sectioning. In addition, there were numerous moderately electron-dense round structures with a diameter of 30–100 nm limited by a unit membrane similar to that surrounding the virus particles (Figs. 5 and 6).

In areas with abundant viral particles, degenerative changes of FDC can be observed. Focal loss of cytoplasmic matrix (Fig. 3), severe swelling of mitochondria, or complete cytolysis (Fig. 6a and 6b) were regularly found. In addition, erythrocytes, some polymorphonuclear leukocytes, and lymphocytes with pyknotic nuclei and disintegrated cytoplasm can be recognized in the vicinity of virus particles containing areas.

The retrovirus particles were unevenly distributed. Each block contained at least one heavily infected focus extending over two or more meshes of the grid. Occasional virus particles were present in areas between these foci, and ultrastructural changes of FDC were not evident.

In 6 cases, macrophages contained retrovirus particles located in intracytoplasmic

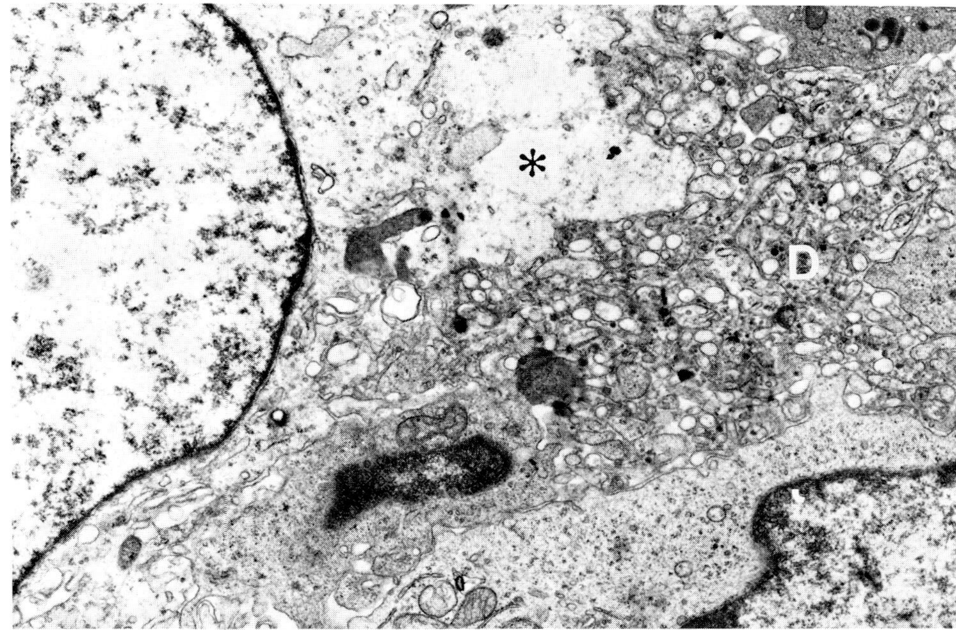

Figure 3. Increased number of dendrites (D) in longstanding lymphadenopathy. Focal disintegration (asterisk) of cytoplasmic matrix of a FDC. Original magnification ×7,000.

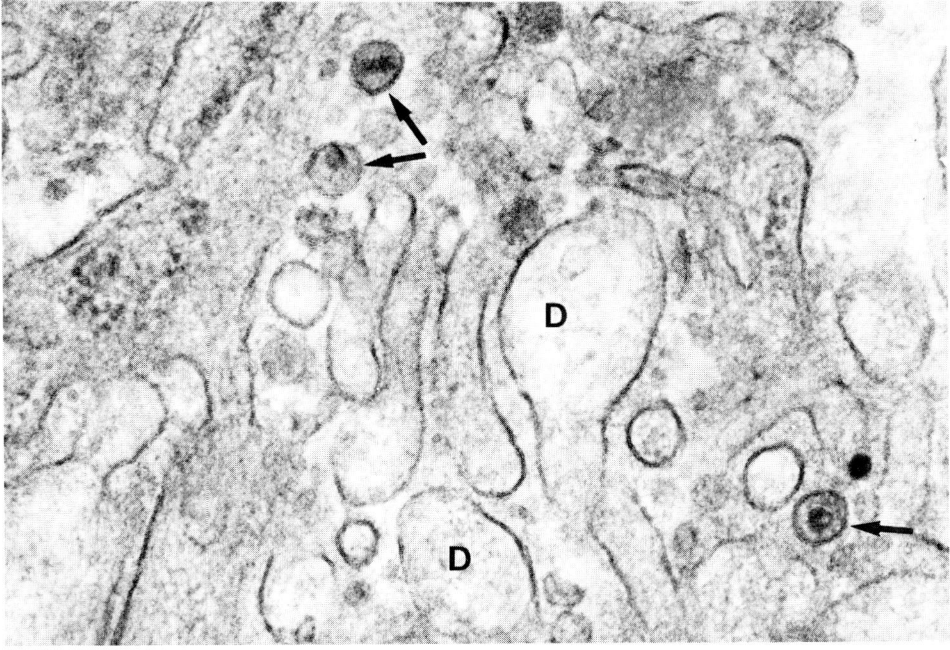

Figure 4. Many extracellular retrovirus particles (arrows) in longstanding lymphadenopathy. The dendrites (D) are swollen and fragmented. Original magnification ×30,000.

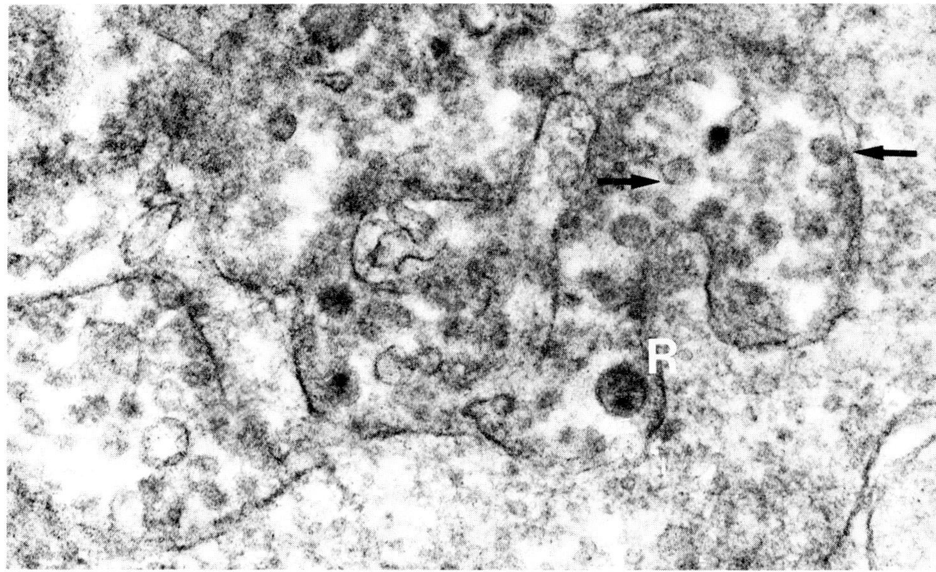

Figure 5. A retrovirus particle (R) and numerous moderately electron dense round structures of differing diameters (arrows) in the interdendritic extracellular space. Longstanding lymphadenopathy. Original magnification ×30,000.

vacuoles (Fig. 7). The structure of these macrophages was well preserved. However, no retrovirus particles were seen in tingible body macrophages.

ULTRASTRUCTURAL CHANGES OF GERMINAL CENTERS IN CASES WITH REPEATED BIOPSIES

In all cases, the same ultrastructural alterations as described in lymph nodes with longstanding lymphadenopathy were observed in the first as well as in the second specimens. Infected foci with numerous retrovirus particles could easily be found even in lymph nodes taken 25 months after the initial biopsy.

VIRUS REPLICATION WITHIN THE GERMINAL CENTERS

Budding of virus particles from the cellular membrane of FDC, macrophages, and lymphocytes (Fig. 8a, b, c) was detected only in samples with longstanding lymphadenopathy. An extensive examination was required to find the budding particles. No budding profiles were present on blasts and degenerating lymphocytes.

DISCUSSION

The present ultrastructural study underlines the importance of GC in the pathogenesis of HIV-1-induced lymphadenopathy. It demonstrates that GC can be infected very early in the course of the disease, that the infection persists for long periods of time, and that active virus replication involving different cell types occurs here.

Retrovirus particles gain access to GC shortly after infection. Lymph nodes removed at the time of seroconversion or shortly thereafter already contain a few virions. The retrovirus particles are located exclusively in the interdendritic extracellular spaces. In this phase of the infection, FDC lack any significant ultrastructural al-

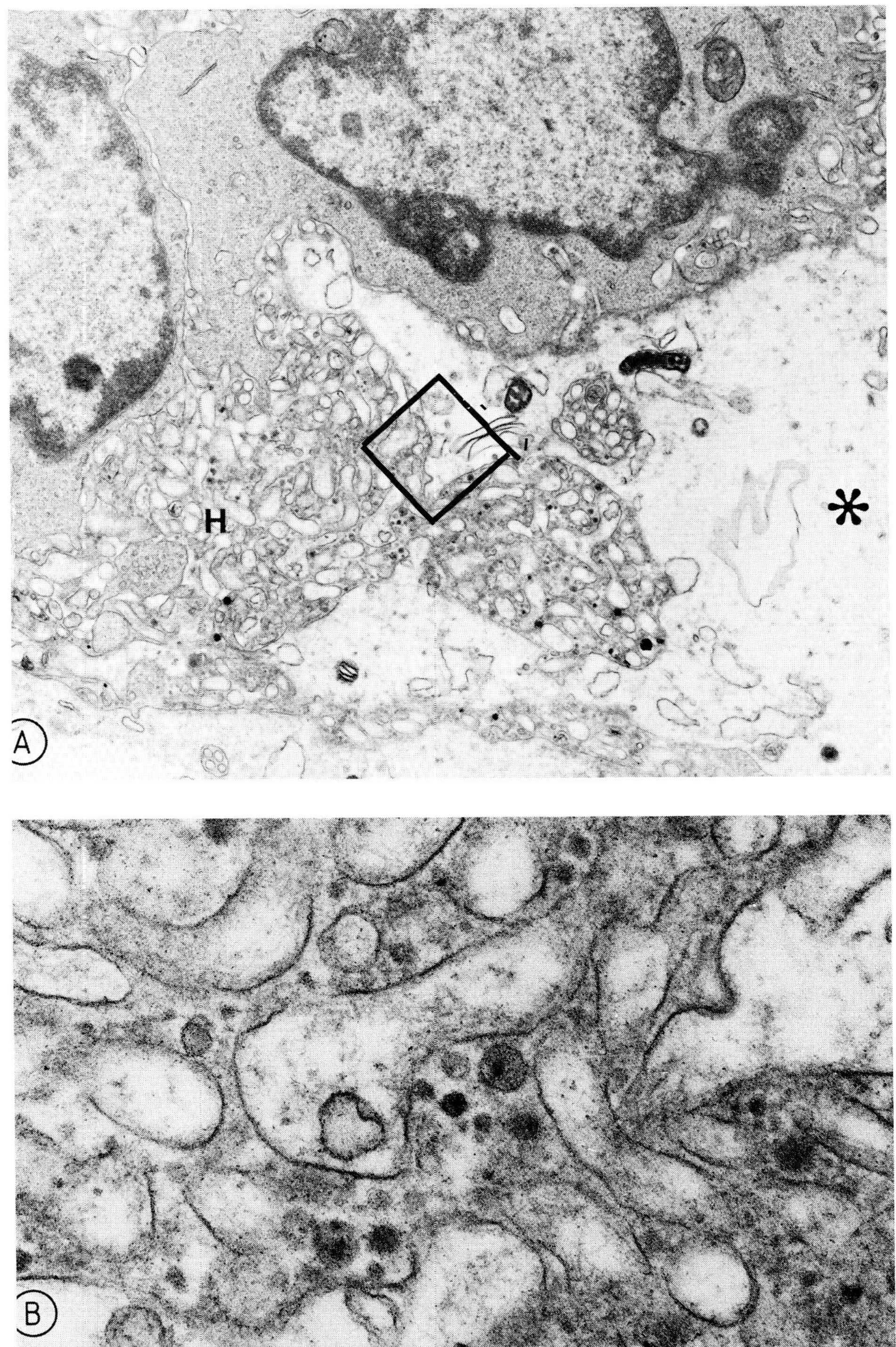

Figure 6. (A) Hypertrophy (H) and cytolysis (asterisk) of FDC in longstanding lymphadenopathy. Note the well preserved ultrastructure of the neighboring lymphocytes. (B): Higher magnification illustrates the presence of small round structures and retrovirus particles. Original magnification (A) ×7,000; (B) ×30,000.

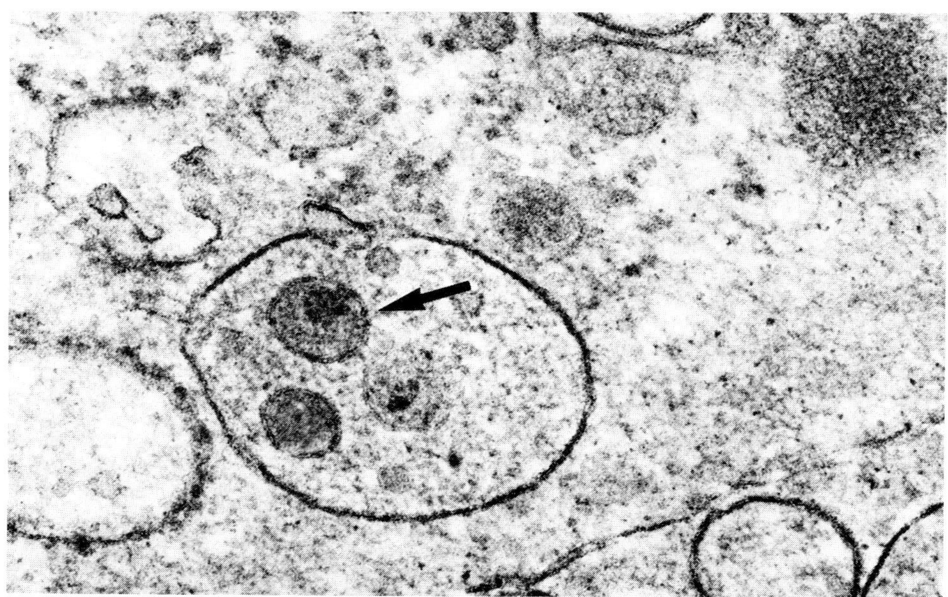

Figure 7. Retrovirus particles (arrow) in an intracytoplasmic vacuole of a macrophage. Longstanding lymphadenopathy. Original magnification ×45,000.

terations. Previous immunohistochemical examinations of these cases revealed no major destruction of the network of FDC and only slight deposition of gag proteins associated with the network.[16] The lack of significant alteration of FDC at early stages of infection suggests that functional impairment is limited. Given the crucial role of FDC in the immune response, these findings further indicate that FDC may also play a major role in the initial infection of GC by HIV-1.

The FDC in organized lymphoid tissues are known to capture, retain, and present antigen to lymphocytes.[22] In HIV-1-induced PGL, there is continuous entrapment of the virus by FDC, which can result in the infection of other cells (FDC, macrophages, lymphocytes) with subsequent replication of HIV-1 in a considerable number of cells within GC. Virus production continues unabatedly and HIV-1 itself, behaving as an antigen, becomes the source of chronic antigenic stimulation. The ultimate result is hypertrophy and hyperplasia of GC as well as

the FDC themselves. A similar phenomenon can be elicited by antigenic stimulation in experimental animals.[23-26]

Germinal centers are rich in cells bearing the CD4 receptor. Lymphocytes with a high density of the CD4 molecule can represent as much as 25% of the total cell population.[27] Present also are macrophages and a smaller number of FDC, both of which are cell types expressing the CD4 molecule in lower concentrations.[28] Although the number of FDC is not high, their surface area exceeds that of any other cell types in the follicles because of their ramified cell processes. It has been estimated that in mice immunized with sheep erythrocytes, FDC account for approximately only 2% of the total cell population. Their surface area, however, was found to be 10 times greater than that of the lymphoid cells.[26]

Antigens trapped by and retained on FDC are generally complexed with antibody.[24,26] However, in view of the limited ability of anti-HIV antibody to neutralize the virus,[29-31] it is likely that some virions found

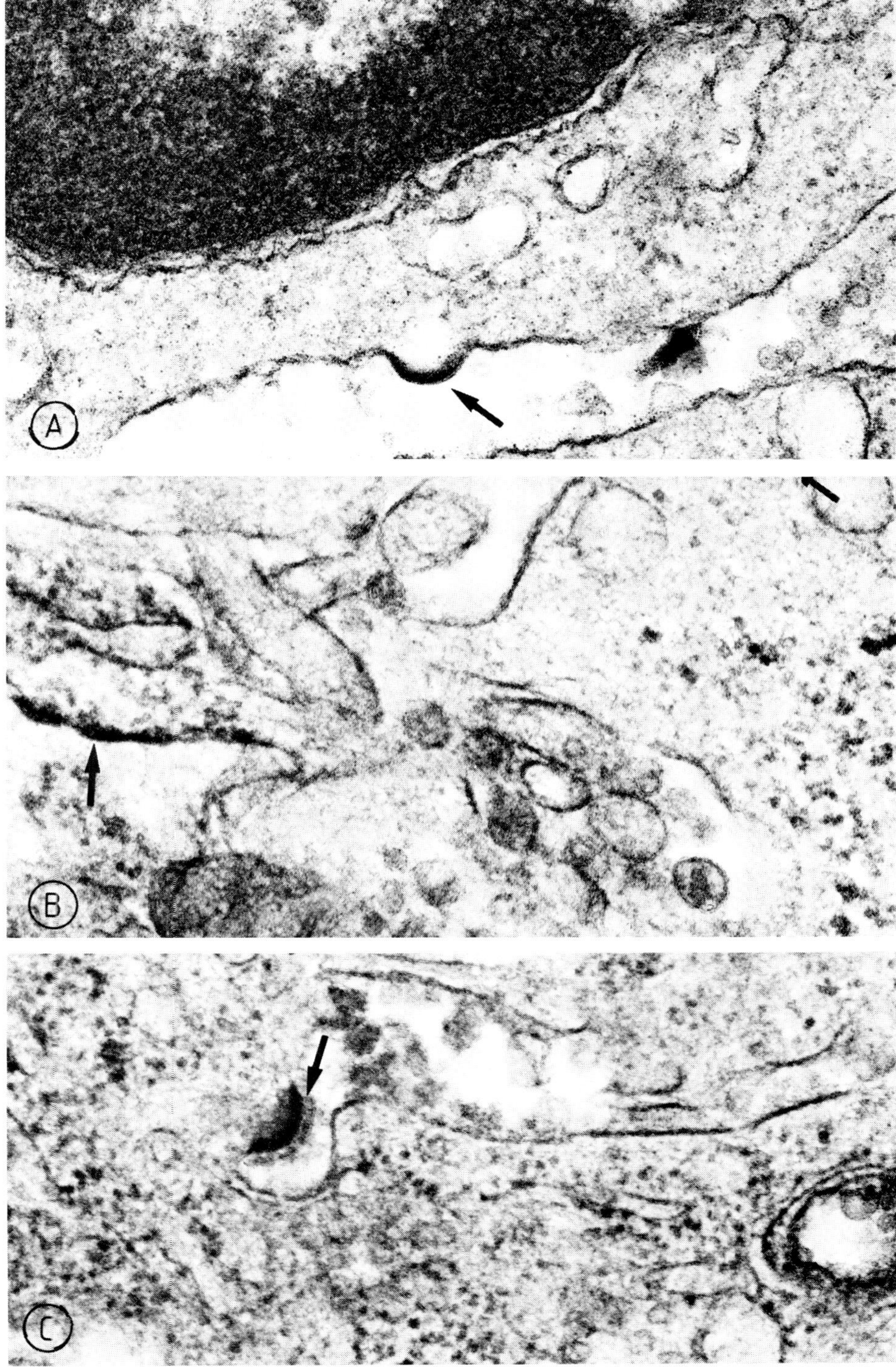

Figure 8. Budding of virus particles (arrows) from the cellular membrane of a lymphocyte (A), an FDC (B), and a macrophage (C). Original magnification (A) ×30,000; (B) ×30,000, and (C) ×45,000.

in the GC remain infectious. Because of the migratory capability of lymphocytes and macrophages, the presence of budding virions on the surface of these cells while residing in the GC is not evidence of infection. Follicular dendritic cells, however, are thought to be nonmigratory as well as long-lived.[32] Therefore, the presence of budding particles on the surface of FDC suggests that HIV-1 infection of permissive cells actually occurs within the GC.

Free retrovirus particles persist in the GC for a long time. To our knowledge, there are no data in the literature dealing with the question of how long a lymph node can harbor HIV-1. In our limited number of cases, repeated biopsies demonstrated the persistence of many free virions for up to 2 years.

Destruction of different cell types in HIV-1 induced lymphadenopathy is evidenced by the presence of degenerating FDC[10,12,14–16,33–39] and lymphocytes in the GC. This can be a consequence either of the cytopathic effects of HIV-1, or of an autoimmune-like process possibly related to the recognition of HIV-antigens presented by FDC.[40] Surprisingly, although these alterations lead to follicular disintegration and involution, the process is a slow one. In most patients, the histologic features of the lymph node(s) remain quite constant for a number of years. Likewise, immunologic parameters and the general clinical picture remain stable. Obviously, the immunologic mechanism(s) involved in the balance between virus and host are complex and not fully understood. Several factors must be considered.

In vitro studies have suggested that non-lymphoid target cells are less sensitive to the cytopathic effects of HIV-1 than CD4$^+$ lymphocytes, in spite of the fact that the magnitude and longevity of virus production in the former exceeds that of the latter.[2,3,5,6] The interaction between HIV-1 and its host FDC or macrophage in the GC could be similar. In addition, the numerous round, moderately electron dense structures of differing diameters seen in the nodes taken from patients with longstanding lymphadenopathy might represent degenerating virions, defective or biologically inactive particles. Such particles could compete with infectious virions for the CD4 receptor on susceptible target cells.

The immunologic equilibrium in the GC is also a factor to be considered. It is known that immune complexes held on FDC can dissociate when the equilibrium between antigen, immune complexes, and free specific antibody changes.[22,24,41] Experimental evidence from other systems suggests that a decrease in the amount of antibody-complexed antigen localized on the FDC can result in the initiation of a new cycle of antibody production, since the antigen is now made accessible as an immune stimulus.[22,24,41] If this mechanism is involved, fluctuation in antibody levels, either in the circulation or locally, may lead to dissociation of virus-antibody complex, thereby making free virions available to CD4$^+$ target cells.

The infection of GC is of significance in the pathogenesis of the disease for another reason. The cellular diversity of the GC offers the virus an opportunity to infect target cells of different origin. Indeed, the finding of budding profiles on lymphocytes, macrophages, and FDC indicates that several cell types are involved in virus production. It has become apparent that circulating monocytes, being both migratory and highly susceptible and permissive hosts for HIV-1, can spread virus throughout the body.[2–6] Because virus can be sequestered within intracytoplasmic vacuoles, the entry as well as the residence of such cells with vacuolized virus in the GC can set the stage for very efficient transmission of virus from these cells to other susceptible host cells. Indeed, in vitro studies have shown that the infection of CD4$^+$ lymphocytes is greatly enhanced when the T cells are exposed to virus-infected autologous macrophages instead of to cell-free HIV-1 of comparable virus titer.[42] Quite possibly, a genomic shift may occur at the time of virus transmission to a novel host. The GC may be one of the anatomic sites where the virus acquires preferential tropism for a given target cell type.

Conceivably, antiviral agents could alter the level of cell-free virus, and consequently, effect the degree of HIV-1 persistence in lymph nodes of patients with PGL. Favorable clinical response could be an outcome of such treatment.

SUMMARY

Germinal centers play an important role in the pathogenesis of HIV-1-induced lymphadenopathy. Cell-free retrovirus particles, gag proteins of HIV-1, and cells expressing viral RNA can be detected in these areas of the lymph node. In the present study, the ultrastructural changes and the interactions of virus with different cell types of the germinal centers were investigated. We compared the alterations of lymph nodes obtained shortly after seroconversion with those seen in longstanding lymphadenopathy. The results demonstrated that germinal centers were already infected in the early phase of the disease. However, the number of cell free virions was low. During the course of the disease, large amounts of cell free virions accumulated in the germinal centers. The persistence of germinal center infection for up to 2 years was demonstrated by detecting retrovirus particles in repeated biopsy specimens. In addition, the presence of numerous small, moderately electron dense structures that might represent defective particles of HIV-1 and influence the course of the disease were described. HIV-1 was found to replicate in lymphocytes, macrophages, and follicular dendritic cells. Quite possibly, a genomic shift may occur at the time of transmission of the virus to a novel target cell, thus, germinal centers may be one of the anatomic sites where HIV-1 acquires the ability to develop into a variant with preferential tropism for a given cell type.

ACKNOWLEDGMENTS

We thank Ms. Ulrike Fritzsche, Ms. Brigitte Krüger, Ms. Angela Pries, and Ms. Traute Thiede for their excellent assistance.

REFERENCES

1. Harper ME, Marselle LM, Gallo RC, Wong-Staal, F: Detection of lymphocytes expressing human T-lymphotropic virus type III in lymph nodes and peripheral blood from infected individuals by in situ hybridization. Proc Natl Acad Sci USA 1986; 83:772–776
2. Gartner S, Markovits P, Markovitz DM, et al: Virus isolation from and identification of HTLV-III/LAV-producing cells in brain tissue from a patient with AIDS. JAMA 1986; 256:2365–2371
3. Gartner S, Markovits P, Markovitz DM, et al: The role of mononuclear phagocytes in HTLV-III/LAV infection. Science 1986; 233:215–219
4. Ho DD, Rota T, Hirsch MS: Infection of monocyte/macrophages by human T lymphotropic virus type III. J Clin Invest 1986; 77:1712–1715
5. Popovic M, Read-Connole E, Gartner S: Biological properties of HTLV-III/LAV: A possible pathway of natural infection in vivo. Ann Inst Pasteur 1986; 137D:413–417
6. Popovic M, Read-Connole E, Gartner S: HTLV-III/LAV infection of mononuclear phagocyte cells *in vivo* and *in vitro*. UCLA Symp Molec Cell Biol. New Series 1987; 43:161–176
7. Tschachler E, Groh V, Popovic M, et al: Epidermal Langerhans cells: A target for HTLV-III/LAV infection. Invest Dermatol 1987; 88:233–237
8. Armstrong JA, Horne R: Follicular dendritic cells and virus-like particles in AIDS-related lymphadenopathy. Lancet 1984; 2:370–372
9. Armstrong JA, Dawkins RL, Horne R: Retroviral infection of accessory cells and the immunological paradox in AIDS. Immunology Today 1985; 6:121–122
10. Tenner-Racz K, Racz P, Dietrich M, Kern P: Altered follicular dendritic cells and virus-like particles in AIDS and AIDS-related lymphadenopathy. Lancet 1985; 1:105–106
11. Diebold J, Marche CL, Audouin J, et al: Lymph node modification in patients with the acquired immunodeficiency syndrome (AIDS) or with AIDS-related complex (ARC). A histological, immunohistological and ultrastructural study. Pathol Res Pract 1985; 180:590–611
12. Racz P, Tenner-Racz K, Kahl C, et al: The spectrum of morphologic changes in lymph nodes from patients with AIDS or AIDS-related complex. Progr Allergy 1986; 37:81–181
13. Warner TF, Crass B, Gabel C, et al: Diagnosis of HTLV-III infection by ultrastructural examination of germinal centers in lymph nodes. A case report. AIDS Res 1986; 2:43–50
14. Tenner-Racz K, Racz P, Bofill M, et al: HTLV-III/LAV viral antigens in lymph nodes of homosexual

men with persistent generalized lymphadenopathy and AIDS. Am J Pathol 1986; 123:9–15

15. Tenner-Racz K, Racz P, Kern P, Dietrich M: Prognostic and diagnostic value of lymph node biopsy in AIDS and persistent generalized lymphadenopathy. In: Staquet M, Hemmer R and Baert H, eds. Clinical Aspects of AIDS and AIDS-related Complex. Oxford, Oxford University Press, 1986; 125–136

16. Tenner-Racz K, Racz P, Dietrich M, et al: Monoclonal antibodies to human immunodeficiency virus: Their relation to the patterns of lymph node changes in persistent generalized lymphadenopathy and AIDS. AIDS 1987; 1:95–104

17. Tenner-Racz K, Racz P, Gluckman JC, Popovic M: Cell-free HIV in lymph nodes of patients with persistent generalized lymphadenopathy and AIDS. N Engl. J. Med 1988; 318:49–50

18. Baroni CD, Pezzella F, Mirolo, et al: Immunohistochemical demonstration of p24 HTLV-III major core protein in different cell types within lymph nodes from patients with lymphadenopathy syndrome (LAS). Histopathology 1986; 10:5–13

19. Biberfeld P, Chayt KJ, Marselle LM, et al: HTLV-III expression in infected lymph nodes and relevance to pathogenesis of lymphadenopathy. Am J Pathol 1986; 125:436–442

20. Hanna MG, Szakal AK, Tyndall RL: Histoproliferative effect of Rauscher leukemia virus on lymphatic tissue: Histological and ultrastructural studies of germinal centers and their relation to leukemogenesis. Cancer Res 1970; 30:1748–1763

21. Hoover EA, Mullins JI, Quackenbush SL, Gasper PW: Pathogenesis of feline retrovirus-induced cytopathic disease: Acquired immune deficiency syndrome and aplastic anemia. In: Salzman LA, ed. Animal Models of Retrovirus Infection and Their Relationship to AIDS. Orlando, Academic Press Inc., 1986; 59–74

22. Tew JG, Phipps RP, Mandel TE: The maintenance and regulation of the humoral response: Persisting antigen and the role of follicular antigen-binding dendritic cells as accessory cells. Immunol Rev 1980; 53:175–201

23. Hanna MG, Szakal AK: Localization of I^{125}-labeled antigen in germinal centers of mouse spleen: Histologic and ultrastructural autoradiographic studies of the secondary immune reaction. J Immunol 1968; 101:949–962

24. Mandel TE, Phipps RP, Abbot AP, Tew JC: The follicular dendritic cell: Long term antigen retention during immunity. Immunol Rev 1980; 53:29–59

25. Mandel TE, Phipps RP, Abbot AP, Tew JC: Long-term antigen retention by dendritic cells in the popliteal lymph nodes of immunized mice. Immunology 1981; 43:353–362

26. Radoux D, Heinen E, Kinet-Demoel C, et al: Precise localization of antigens on follicular dendritic cells. Cell Tissue Res 1984; 253:267–274

27. Dvoretsky P, Wood GS, Levy R, Warnke RA: T-lymphocyte subsets in follicular lymphomas compared with those in non-neoplastic lymph nodes and tonsils. Hum Pathol 1982; 13:618–625

28. Wood GS, Turner RR, Shiurba RA, et al: Human dendritic cells and macrophages: In situ immunophenotypic definition of subsets that exhibit specific and morphologic characteristics. Am J Pathol 1985; 119:73–82

29. Clavel F, Klatzmann D, Montagnier L: Deficient neutralizing capacity of sera from patients with AIDS or related syndromes. Lancet 1985; 1:879–880

30. Robert-Guroff M, Brown M, Gallo RC: HTLV-III neutralizing antibodies in patients with AIDS and AIDS-related complex. Nature 1985; 316:72–74

31. Weiss RA, Clapham PR, Cheinsong-Popov R, et al: Neutralization of human T-lymphotropic virus type III by sera of AIDS and AIDS-risk patients. Nature 1985; 316:69–72

32. Fossum S, Ford WL: The organization of cell populations within lymph nodes: Their origin, life history and functional relationships. Histopathology 1985; 9:469–499

33. Biberfeld P, Porwit-Ksiazek A, Böttiger B, et al: Immunohistopathology of lymph nodes in HTLV-III infected homosexuals with persistent adenopathy or AIDS. Cancer Res 1985; 45:465–470

34. Cameron PU,, Dawkins RL, Armstrong JA, Bonifacio E: Western blot profiles, lymph node ultrastructure and viral expression in HIV-infected patients: A correlative study. Clin Exp Immunol 1987; 68:465–478

35. Janossy G, Pinching AJ, Bofill M, et al: An immunohistochemical approach to persistent lymphadenopathy and its relevance to acquired immune deficiency syndrome. Clin Exp Immunol 1985; 59:257–266

36. Pallesen G, Gerstoft J, Mathiesen L: Stages in LAV/HTLV-III lymphadenitis. I. Histological and immunohistological classification. Scand J Immunol 1987; 25:83–91

37. Pileri S, Rivano MT, Raise E et al: The value of lymph node biopsy in patients with the acquired immunodeficiency syndrome (AIDS) and the AIDS-related complex (ARC): A morphological and immunohistochemical study of 90 cases. Histopathology 1986; 10:1107–1129

38. Racz P, Feller AC, Tenner-Racz K, et al: Human lymphocyte subpopulations in lymphadenopathies in homosexual men. Adv Exp Biol Med 1985; 186:1069–1076

39. Wood GS, Garcia CF, Dorfman RF, Warnke RA: The immunohistology of follicle lysis in lymph node biopsies from homosexual men. Blood 1985; 66:1092–1097

40. Klatzmann D, Gluckman JC: HIV infection: facts and hypotheses. Immunol Today 1986;7:291–296

41. Donaldson SL, Kosco MH, Szakal AK, Tew JG: Localization of antibody-forming cells in draining lymphoid organs during long-term maintenance of the antibody response. J Leuk Biol 1986; 40:147–157

42. Buchow HD, Gartner S, Gallo RC, Popovic M: *In vitro* studies of HTLV-III/LAV transmission from monocyte/macrophages to autologous T cells. In: Abstract Volume of III International Conference on AIDS, June 1–5, Washington, D.C., 1987; 82

3

Ultrastructural Markers and Interferon Levels in HIV-Positive Individuals Treated with D-Penicillamine

Jan Marc Orenstein
Richard S. Schulof

IN THE UNITED STATES ALONE, an estimated 1–1.5 million people are infected with the human immunodeficiency virus (HIV). Widely differing predictions have been made to the percentage of infected individuals who will progress to develop AIDS. Whatever the percentage, it is important to identify those individuals as soon as possible after infection. Presently, it appears that any drug treatment used to suppress viral replication will have to be taken for life and will not be without significant side effects. Treatment should, therefore, be confined only to those individuals with the highest risk of progression, and commence at the most appropriate time. Considerable effort has gone into identifying a surrogate marker or predictor. The candidates include the absolute number of circulating T-helper lymphocytes (T-4, CD4), impaired lymphokine production, presence of circulating acid-labile α-interferon (IFN), and the presence of ultrastructural markers.[1–15]

The two ultrastructural markers that have received the most attention are the tubuloreticular inclusion (TRI) and the cylindrical confronting cisternae (CCC). TRI was first described in the 1960s, especially associated with viral infections and systemic lupus ery-thematosus (SLE) for which it was initially considered a marker.[16] The relationship to elevated α-IFN in these conditions was subsequently documented; and the in vitro induction, first with the halogenated pyrimidine, BUdR (an inducer of α-IFN).[16,17] and then directly with α-IFN, was demonstrated.[18–22] Philip Grimley coined the term "interferon footprint" for TRI.[23] Sidhu and associates first noted TRI in HIV-infected individuals in 1983,[2] about the same time that the acid-labile form of α-IFN was reported to be elevated in the majority of AIDS patients and a portion of patients with AIDS-related conditions.[9–11] On its own, α-IFN, has been championed as a predictor of progression to AIDS.[10–12,15] TRI are observed in the rough endoplasmic reticulum (RER) of lymphocytes, endothelial cells, and monocytes/macrophages and appear as complex networks of apparently branching tubules measuring 20–25 μm in thickness (Fig. 1).[3,6,7,24,25]

The CCC, also an inclusion of the RER, was first described in 1978,[26] in a case of multiple sclerosis and soon after in hepatocytes of chimpanzees injected with serum from humans with non-A, non-B hepatitis (NANB).[27,28] Initially, CCC were felt to be a

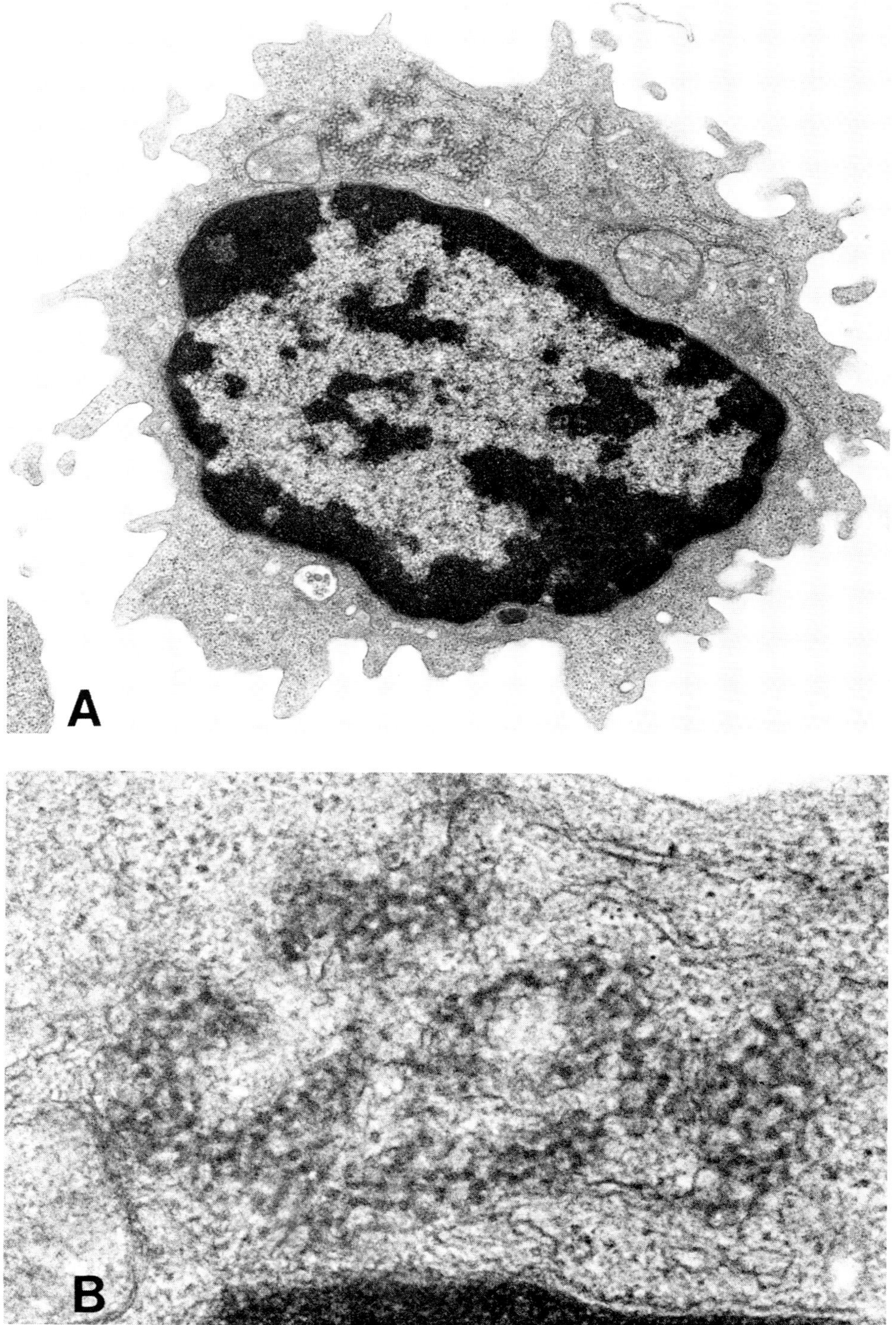

Figure 1. (A) Electron micrograph of a typical peripheral blood lymphocyte containing a TRI. Original magnification ×19,000. (B) An enlargement of the TRI in Fig. 1A, showing the branching appearance. Original magnification ×84,000.

marker for this particular form of hepatitis, but subsequently, CCC have never been observed in humans with any type of hepatitis. CCC were next described in a patient with HTLV T-cell leukemia[29] and then in HIV-infected individuals.[2,3] CCC were only recognized in SLE patients in 1984,[30] and shown to be inducible with α-IFN in vitro in 1987,[31] although the close association of TRI and CCC was well known from ultrastructural studies, (e.g., CCC are never seen in the absence of TRI in a patient and can be seen in continuity in the same cell).[7,25] CCC were first referred to as test tube and ring-shaped forms, a description of the appearance of a cylinder in varying planes of sectioning.[32,33] CCC appear to be formed by the fusion of two apposing membranes of pairs of confronting cisternae of endoplasmic reticulum (Fig. 2).

These inclusions have been shown to be present in cells from virtually all AIDS patients and a significant proportion of patients with AIDS-related conditions such as lymphadenopathy syndrome (LAS) and AIDS-related complex (ARC), and they can appear before other signs of clinical progression.[6,7,34] TRI are regularly detected before CCC and increase in percentage before CCC are observed. The percentage of patients positive for the ultrastructural markers[6,7,34] and circulating α-IFN increases from asymptomatic patients to those with LAS, ARC, and finally, to patients with clearly evident cases of AIDS.[8-12,35] Once patients are TRI positive for several weeks, they invariably remain so until AIDS develops. Once CCC appear, they have rarely been seen to disappear and indicate that the individual is closer to a diagnosis of AIDS. As with SLE, the presence of circulating α-IFN is highly predictive of the presence of TRI.[22,36-38] In both HIV infection and SLE, however, lymphocytes containing TRI can be detected in the peripheral circulation before α-IFN is evident.

D-penicillamine, an analogue of cysteine, interacts with proteins and peptides to crosslink disulfide groups. It is a synthetic oral chelator that is used in the treatment of Wilson's disease, cystinuria, and rheumatoid arthritis. In vitro, it has recently been shown to display dose-related inhibition of HIV replication. Initial in vivo studies have likewise demonstrated an inhibitory effect or viral replication.[39] D-penicillamine has been proposed to function through cross-linking specific cysteine-rich viral proteins important for HIV replication.

Our interest in the induction and significance of the ultrastructural markers and their relationship to α-IFN led the authors to evaluate their presence in patients treated with D-penicillamine.

MATERIALS AND METHODS

Ten HIV-positive subjects with lymphadenopathy were selected; all had T4:T8 lymphocyte ratios of less than 1.0, absolute T4 levels of less than $500/mm^3$, and depressed mixed lymphocyte responses (MLR).[23] Every 2 weeks, while on D-penicillamine, and 2, 4, and 6 weeks after discontinuation, the subjects were monitored for T-lymphocyte levels and MLR activity. HIV expression was assayed by measuring reverse transcriptase activity and p15 and p25 core proteins in the subjects' phytohemagglutinin (PHA)-stimulated peripheral blood lymphocytes cocultured with permissive H-9 cells.[40] The first five subjects received daily oral 250 mg of D-penicillamine b.i.d. for 1 week, 250 mg q.i.d. for 1 week, and then 500 mg q.i.d.. Based on drug tolerance of the first group, the second five subjects omitted the 500 mg/day dose. Six weeks after the initial five individuals were begun on therapy, the trial was stopped when it was determined that the MLR was depressed. Therefore, instead of the scheduled 3 months of therapy, the first five subjects received 6 weeks; the second 2 subjects, 4 weeks; and the final three subjects, only 2 weeks of treatment. Follow-up information is available for several of the individuals.

Buffy coat lymphocytes were prepared for

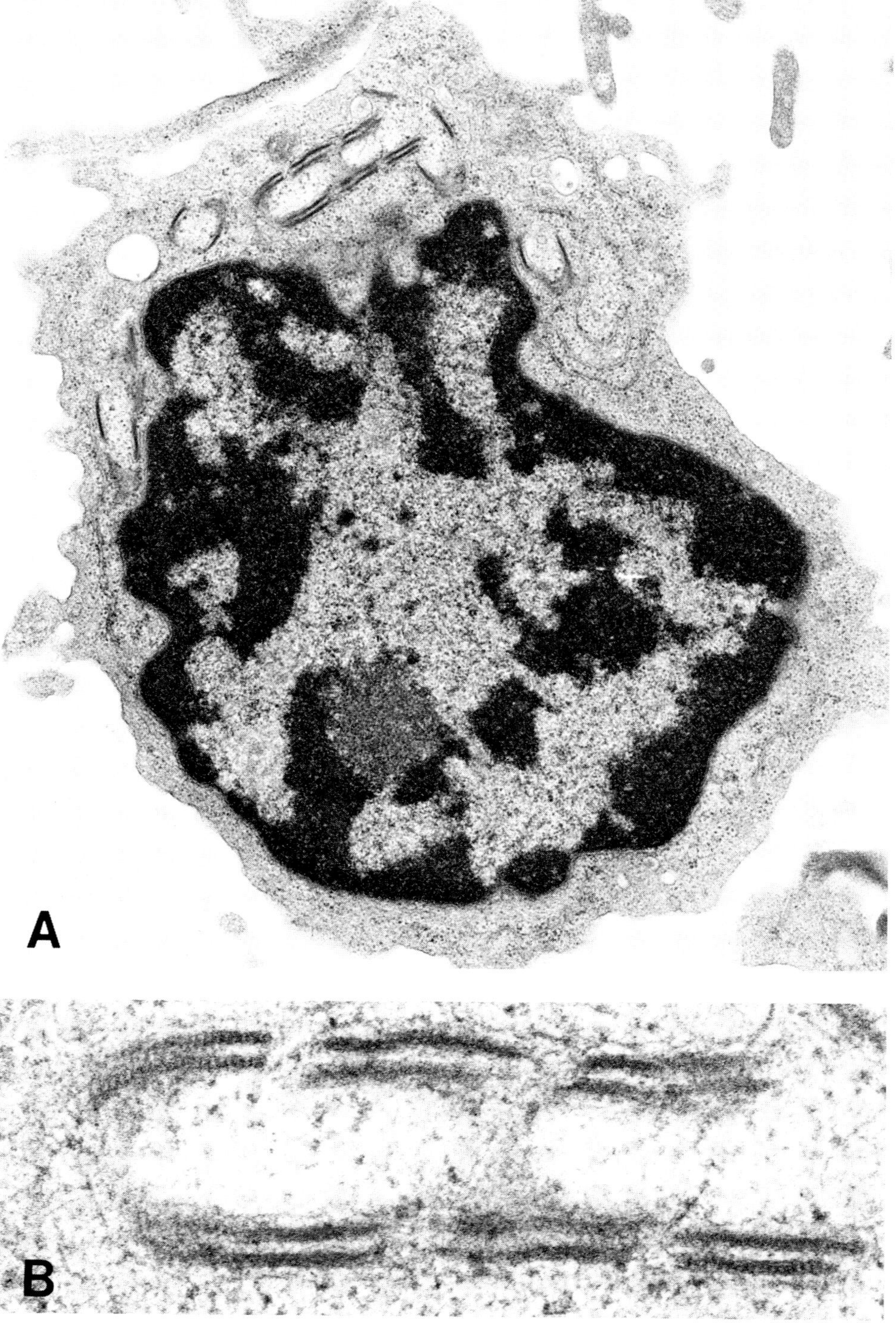

Figure 2. (A) Electron micrograph of a peripheral blood lymphocyte containing several profiles of CCC. Original magnification ×25,000. (B) The enlarged CCC in Fig. 2A is doubled and shows the characteristic periodicity. Original magnification ×110,000.

transmission electron microscopy (TEM) as previously described.[6] The percent of lymphocytes positive for TRI and CCC was based on screening 100 consecutive lymphocytes in each buffy coat preparation. The markers observed in monocytes within the preparations were not included in the final tabulations, although they were frequently equal in number to the level seen in lymphocytes. Serum IFN was determined as previously described in the literature.[10,11,20,34] Samples ≥ 8 IU/ml of IFN were considered IFN-positive, ≤ 4 IU/ml were considered negative, and samples that ranged in between were considered marginal. Previous experience with HIV-positive individuals indicated that when IFN fractionation is performed, elevation in total IFN is predominantly due to the acid-labile form of α-IFN.

RESULTS

D-penicillamine treatment led to at least some suppression of HIV replication in all ten subjects, as indicated by decreasing levels of reverse transcriptase (RT) (Table 1) and core antigen.[39] Complete inhibition of viral expression was seen in four of the first five individuals (all but patient #1) receiving 6 weeks of therapy; two of the four (patients #s 2 & 4) were still negative 48 weeks following discontinuation of therapy. Another individual patient (#8) became HIV-negative after the follow-up and remained negative at 48 weeks. These three subjects have remained clinically and immunologically stable in the interim with T4 counts above 300 mm³. As for the incomplete or unsustained responders, AIDS developed in subjects #1 and #10, 5 and 10 months after therapy, respectively; and ARC developed in subjects #3 and #5. Two others, (patients #s 7 & 9) have developed nonspecific clinical symptoms (e.g., fatigue) with falling T4 counts. Subject #6 was lost to follow-up.

A total of 65 peripheral blood specimens were evaluated for ultrastructural markers and total serum IFN (Table 1).[41] The table indicates the specimens that were positive and negative for TRI, CCC, and IFN. A total of 7, 1, and 4 subjects were TRI, CCC, and IFN-positive at week zero of the study, respectively. One subject (patient #6) became IFN-positive, and 3 CCC-positive (patients #s 3,5,7) during therapy.

Five of the 10 subjects displayed features that heretofore had rarely been observed in untreated individuals, namely, the disappearance of TRI and, especially, CCC after their prolonged presence. From week zero to the end of therapy, subject #1 had four consecutive TRI-positive specimens, with rising percentages. At 2 weeks post therapy, the percentage of TRI fell and they were not detected at week four post therapy. The next two specimens were TRI/CCC-positive and AIDS was diagnosed 14 weeks after the first TRI/CCC-positive specimen. Subject #3 went from TRI-positive to TRI/CCC-positive after 2 weeks on therapy, remained so while on therapy (three specimens), then reverted to just TRI-positive, and again to TRI/CCC-positive during follow-up when he progressed to ARC. Subject #5 started TRI-positive, became TRI/CCC-positive, reverted to only TRI-positive, and then TRI/CCC-positive, and progressed to ARC. Subject #7 started TRI-positive, became TRI/CCC-positive, then only TRI-positive, and finally, totally marker-negative until becoming TRI/CCC-positive again during the follow-up. Subject #8 started TRI-positive and became negative during follow-up.

Seven subjects had elevated IFN levels at some time during the study. In three (patients #s 5,6,9), the elevations were only transient. Although there was some depression in the levels in three others, none became negative. The levels in the other subject (#10) who developed AIDS rose steadily. Thus, both subjects who developed AIDS were TRI, CCC, and IFN-positive during the study.

Subjects #s 3, 4, 5, 7, and 9 had additional samples analyzed for ultrastructural markers in the follow-up period, subsequent

TABLE I

Effect of D-Penicillamine on ten HIV-Positive Subjects with Lymphadenopathy Syndrome

| | Weeks on D-Penicillamine | | | | | | | | | | |
| | 0 | | 2 | | | 4 | | | 6 | | |
#	TEM	IFN	TEM	IFN	RT	TEM	IFN	RT	TEM	IFN	RT
1	1/0	18	4/0	16	100	5/0	25	53	8/0	16	27
2	0/0	4	—	7	63	0/0	4	0	3/0	4	0
3	4/0	4	3/2	4	100	2/1	4	100	3/3	4	30
4	0/0	4	0/0	7	100	0/0	4	30	0/0	4	0
5	6/0	6	2/1	—	58	8/0	4	21	9/3	16	0
6	5/0	4	3/0	18	70	2/0	4	10	—	—	—
7	4/0	10	11/1	12	33	1/1	7	10	—	—	—
8	1/0	16	1/0	12	57	—	—	—	—	—	—
9	0/0	4	0/0	4	0	—	—	—	—	—	—
10	16/3	12	—	16	10	—	—	—	—	—	—

TEM = %TRI/%CCC

IFN = Total interferon, International units/ml: ≤4 = (−); >4 <8 = (+/−); ≥8 = (+).

Drug stopped for last 5 subjects because T-cell function (MLR) depressed in first 5.

RT = Reverse transcriptase activity expressed as % of week *0* level set as 100%.

Follow-up = status last evaluation; interferon levels not determined during follow-up.

to the 12-week post D-penicillamine treatment period of the study. No further samples were available for subjects #2, 6, and 8. Subjects #3 and #5 remained TRI-positive in five and four additional specimens respectively, and then became TRI/CCC-positive. During the interval, their T4 counts fell and they developed ARC. Subject #4 was TRI and RT-negative at 24 and 48 weeks respectively. Subject #7 had eight additional samples analysed during the follow-up period after an initial negative sample; the next five were TRI-positive, and the last two were TRI/CCC-positive, during which time he developed fatigue and muscle aches with a T4 count that fell to 20. Subject #9 had nine additional specimens analyzed during the follow-up period; single TRI were seen in specimens 1, 4, and 7; 3% TRI were observed in specimen 8. The ninth specimen contained TRI and CCC, and during the period he developed fatigue and headaches and the T4 count fell to 144.

It was found that if the specimen was positive for IFN, there was an 81% (22/27) chance that it was also positive for at least TRI, when comparing all samples evaluated for both ultrastructural markers and IFN levels. Conversely, when the specimen was TRI-positive, there was a 54% (22/41) chance that it was also IFN-positive.

DISCUSSION

It is difficult to decipher the complicated relationships between the ultrastructural markers, IFN levels, and HIV induction in a pilot study of this size. The observations in this trial of D-penicillamine, however, are consistent with those of other reports. For example, naltrexone, an opiate antagonist, was given orally to 38 AIDS patients and one ARC patient.[42,43] As compared to a matched control group on placebo, 23 patients on naltrexone showed a significant drop in serum α-IFN levels over a 12-

TABLE I
Effect of D-Penicillamine on ten HIV-Positive Subjects with Lymphadenopathy Syndrome
(Continued)

						Weeks Post D-Penicillamine					
2			4			6			12		Follow-up
TEM	IFN	RT	TEM	IFN	RT	TEM	IFN	RT	TEM	IFN	
3/0	16	100	0/0	10	100	10/1	10	100	9/2	6	AIDS wk 20
0/0	5	0	0/0	4	0	2/0	4	0	2/0	4	RT − wk 48, no TEM
1/0	4	0	1/0	4	10	7/0	4	0	1/0	4	ARC RT + TRI/CCC + wk 51
0/0	4	0	0/0	4	0	0/0	4	0	0/0	4	RT − wk 48, TRI − wk 24
7/2	8	100	5/0	6	100	5/0	8	100	5/1	6	ARC RT + TRI/CCC + wk 58
2/0	4	60	—	—	—	—	—	—	—	—	Lost to follow up
2/0	18	25	1/0	9	15	0/0	8	0	0/0	8	RT + TRI/CCC + wk 47
1/0	8	50	0/0	8	60	0/0	—	25	—	—	RT − wk 48, no TEM
0/0	6	35	0/0	6	40	0/0	6	35	0/0	10	RT + TRI/CCC + wk 58
18/4	32	100	11/3	32	100	8/1	32	—	—	—	AIDS wk 40

month period (from mean of 144 to 11 IU/ml). The 23 responders had significantly fewer opportunistic infections (8 versus 16) and deaths (4 versus 13) as compared to the 16 nonresponders. The effect of naltrexone on the recovery of HIV was not evaluated. The acid-labile form of α-IFN is thought to down-regulate the immune system, perhaps by interacting with the opiate receptors. Its presence might add to, or even amplify the immunosuppression caused by HIV. Recently, two AIDS patients with elevated serum α-IFN levels were treated with anti-α IFN immunoglobulin.[44] The α-IFN became undetectable, the patients gained weight, and there was an increase in their "sense of well being".

The detection of circulating α-IFN is highly correlated with the presence of ultrastructural markers in circulating lymphocytes in HIV-positive subjects, as it is in individuals with SLE.[22,34,36,37] The converse is not as highly correlated a phenomenon,

perhaps reflecting an initial local, compartmentalized α-IFN induction of TRI in migrating mononuclear cells preceding the detection of circulating IFN. This would explain why TRI are often detected prior to the appearance of serum IFN. The presence of CCC-positive lymphocytes correlates with higher percentages of TRI and a greater likelihood of detecting circulating IFN, perhaps due to greater IFN stimulation and evolution of the HIV infection. The presence of TEM markers inversely correlates with T4 levels, which has also been shown to correlate with the clinical status of the infection.[6,14]

Transient TRI-positivity has occasionally been observed in untreated patients followed over a long period of time,[34] however, this has usually been a single sample, at a very low percentage, and never accompanied by CCC. In the majority of instances, once TRI-positive, these individuals remained positive. Only four of the 26 subjects who were previously followed by us with multiple evaluations were observed to become CCC-negative after being CCC-positive in one or two specimens.[34] All remained TRI-positive and three converted back to CCC-positive before developing AIDS. The fourth individual had not converted back to CCC-positive by the time of the last available specimen, 13 months before AIDS was diagnosed. Similar persistence has been noted for α-IFN levels. Therefore, the fluctuations in both ultrastructural markers observed in our present 10 subjects treated with D-penicillamine would appear to be related to the drug, a known inhibitor of HIV replication.[39]

From the presence of both TRI and CCC, it can be expected that at least four more subjects in this study will most likely progress to AIDS in addition to the two already so diagnosed. The total may be even higher, since specimens were not available for the other four subjects. It is unclear if the therapy with D-penicillamine altered the natural progression of the HIV infection in these subjects.

The IFN levels appeared to be less clearly affected by the therapy. In this study, however, even the positive IFN levels were relatively low as compared to those recorded (e.g., the naltrexone studies[42,43]), and for AIDS and ARC patients in general.[12] Thus, single elevations and fluctuations would be difficult to interpret. Other factors may come into play with IFN, such as half-life in the peripheral circulation, as compared to that of the markers and the kinetics of induction of the markers by α-IFN. Nevertheless, relatively low elevations of IFN may be significant, as long as they persist. Abnormal levels, although relatively low, were present for at least 26 and 46 weeks before AIDS was diagnosed in subjects #1 and #10, respectively.

The inducer of α-IFN in HIV-infected individuals is unclear. In our experience, HIV infection of neither H-9 lymphocytes nor U-937 promonocytes[45] induced ultrastructural markers until α-IFN was added to the culture. Neither γ-IFN, phytohemagglutinin, nor pokeweed mitogen alone induced marker production, and furthermore, they did not block the induction of markers when α-IFN was subsequently added. A wide variety of cultured cells have been induced to form TRI with α-IFN, including normal peripheral B and T lymphocytes.[17-19,46] To date, however, CCC have only been induced by α-IFN in Daudi cells, a lymphoblastoid cell line infected with Epstein-Barr virus (EBV), which does not contain TRI without stimulation.[31] TEM observations on material from HIV-infected individuals and in vitro induction experiments appear to indicate that CCC and TRI are likely to be part of a spectrum of membrane changes induced by α-IFN, a known inhibitor of membrane metabolism.[47,48] The spectrum of changes also includes paired cisternae and annulate lamellae.[46,49,50] CCC represent the most highly structured member of the group, with a uniformity of width, a rigidity, and a periodicity not shared by other members (Fig. 2). The appearance of CCC may require higher or, more prolonged stimulation by α-IFN, plus the presence of other factors. Members of the Herpes group of DNA viruses, such as cytomegalovirus, have been proposed as cofactors in the evolution of HIV infection to AIDS, and they are potent stimulators of α-IFN.[14,51] The appearance of TRI may reflect the presence of a subclinical opportunistic infection that, when manifest, equates with a diagnosis of AIDS. However, HIV may still be a factor in the induction of α-IFN through HIV-related immune complexes and/or combinations with other factors. It is perhaps paradoxical that α-IFN, which is elevated in AIDS patients, is a potent inhibitor of retroviral replication, in vivo and in vitro.[47,48,52,53]

Attempts are being made to find a treatment plan that preserves the viral-inhibitory effect of D-penicillamine, while eliminating its immunosuppressive effect. Lower drug levels and combination therapy with other agents are presently being tested or anticipated.

ACKNOWLEDGMENTS

We are grateful to Drs. Olivia T. Preble and Philip Grimley, Department of Pathology, uniformed Services University for the Health Sciences, Bethesda, Maryland, for performing the interferon evaluations and collaboration on in vitro interferon studies, respectively. We acknowledge the expert technical assistance of Seth Honig and Julie Sesno.

REFERENCES

1. Orenstein JM, Schulof RS, Simon GL: Ultrastructural markers in acquired immune deficiency syndrome (letter). Arch Pathol Lab Med 1984; 108:857–859
2. Sidhu GS, Stahl RE, El-Sadr, et al: Ultrastructural markers in AIDS (letter). Lancet 1983; 1:990–991
3. Orenstein JM: Ultrastructural markers in AIDS (letter). Lancet 1983; 2:284–285
4. Murray HW, Welte K, Jacobs JL, et al: Production of and in vitro response to interleukin 2 in acquired immunodeficiency syndrome. J Clin Invest 1985; 76:1959–1964
5. Ewing Jr EP, Spira TJ, Chandler FW, et al: Ultrastructural markers in AIDS (letter). Lancet 1983; 2:285
6. Orenstein JM, Simon GL, Kessler CM, et al: Ultrastructural markers in circulating lymphocytes of subjects at risk for AIDS. Am J Clin Pathol 1985; 84:603–609
7. Sidhu GS, Stahl RE, El-Sadr W, et al: The acquired immunodeficiency syndrome: An ultrastructural study. Hum Pathol 1985; 16:377–386
8. Abbott SR, Buimovici-Klein E, Cooper LZ, et al: Rapid detection of immunoreactive interferon-α in AIDS (letter). Lancet 1984; 1:564
9. Buimovici-Klein E, Lange M, Klein RJ, et al: Is presence of interferon predictive for AIDS? (letter) Lancet 1983; 2:344
10. Eyster ME, Goedert JJ, Poon M-C, et al: Acid-labile alpha interferon. A possible preclinical marker for the acquired immunodeficiency syndrome in hemophilia. N Engl J Med 1983; 309:583–586
11. DeStefano E, Friedman RM, Friedman-Kien AE, et al: Acid-labile human leukocyte interferon in homosexual men with Kaposi's sarcoma and lymphadenopathy. J Infect Dis 1982; 146:451–455
12. Buimovici-Klein E, Lange M, Klein RJ, et al: Long-term follow-up of serum-interferon and its acid-stability in a group of homosexual men. AIDS Res 1986; 2:99–108
13. Grimley PM, Kang Y-H, Frederick W, et al: Interferon-related leukocyte inclusions in acquired immune deficiency syndrome: Localization in T-cells. Am J Clin Pathol 1984; 81:147–155
14. Polk BF, Fox R, Brookmeyer R, et al: Predictors of the acquired immunodeficiency syndrome developing in a cohort of seropositive homosexual men. N Engl J Med 1987; 316:61–66
15. Buimovici-Klein E, Sonnabend JA, Lange M, et al: Predictors of AIDS in homosexual men. N Engl J Med 1987; 317:245
16. Grimley PM, Schaff Z: Significance of tubuloreticular inclusions in the pathobiology of human diseases. Pathobiol Ann 1976; 6:221–257
17. Grimley PM, Barry DW, Schaff Z: Induction of "virus-like" tubular structures in the endoplasmic reticulum of human lymphoid cells treated with 5-bromodeoxyuridine (BrdU) (abstract). Fed Proc 1973; 32:964
18. Rich SA: Human lupus inclusions and interferon. Science 1981; 213:772–775
19. Grimley PM, Rutherford MN, Kang Y-H, et al: Formation of tubuloreticular inclusions in human lymphoma cells compared to the induction of 2'-5'-oligoadenylate synthetase by leukocyte interferon in dose-effect and kinetic studies. Cancer Res 1984; 144:3480–3488
20. Preble OT, Black RJ, Friedman RM, et al: Systemic lupus erythematosus presence in human serum of an unusual acid-labile leukocyte interferon. Science 1982; 216:429–431
21. Grimley PM, Davis GL, Kang Y-H, et al: Tubuloreticular inclusions in peripheral blood mononuclear cells related to systemic therapy with α-interferon. Lab Invest 1985; 52:638–649
22. Grimley PM, Kang Y-H, Masur H, et al: Tubuloreticular inclusions in patients with AIDS: Interferon-related effect in circulating T-cells and monocytes. In: Friedman-Kein AE and Laubenstein LJ, eds. AIDS: The Epidemic of Kaposi's Sarcoma and Opportunistic Infections. New York, Masson Publishing Co. 1984; 181–192
23. Grimley PM, Kang Y-H, Silverman RH, et al: Blood lymphocyte inclusions associated with alpha interferon (abstract). Lab Invest 1983; 48:30A
24. Ghadially FN: Ultrastructural Pathology of the Cell and Matrix, 2nd ed. England, Butterworths 1982; 398–405
25. Kostianovsky M, Orenstein JM, Schaff Z, et al: Cytomembranous inclusions observed in acquired immunodeficiency syndrome. Clinical and experimental review. Arch Pathol Lab Med 1987; 111:218–223
26. Prineas JW, Wright RG: Macrophages, lymphocytes, and plasma cells in the perivascular compartment in chronic multiple sclerosis. Lab Invest 1978; 38:409–421
27. Jackson D, Tabor E, Gerety RJ: Acute non-A, non-B hepatitis: Specific ultrastructural alterations in endoplasmic reticulum of infected hepatocytes. Lancet 1979; 1:1249–1250
28. Pfeifer U, Thomssen R, Legler K, et al: Experimental non-A, non-B hepatitis: four types of cytoplasmic alterations in hepatocytes of infected chimpanzees. Virchows Arch (Cell Pathol) 1980; 33:233–243
29. Shamoto M, Murakami S, Zenke T: Adult T-cell leukemia in Japan: An ultrastructural study. Cancer 1981; 47:1804–1811

30. Hammar SP, Bockus D, Remington F, et al: More on ultrastructure of AIDS lymph nodes (letter). N Engl J Med 1984; 310:924
31. Bockus D, Remington F, Luu J, et al: Induction of cylindrical confronting cisternae (CCC) in Daudi lymphoblastoid cells by recombinant α-interferon (r α-IFN) (abstract). Lab Invest 1986; 54:7A
32. Ghadially FN. Ultrastructural Pathology of the Cell and Matrix, 2nd ed. England, Butterworths. 1982; 372–377
33. Ghadially FN, Senoo A, Fuse Y, et al: A serial section study of tubular confronting cisternae (so-called 'test-tube and ring-shaped forms') in AIDS. J Submicrosc Cytol 1987; 19:175–183
34. Orenstein JM, Preble OT, Kind P, et al: The relationship of serum alpha-interferon and ultrastructural markers in HIV-seropositive individuals: correlation with prognosis. Ultrastruct Pathol 1987; 11:673–679
35. Preble OT, Rook AH, Quinnan GV, et al: Role of interferon in AIDS. Ann N Y Acad Sci 1984; 437:65–75
36. Preble OT, Friedman RM: Interferon-induced alterations in cells: Relevance to viral and nonviral diseases. Lab Invest 1983; 49:4–18
37. Preble OT, Rook AH, Steis R, et al: Interferon-induced 2′-5′ oligoadenylate synthetase during interferon-α therapy in homosexual men with Kaposi's sarcoma: Marked deficiency in biochemical response to interferon in patients with acquired immunodeficiency syndrome. J Infect Dis 1985; 152:457–465
38. Ytterberg SR, Schnitzer TJ: Serum interferon levels in patients with systemic lupus erythematosus. Arth Rheum 1982; 25:401–406
39. Schulof RS, Scheib RG, Parenti DM, et al: Treatment of HTLV-III/LAV-infected patients with D-penicillamine. Arzneim-Forsch/Drug Res 1986; 36:1531–1534
40. Sarin PS, Taguchi Y, Sun D: Inhibition of HTLV-III/LAV replication by Foscarnet. Biochem Pharmacol 34:4075, 1985
41. Orenstein J, Schulof R, Parenti D, et al: Effect of D-penicillamine on interferon levels and TEM markers in HIV-infected individuals (abstract). Lab Invest 1987 56:57A
42. Bihari B, Drury F, Ragone V, et al: Low dose naltrexone in the treatment of AIDS. Presented at the III International Conference on AIDS, Washington, D.C., June 1–5, 1987; p. 148, abstract WP227
43. Bihari B, Drury F, Ragone V, et al: Alpha interferon, a marker and secondary pathogenic factor in AIDS. Presented at the III International Conference on AIDS, Washington, D.C., June 1–5, 1987; p. 184, abstract THP124
44. Bellanti JA, Skurkovich SV, Peters SM, et al: Preliminary clinical trial of anti-alpha IFN in patients with AIDS: A possible approach for immune enhancement. Presented at the III International Conference on AIDS, Washington, D.C., June 1–5, 1987; p. 18, abstract MP18
45. Sundstrom C, Nilsson K: Establishment and characterization of human histiocytic lymphoma line (U-937). Int J Cancer 1976; 17:565–577
46. Kuyama J, Kanayama Y, Mizutani H, et al: Formation of tubuloreticular inclusions in mitogen-stimulated human lymphocyte cultures by endogenous or exogenous alpha-interferon. Ultrastruct Pathol 1986; 10:77–85
47. Hirsch MS, Kaplan JC: Prospects of therapy for infections with human T-lymphotropic virus type III. Ann Intern Med 1985; 103:750–755
48. Pitha PM, Bilello JA, Riggin CH: Effect of interferon on retrovirus replication. Texas Rep Biol Med 1981; 41:603–609
49. Kuyama J, Kanayama Y, Katagiri S, et al: Tubuloreticular inclusions and paired cisternae induced in human lymphocytes cultured with *Staphlococcus aureus* Cowan 1. Ultrastruct Pathol 1985; 8:155–163
50. Hiraoka A, Rosner MC, Golomb HM: In vitro response from three patients with hairy cell leukemia to recombinant leukocyte interferon. Virchows Arch (Cell Pathol) 1985; 49:73–82
51. Gendelman HE, Phelps W, Feigenbaum L, et al: Trans-activation of the human immunodeficiency virus long terminal repeat sequence by DNA viruses. Proc Natl Acad Sci USA 1986; 83:9759–9763
52. Yamamoto JK, Barre-Sinoussi, Bolton V, et al: Human alpha- and beta-interferon but not gamma- suppress the in vitro replication of LAV, HTLV-III, and ARV-2. J Interferon Res 1986; 6:143–152
53. Ho DD, Rota TR, Kaplan JC, et al: Recombinant human interferon alfa-A suppresses HTLV-III replication in vitro. Lancet 1985; 1:602–604

4

Lung Biopsy Interpretation in the Acquired Immunodeficiency Syndrome: Experience of the National Institutes of Health with Literature Review

William D. Travis
Ernest E. Lack
Frederick P. Ognibene
Anthony F. Suffredini
James Shelhamer

PULMONARY DYSFUNCTION represents the most common life-threatening complication of the acquired immunodeficiency syndrome (AIDS), and is the immediate cause of death in 55% of all fatal cases.[1] Since the initial recognition of AIDS in 1981, the diagnosis and management of the pulmonary complications have presented a difficult challenge to both clinicians and pathologists. Accurate diagnosis of pulmonary infection in AIDS patients is essential because in many cases this represents a treatable cause of respiratory dysfunction.

Although many of the pulmonary complications of AIDS are familiar to pathologists who work in referral institutions where AIDS is commonly seen, now that AIDS patients are being diagnosed and followed in a much larger number of hospitals around the country, there is a great need to provide information regarding the problems faced in interpreting lung biopsies from these pa-

tients. In addition, there are several pulmonary manifestations of AIDS that are poorly understood such as interstitial diseases including lymphocytic interstitial pneumonitis and nonspecific interstitial pneumonitis.

The most important aspect in the evaluation of pulmonary biopsies in AIDS patients is to develop a systematic approach to looking for the various types of processes known to occur: (1) infections, (2) interstitial pneumonitis, and (3) neoplasms (Table 1). It is helpful to develop a mental check list of organisms to be considered and to always look for subtle infiltrates by Kaposi's sarcoma. If one organism is identified, the search should continue for others, since pneumonitis in AIDS is frequently caused by multiple infectious agents. Although the associated inflammatory response can be helpful in deciding which type of organism to consider and in choosing where to focus attention when examining the special stains,

TABLE I
Pulmonary Complications of the Acquired Immune Deficiency Syndrome

I. INFECTIONS
  A. *Pneumocystis carinii*
  B. Viral infection
    Cytomegalovirus
    Herpes simplex
    (Epstein-Barr virus)
  C. Mycobacterial infection
    M. avium-intracellulare
    M. tuberculosis
    Other atypical mycobacteria
  D. Bacterial infection*

Streptococcus pneumoniae	*Pseudomonas aeruginosa*
Hemophilus influenzae	*Group B streptococcus*
Nocardia asteroides	*Branamella catarrhalis*
Legionella species	*Staphylococcus aureus*

  E. Fungal infection
    Cryptococcus neoformans
    Coccidioides immitis
    Histoplasma capsulatum
    Candida species
    Aspergillus species
  F. Parasitic infection
    Strongyloides stercorales
  G. *Cryptosporidium*
  H. *Toxoplasma gondii*
II. INTERSTITIAL PNEUMONITIS
  A. Lymphocytic Interstitial Pneumonitis
  B. Nonspecific Interstitial Pneumonitis
  C. Alveolar Proteinosis
  D. Drug Reactions
    Eosinophilic Pneumonia
III. KAPOSI'S SARCOMA AND OTHER MALIGNANCIES
  A. Kaposi's Sarcoma
  B. Malignant Lymphoma
  C. Solid Malignancies

*See text for more complete listing

it is important to remember that pulmonary infections in AIDS may be accompanied by a minimal histologic response or an exuberant one that overshadows the underlying infection. Certain unusual infections such as toxoplasmosis, cryptosporidiosis, or strongyloidiasis are easily overlooked and should be considered. With certain endemic infections such as coccidioidomycosis,[2] histoplasmosis,[3] or strongyloidiasis,[4] it may be helpful to keep in mind the exposure history of the patient. If no infectious agents or neoplasms are identified, a form of interstitial pneumonitis should be considered.

Bronchoscopy with transbronchial biopsy and/or bronchoalveolar lavage is a well established approach to the diagnosis of common pulmonary infections with a diagnostic yield of up to 95%.[5-15] Nonbronchoscopic bronchoalveolar lavage is another useful approach with a diagnostic sensitivity of 88% for *Pneumocystis carinii* pneumonitis

(PCP).[16] The sensitivity of transbronchial biopsy and bronchoalveolar lavage for the diagnosis of the uncommon pulmonary infections in AIDS is less well defined. Other techniques such as percutaneous needle lung aspiration may provide a high diagnostic yield for pulmonary infections (88%), however, the frequent complication of pneumonthorax (44%) makes it a risky procedure for patients who have significant pulmonary dysfunction.[17] The following review will focus on the pulmonary pathology of AIDS utilizing case material accrued at the National Institutes of Health (NIH) prior to August 1987 and will also update the recent literature.

PATHOLOGY OF PULMONARY INFECTIONS

Pneumocystis Carinii

Pneumocystis carinii pneumonia (PCP) was a hallmark of the initial reported cases of AIDS,[18,19] and currently, it remains the most frequent serious pulmonary complication of this syndrome. It was found at presentation in 64% of AIDS patients and at least once in 80% of all cases reported in the first National Heart Lung and Blood Institute conference on the pulmonary complications of AIDS.[9] Moreover, the recognition of PCP is an important criteria for the diagnosis of AIDS.[20-22] PCP usually presents radiographically as diffuse bilateral pulmonary infiltrates; however, AIDS patients have also been reported to have solitary cavitating and noncavitating nodules,[23] and predominant upper lobe involvement resembling the radiographic appearance of tuberculosis.[24] Although *Pneumocystis carinii* infection is usually restricted to the lung, extrapulmonary spread to the eye, ear, skin, adrenal, spleen, and bone marrow have recently been described in AIDS patients.[25-28]

Special stains are necessary to confirm the presence of *Pneumocystis carinii,* although in some cases where the organisms are very numerous, one can be confident of the diagnosis based upon examination of hematoxylin and eosin (H&E) stained sections. Several methods can be used to stain the organism, including Giemsa, cresyl violet, toluidine blue, and methenamine silver.[29] Recent reports have recommended various methods to facilitate the diagnosis of PCP. These include the use of touch preparations of lung biopsies,[30,31] and various staining methods such as modification of the methenamine silver stain for more rapid processing,[32] fluorescence of *Pneumocystis carinii* in Papanicolaou smears of bronchial washings,[33] and Wright's stain.[30] Monoclonal antibodies have also recently been shown to be promising in the diagnosis of PCP.[34,35]

The histologic features of PCP are well known; however, cases with an atypical histologic reaction occasionally cause difficulties in diagnosis. A striking lymphoplasmacytic interstitial pneumonitis may accompany PCP giving a resemblance to lymphocytic interstitial pneumonitis (LIP)[36] (Fig. 1). This has been recognized, since the initial descriptions of human PCP, as *interstitial plasma cell pneumonia* among children in European orphanages.[37] Other atypical pathologic manifestations of PCP include diffuse alveolar damage,[38] interstitial fibrosis,[39] necrotizing cavitary nodules,[23,24] endobronchial lesions,[40] and granulomatous inflammation.[39,41]

A characteristic feature of PCP is an eosinophilic, foamy, intraalveolar exudate. Recognition of these exudates should raise the suspicion of PCP in H&E stained sections. Although the *Pneumocystis carinii* organisms are usually distributed diffusely in biopsy sections, occasionally, they will be very limited in number making it necessary to carefully examine histologic sections. In this situation, the location of an intraalveolar exudate seen on routine sections may provide a helpful clue to where to look on the special stains. This exudate can resemble pulmonary alveolar proteinosis. In H&E stained sections, however, the exudate of

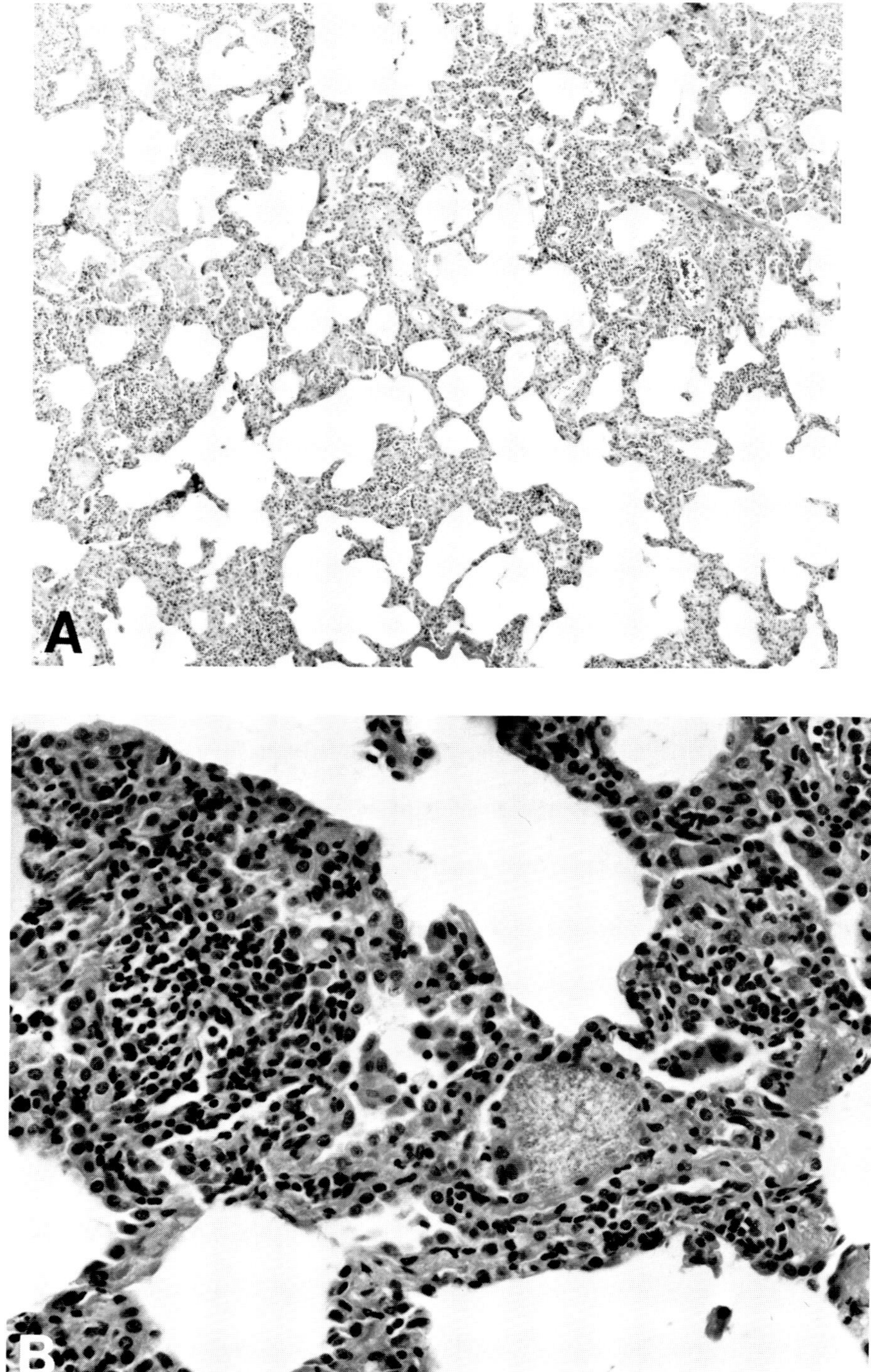

Figure 1 (A).   This example of *Pneumocystis carinii* pneumonia is characterized by a prominent lymphoplasma-cytic interstitial infiltrate, which overshadows the focal characteristic intraalveolar exudate of PCP (H&E, original magnification ×60). (B) Higher power shows one alveolar space containing a typical exudate of PCP. The adjacent interstitium is infiltrated with numerous lymphocytes and plasma cells (H&E, original magnification ×250).

PCP appears more foamy, in contrast to the evenly granular intraalveolar material in alveolar proteinosis. Although pulmonary alveolar proteinosis has been reported in AIDS patients,[42] PCP should be ruled out in all cases by careful examination of special stains for organisms.

The cyst form of *Pneumocystis carinii* is 4–6 μm in diameter and is usually spherical, ovoid, or cup-shaped. The majority of the cysts have single or paired, discrete, darkly staining foci that represent focal thickening of the cyst wall.[29,43] The morphologic differential diagnosis of the cysts of *Pneumocystis carinii* includes *Torulopsis glabrata, Histoplasma capsulatum, Candida albicans, Cryptococcus neoformans,* and *Coccidioides immitis.*[43]

Recent progress in the diagnosis of PCP has led to the use of sputum cytology as an initial investigative tool for AIDS patients with pneumonitis. Although not all cases of PCP are detected by this method, it spares these patients the need for bronchoscopy.[34,44,45] Recent studies indicate that the use of induced liquified sputum may improve the sensitivity of PCP diagnosis to 78%,[45a] and with immunofluorescence it may increase to 92%.[34] Plastic embedding has been recommended for evaluation of PCP in transbronchial biopsies from AIDS patients, but it remains to be proven whether this special processing technique provides a diagnostic advantage over routine paraffin sections.[46] With 0.9 μm thick methacrylate sections stained by silver methenamine and counterstained with toluidine blue, both the sporozoites and cysts of *Pneumocystis carinii* can be sharply visualized by light microscopy.[46] Electron microscopy has provided important information regarding structure of the organism, and hence, insight into its taxonomy and classification. The procedure, however, provides little diagnostic information that is not available by light microscopy.[43,47]

In up to 32% of cases, PCP coexists with other pulmonary infections, most commonly cytomegalovirus (CMV) and *Mycobacterium avium-intracellulare,* followed by *M. tuberculosis.*[9] For this reason, it is important to continue to look for other organisms even after *Pneumocystis* is detected.

Viral Infections

Cytomegalovirus (CMV) is the most frequent cause of viral pneumonia in AIDS patients. It represented the sole infective agent isolated from the lung in 4.1% of AIDS patients reported in the first National Heart Lung Blood Institute workshop on the pulmonary complications of AIDS. It presents most frequently, however, in association with *Pneumocystis carinii,* followed by other organisms such as *M. avium-intracellulare,* and *Cryptococcus neoformans.*[9] CMV with or without associated infection was found in 17% of all AIDS patients with pulmonary complications.[9] CMV pneumonitis usually presents as a diffuse bilateral interstitial process; however, it can rarely cause a localized pneumonitis in immunocompromised hosts.[48] At autopsy, CMV pneumonitis has been reported in up to 58% of AIDS patients.[49–51,51a]

CMV induces a characteristic viral cytopathic effect. As the name implies, the infected cells are enlarged, with a prominent, amphophilic to deeply basophilic intranuclear inclusion separated from the prominent nuclear membrane by a lucent halo. The cytoplasm of infected cells often contains a variable number of small indistinct basophilic inclusions.[52] CMV inclusions may be found in Type II alveolar pneumocytes, in alveolar macrophages, in endothelial cells, and in bronchial epithelial cells. Rarely, CMV pulmonary infection can be associated with necrotizing pulmonary vasculitis.* When only nuclear inclusions are found, it may be difficult to distinguish CMV from other nuclear viral inclusions such as herpes simplex. It should be recognized that the cytoplasmic inclusions of CMV stain positively with the Gomori's methenamine silver and the periodic-acid-

---

*W. Travis, unpublished observations.

Schiff stains, but the nuclear inclusions do not.[53] Hyperplastic and atypical reactive type II pneumocytes, typically seen in diffuse alveolar damage, radiation, and chemotherapy-associated pulmonary toxicity can also be confused with CMV infected cells.

The histologic response associated with cytomegalovirus infection may resemble diffuse alveolar damage or a chronic interstitial pneumonitis.[51] Occasionally, CMV inclusions are found in lung biopsies where there is a minimal histologic reaction. The significance of CMV inclusions in this situation is unknown.[51,54] It is also frequently difficult to assess the contribution of CMV to pulmonary disease when there is concomitant infection due to other opportunistic organisms.

Although CMV pneumonitis has been clearly shown to be a cause of respiratory failure and death, its prevalence and severity is probably underestimated in AIDS patients.[49-51,55-58] It is difficult to assess the frequency of CMV pneumonitis in AIDS patients for several reasons. Part of the problem lies in the different criteria for diagnosis. If positive cultures from bronchoalveolar lavage are used, the frequency of CMV pneumonitis will be much higher than if traditional light microscopic viral inclusions in lung biopsies are required for the diagnosis. The effect of methodology on diagnostic criteria and the frequency of the diagnosis of CMV pneumonitis must be kept in mind as more sensitive techniques, such as monoclonal antibodies and in situ hybridization techniques are applied. Another problem relates to the small amount of tissue obtained by transbronchial biopsy and cases of CMV pneumonitis that may be overlooked compared to the number detected by open lung biopsy.

Pulmonary infection in AIDS by other viral agents is rare. Herpes simplex virus pneumonitis is unusual in AIDS and only a few cases have been reported.[9,56,59,60] The rarity of disseminated herpes simplex infection in AIDS may be due to the effectiveness of acyclovir therapy in patients who present with localized mucocutaneous herpetic infections.[60] Rare cases of measles pneumonitis have occurred in HIV-infected children.[61] So far, human immunodeficiency virus (HIV) has not been shown to be a direct cause of pneumonitis in AIDS patients, although some have proposed that it may play a role in the development of lymphocytic interstitial pneumonitis.[62,63] Similarly, Epstein-Barr virus (EBV) has been proposed as an opportunistic infectious agent in AIDS patients who have lymphocytic interstitial pneumonitis[64-68] or pulmonary lymphoproliferative disorders.[69-71] There may be other viral pulmonary infections that are currently unrecognized due to the lack of morphologically recognizable cytopathic effects or proper methods for in vitro isolation.

Mycobacterial Infections

After *Pneumocystis carinii* and CMV, *Mycobacterium avium-intracellulare* (MAI) is the third most common infectious agent found in AIDS patients with pulmonary disorders.[9] It was cultured in 17% of patients during life from one large series of AIDS cases.[9] Since MAI is often disseminated in AIDS patients,[72] when pulmonary infection is detected, other sites of involvement should be anticipated. Although MAI pulmonary infection is relatively common in AIDS, death due to MAI infection and respiratory failure is unusual.[73,74]

Mycobacterium tuberculosis (MTB) pneumonia was rarely seen during the first few years of the AIDS epidemic.[9] In the last few years, however, tuberculosis has emerged as an important cause of pulmonary disease in AIDS patients.[74-82] One study recently reported that the rate of tuberculosis is 100 times greater in AIDS patients than in the general population.[77]

Several clinical aspects distinguish AIDS patients who develop MTB infection. Several groups of AIDS patients have been shown to be particularly prone to tuberculosis including Haitians,[80-82] intravenous drug abusers,[76,82,83] and patients from Africa.[84] However, recent evidence indicates that tuberculosis is an important complication of AIDS in United States born homosexuals as well.[75] In many cases, tuberculosis precedes the diagnosis of AIDS.[80,83,84] These patients also have frequent extrathoracic disease, nonapical pulmonary tuberculosis, and infrequent cavitation. Mediastinal and hilar lymphadenopathy are also common. As a result, the radiographic appearance of pulmonary tuberculosis in AIDS patients often resembles primary tuberculosis rather than reactivation tuberculosis.[75,81]

Mycobacterial infections in AIDS are frequently diagnosed in specimens obtained from extrapulmonary sites such as the urine, blood, lymph node, bone marrow, or liver.[77] The role MAI plays in pulmonary dysfunction is unclear for those patients in whom organisms from respiratory secretions are recovered, but there is no histologic evidence of lung involvement on transbronchial or open lung biopsy. In this situation, the organisms may be derived from blood contamination in a bacteremic patient and may not indicate pulmonary infection. For the diagnosis of pulmonary MAI infection we require the presence of acid-fast organisms in tissue sections or the presence of an appropriate histologic reaction, in addition to identification of MAI by culture of respiratory secretions. The distinction of MAI from other mycobacteria is important since MAI appears to be resistant to antimicrobial therapy.[85]

The histologic reaction associated with MTB or MAI infections in the lungs of AIDS patients can be either granulomatous or nongranulomatous.[72,74,76,86-89] Granulomas may be caseating, noncaseating, or both.[87] The lack of granuloma formation in some cases is thought to correlate with a rapid spread of pulmonary disease, decreased T-helper and suppressor lymphocytes, and defective T-cell mediated macrophage activation.[72,87,88] In the absence of granulomas, the histologic reaction asso-

ciated with mycobacterial infection is commonly that of a histiocytic pneumonia.[74,87,88] The macrophages become stuffed with innumerable organisms resulting in the production of "striated histiocytes" that recently have been suggested as a morphologic hallmark of MAI infection.[74] For this reason, lung biopsies should be examined carefully with special stains for mycobacteria even in the absence of granulomas, and especially, when foamy macrophages or "striated histiocytes" are seen. Identification of mycobacteria in histologic sections requires the use of acid-fast stains such as the Ziehl-Neelson or Fite stains. With MAI infection, the numerous organisms stuffing macrophages may be seen with H&E sections or with other stains such as PAS and methenamine silver stains.

Bacterial Infections

Bacterial pneumonia is relatively uncommon in AIDS and this is shown by the 3–4% incidence from two large series of patients.[9,90] In some institutions, however, the frequency of bacterial pneumonia is considerably higher in AIDS and AIDS-related complex patients than in patients without HIV infection.[91] The following bacterial pathogens have been reported: most commonly, *Streptococcus pneumoniae*,[90,91] and *Hemophilus influenzae*,[90,91] followed by *group B Streptococcus*,[90] *Branhamella catarrhalis*,[90,91] *Pseudomonas aeruginosa*,[49,55,56] *Klebsiella pneumoniae*,[49,56] *Enterobacter cloacae*,[56] *Staphylococcus aureus*,[49,55,91] *Mycoplasma pneumoniae*,[91] *Nocardia asteroides*,[92,93] and *Legionella species*.[9,56,90] Recent reports indicate that *Legionella pneumoniae* appears to be seen less frequently than in the early years of AIDS epidemic.[78]

It is thought that abnormalities in the B-cell immune system may be the underlying cause for the increased susceptibility of some AIDS patients to pneumococcal and *Haemophilus* infections.[90,94,95] According to a recent study in AIDS and ARC patients, community-acquired bacterial infections could be distinguished from nosocomial infections.[91] Community-acquired bacterial infections were typically caused by encapsulated organisms, presented early in the clinical course of the disease, and were responsive to therapy. In contrast, nosocomial infections were due mostly to gram-negative bacilli, occurred late in the course of disease, often in association with leukopenia, and were frequently unsuspected, undertreated, and often fatal.[91]

There are rare reports of lung abscess due to bacterial infections in AIDS patients. *Rhodococcus equi* (formerly Corynebacterium equi), a rare pathogen in humans, was the cause of lung abscess[96] and pneumonia.[96a]

Fungal Infections

Although several studies indicate that 58–81% of AIDS patients develop a fungal infection at least once during the course of their disease,[97] fungal pneumonias are relatively uncommon. Pulmonary fungal infections were found in less than 2% of a large series of patients reported in the First National Heart Lung and Blood Institute Workshop on the pulmonary complications of AIDS.[9] The most frequent pulmonary fungal infections seen in AIDS patients are cryptococcosis, histoplasmosis, coccidioidomycosis, aspergillosis, and candidiasis.[97] Zygomycosis was listed among the infections that comprised the original case definition for AIDS,[20] however, it has subsequently been removed from this list due to the apparent rarity of infection by this organism in AIDS patients.[21,22] One AIDS patient was found to have invasive *Geotrichum* pneumonia at autopsy, however, this case appears to be unique.[98]

Recent studies suggest that recognition of unexpected fungal infections in patients with the AIDS-related-complex (ARC) may herald the onset of full-blown AIDS.[99-101] The reasons for this are not known, although some have speculated that fungal infection may contribute to the development of AIDS by activating T lymphocytes already infected with HIV.[97] In addition, fungal infections have been shown to induce an immunosuppressive effect on the affected host.[97]

Cryptococcosis

Cryptococcus neoformans infection occurs in 6–13% of living AIDS patients[102-106] and most frequently affects the brain and meninges. The lung, however, is the second most common organ affected, and pulmonary involvement can be found in 31–60% of AIDS patients with cryptococcal infection.[103,103a,105,106] In up to 8% of AIDS patients with cryptococcal infection, the lung is the only organ involved.[106] If pulmonary cryptococcosis is diagnosed, however, the possibility of disseminated infection should be investigated, since the majority of these patients have other sites of infection.[103,103a,105,106] In addition, cryptococcal infection in the lung is frequently associated with other pulmonary infections.[103,105,106] Although pulmonary involvement may be found at autopsy in a relatively high percentage of AIDS patients who die with cryptococcal infection, respiratory failure is seldom the primary cause of death.[103,105]

Thoracic cryptococcosis in AIDS may rarely present with massive mediastinal lymph node[107] or pleural[108] involvement.

Several different histologic patterns have been described in pulmonary cryptococcosis including peripheral granulomas, granulomatous pneumonia, intracapillary/interstitial infiltration, and massive pulmonary involvement.[109] In AIDS patients, the major pattern observed is the interstitial pattern.[103] The minimal inflammatory response and absence of well developed granulomas in many of these cases make it easy to overlook the organisms. In histologic sections, cryptococcus appears as round to oval shaped yeast forms, 4–7 μm in diameter (Fig. 2). Cryptococcus can be recognized on H&E

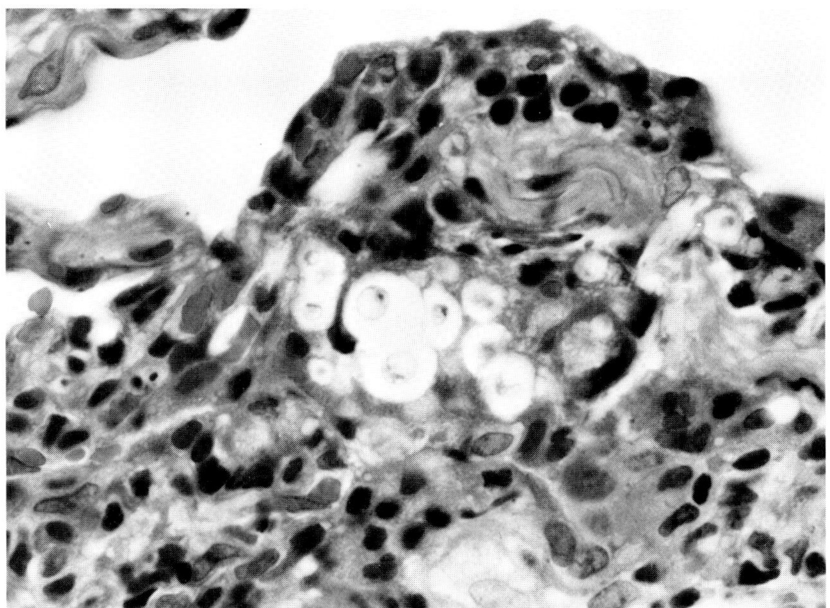

Figure 2. Multiple round to oval yeast forms each with a very thick capsule are compatible with *Cryptococcus* in this transbronchial biopsy. Although the surrounding alveolar walls are compressed, the organisms appear to be within the interstitium (H&E, original magnification ×860).

stained sections, but it is better demonstrated with PAS, methenamine silver, or mucicarmine stains. Other fungi will also stain with PAS and methenamine silver, however, mucicarmine staining of the thick capsule is unique to cryptococcus. In addition, the narrow-based budding of cryptococcus contrasts with the broad-based buds of the yeast forms of blastomycosis.[110,111] With poorly capsulated forms of cryptococcus, problems can occur in the morphologic differential diagnosis with *Candida*,[103] *Blastomyces,* or *Histoplasma*[110,111] In such cases, the Fontana-Masson stain may be useful in distinguishing *C. neoformans.*[112]

Although the presence of cryptococcus in bronchoalveolar lavage is generally considered indicative of pulmonary infection,[111] transbronchial biopsy is thought to be more sensitive for establishing the diagnosis.[5,103]

Coccidioidomycosis

Coccidioides immitis infection in AIDS typically occurs in patients with exposure in endemic areas such as the southwestern United States.[113-116] *Coccidioides immitis* infection was found in 26% of AIDS patients in a recent study from Arizona, which is a much higher incidence than observed in other immunocompromised patients in that region.[2] A review of cases of fungemia due to *Coccidioides immitis* in Arizona, revealed that AIDS was the underlying condition in 20% of cases.[114] The clinical picture of coccidioidomycosis in AIDS patients is characterized by diffuse nodular involvement of the lungs and evidence of extrapulmonary disease.[2] Recognition of this clinical picture in association with coccidioidomycosis has recently been added as a diagnostic criteria for AIDS in patients who have no other apparent cause for immunosuppression.[2,22]

Few details have been reported about the pathologic manifestations of *Coccidioides immitis* infection in AIDS patients. However, well formed granulomas with or without caseating necrosis have been described in several reports,[2,113] and autopsies have revealed disseminated organ involvement.[115] It is likely, although not yet documented, that granulomas can be poorly formed or absent in AIDS patients due to the defective T-cell mediated immune response. In histologic sections, *Coccidioides immitis* has a very distinctive morphologic appearance with thick-walled spherules measuring 30–60 µm that are filled with numerous endospores.[110,111] These organisms can be visualized in routine H&E stained sections; however, they are better seen with the methenamine silver and PAS stains.

Histoplasmosis

Progressive disseminated histoplasmosis (PDH) is a well recognized complication of AIDS and has been observed both in endemic[3,99,117–119] and nonendemic[120] areas. In endemic areas, PDH has been observed in up to 47% of AIDS patients.[99] Since histoplasmosis is uncommon in cities where AIDS is prevalent,[3,97] it took several years for AIDS to spread to endemic areas, and therefore, disseminated histoplasmosis was not included as one of the diagnostic criteria of AIDS until recently.[21,22] Although the lungs are frequently affected in these patients, the clinical presentation is generally that of a systemic illness with fever, weight loss, and splenomegaly.[118] Chest radiographs may resemble an acute pneumonia or miliary tuberculosis.[120]

The diagnosis of disseminated histoplasmosis in AIDS can be established by recognition of organisms in transbronchial or lymph node biopsies, or in the peripheral blood.[117–119] However, bone marrow biopsy has the highest diagnostic yield and is recommended as the optimal method for detection of PDH.[118] A potentially useful new method for detecting *H. capsulatum* in the serum and urine may improve rapid diagnosis for patients with PDH.[121] In histologic sections *H. capsulatum* is characterized by 2–5 µm round to oval yeast cells usually found within the cytoplasm of macrophages.[110,111] In some cases it may be diffi-

cult to distinguish *H. capsulatum* from *Pneumocystis carinii*.[122] In this situation, cultures may be helpful if *H. capsulatum* grows.[122] Recently described immunodiagnostic techniques for the detection of histoplasmosis[123] and *P. carinii*[34,35] may also provide useful ways to distinguish these organisms.

The histologic reactions associated with progressive disseminated histoplasmosis in AIDS patients are not well documented. Several reports indicate that a granulomatous (caseating or noncaseating) reaction may, or may not be present.[99,117]

In Africa, a different species of histoplasma is prevalent, called *Histoplasma duboisii*.[110] The morphology of *H. duboisii* is different from that of *H. capsulatum* with larger round oval, thick-walled yeast forms that measure 10–15 µm.[110] One AIDS patient from Zaire with a disseminated *H. dubosii* infection has been reported.[125] Organisms were found within histiocytes and multinucleated giant cells, characteristic of anergic infection by *H. dubosii*.[125]

Candidiasis

Although *Candida albicans* is the most common cause of fungal infection in AIDS and ARC patients occurring in 80–90% of cases as oroesophageal candidiasis, it is a relatively uncommon cause of primary fungal pneumonia.[97] In most cases *Candida* pneumonia is discovered at autopsy rather than during life, and it is reported in up to 30% of AIDS patients at autopsy.[1,50,55–57,59,98,122,124] In many cases pulmonary candidiasis is accompanied by other pulmonary infections such as cytomegalovirus and *Pneumocystis carinii,* but respiratory insufficiency due to *Candida* pneumonia alone is seldom the primary cause of death.

Pulmonary involvement by *Candida* is included in the CDC criteria for the diagnosis of AIDS.[20–22] However, the recovery of *Candida* species from bronchial washings or lavage fluid, with the use of smears or cultures, alone is not sufficient for the diagnosis.[57,111] Histologic proof or recognition of characteristic plaques on the bronchial mucosa are required to diagnose pulmonary candidiasis.[22]

Candida species in histologic sections demonstrate pseudohyphae or budding yeast cells that can be seen with H&E stained sections, but are best visualized by staining with PAS or methenamine silver stains. Pulmonary infection may occur as a form of bronchitis, a diffuse pneumonic process, necrotizing abscesses, or in severe cases as an invasive infection.[111] When *Candida* pneumonia becomes severe, necrotizing abscesses may form. Invasive pulmonary candidiasis is characterized by the infiltration of fungal organisms into blood vessels and into the pulmonary parenchyma.

Aspergillosis

Disseminated aspergillosis is rare in AIDS,[55,56,59,97] being observed in only five of 3170 AIDS cases recorded by the Centers for Disease Control (CDC).[97] Pulmonary aspergillosis has been observed in AIDS patients as the initial manifestation of disseminated infection,[59] but it can also occur as a terminal complication.[55,56] In one series pulmonary aspergillosis was found in 9% of patients dying of AIDS.[56] When it occurs, .disseminated aspergillosis is preceded by neutropenia and/or corticosteroid therapy.[126-128] AIDS patients generally have normal granulocyte numbers and function, however, the T-cell mediated immune responses are defective. Although initially included in the CDC's diagnostic criteria for AIDS, disseminated aspergillosis has subsequently been removed from the list of infections considered moderately predictive of AIDS.[128]

An unusual presentation of pulmonary aspergillosis was recently described in an AIDS patient who had a pseudomembranous necrotizing form of bronchial aspergillosis.[127] Aspergillus in histologic sec-

tions is characterized by septate hyphae that are $3-4$ μm in diameter, and show branching at approximately $45°$ angles.[110,111] In invasive pulmonary infections, blood vessel invasion is commonly associated with pulmonary infarction.[111]

Cryptosporidiosis

Although *Cryptosporidium* most commonly infects the intestine and causes diarrhea, there are a few reports of involvement of the respiratory tract in AIDS patients.[129-131] All cases of pulmonary involvement have occurred in patients with diarrhea caused by cryptosporidiosis. Spread to the lungs has been thought to occur by either aspiration or hematogenous spread. Whether or not the *Cryptosporidium* causes significant respiratory compromise is somewhat questionable because each of the reported cases has also had an associated pulmonary process, which would account for the respiratory symptoms.

Demonstration of *Cryptosporidium* in lung biopsy sections is difficult, however, trophozoites have been described lining the bronchial epithelium and within inflammatory exudate in the alveolar spaces.[129-131] In formalin-fixed, H&E stained histologic sections the cryptosporidia trophozoites appear similar to those seen in the gastrointestinal tract: small spherical basophilic staining structures lining the bronchial mucosa or within alveoli. The associated inflammatory reactions described include interstitial pneumonitis, bronchiolitis, and alveolitis. Detection of *Cryptosporidium* in the lung is facilitated by the use of modified cold Kinyoun (MCK) and Hemacolor stains on sputum smears or touch preparations from lung biopsies.[129,131]

Toxoplasmosis

Pulmonary toxoplasmosis is very rare in AIDS patients,[122,132-134] however, pulmonary toxoplasmosis is thought to be increasing in incidence and is probably underdiagnosed.[132] It was found in only one of 441 AIDS patients who had pulmonary disorders.[9] Pulmonary involvement by *Toxoplasma gondii* usually occurs in the context of disseminated infection where the central nervous system is the primary site of infection.

The diagnosis of pulmonary toxoplasmosis requires direct visualization of cysts or tachyzoites in bronchoalveolar lavage or lung biopsy specimens, although the most sensitive method for detecting *Toxoplasma gondii* is by mouse inoculation or growth in cell culture.[132] In histologic sections, the tachyzoites of *Toxoplasma gondii* are $2-6$ μm and appear rounded or oval, while the cysts are filled with hundreds of bradyzoites.[110] Typically, the associated inflammatory reaction in the lung consists of an acute necrotizing pneumonia (Fig. 3).

PATHOLOGY OF INTERSTITIAL LUNG DISEASE

Interstitial lung disease, in the absence of any identifiable infectious agent or neoplasm, is seen in a significant percentage of lung biopsies from AIDS patients. Four basic forms of interstitial pneumonitis have been described in AIDS patients including lymphocytic interstitial pneumonitis (LIP), nonspecific interstitial pneumonitis (NIP), alveolar proteinosis, and eosinophilic pneumonia. Desquamative interstitial pneumonitis (DIP) has been described in AIDS patients, however, it appears to be a nonspecific histologic reaction to other pulmonary processes.

LIP is an important cause of pulmonary disease in pediatric patients with AIDS[66,135,136] and can be found in up to 43% of cases.[137] Pulmonary lymphoid hyperplasia (PLH) is another common cause of interstitial lung disease in children with AIDS[67] and is probably related to LIP.[66] This LIP/PLH complex may be a part of a

B-cell lymphoid hyperplasia that can be found in the lymph nodes, liver, and gastrointestinal tract of these patients.[135] Recently, it has been recognized that LIP is not restricted to children with AIDS; it can also occur in adults.[65,138,139]

Pulmonary PLH/LIP may be one of the initial manifestations of pediatric AIDS. Children with AIDS who present with PLH/LIP usually have a chronic, slowly progressive course with mild exacerbations. They often present with cough, digital clubbing, salivary gland enlargement, generalized lymphadenopathy, and a nodular chest x-ray pattern.[67] Pediatric patients with LIP tend to be slightly older (age range $20-68$ months) than those who develop PCP.

Histologically, LIP is characterized by a diffuse interstitial and peribronchiolar infiltrate consisting of lymphocytes, plasma cells, some with Russel bodies, plasmacytoid lymphocytes, and immunoblasts (Fig. 4). Occasionally, giant cells and granulomas may be seen.[135] In pulmonary lymphoid hyperplasia, the lymphocytes are aggregated in nodular collections adjacent to bronchioles and may form germinal centers. It is not unusual to find both PLH and LIP in the same biopsy.[66] Immunotyping of the lymphocytes in these lesions has yielded variable results: predominantly B cells with polyclonal immunoglobulin staining[64] or predominantly T cells.[138] Lymphocytes retrieved from bronchoalveolar lavage from AIDS patients having pneumonitis due to a variety of causes have been shown to be predominantly T cells.[140]

The etiology of LIP in the context of AIDS is unknown. Identification of HIV and EBV in pulmonary specimens from patients with LIP have led to speculations that LIP may be a response to infection with either HIV, EBV, or both. HIV has been identified in pulmonary alveolar macrophages, lymphocytes in lavage fluid,[63,68] and in biopsy tissue[62] from patients with AIDS and ARC. It is possible that HIV-infected macrophages or lymphocytes express viral RNA and release lymphokines or toxic viral

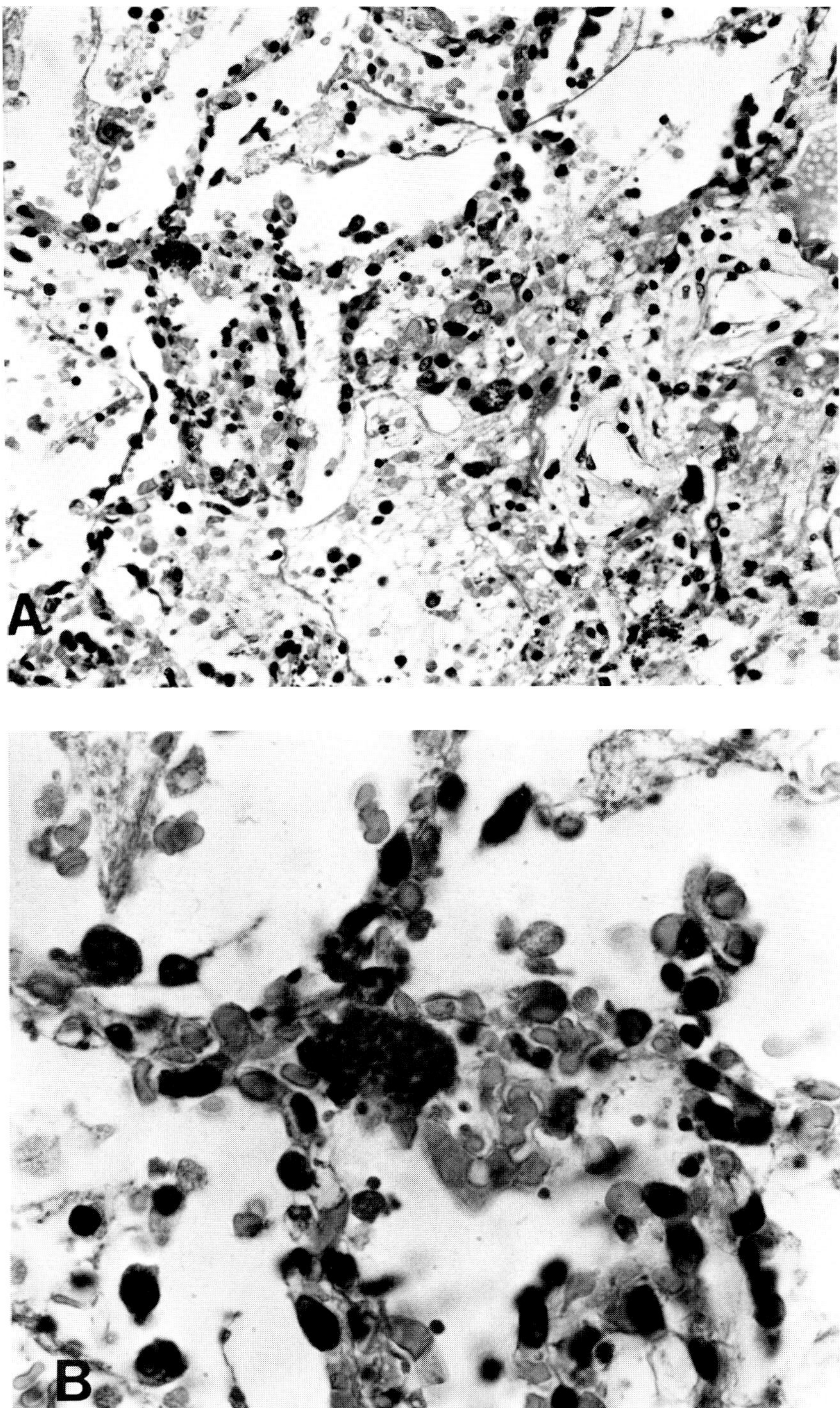

Figure 3 (A). Scattered cysts and tachyzoites of *Toxoplasma gondii* are seen in this lung biopsy, which shows an acute necrotizing pneumonia (H&E, original magnification ×250). (B) A closer view shows a cyst containing multiple tachyzoites (H&E, original magnification ×800).

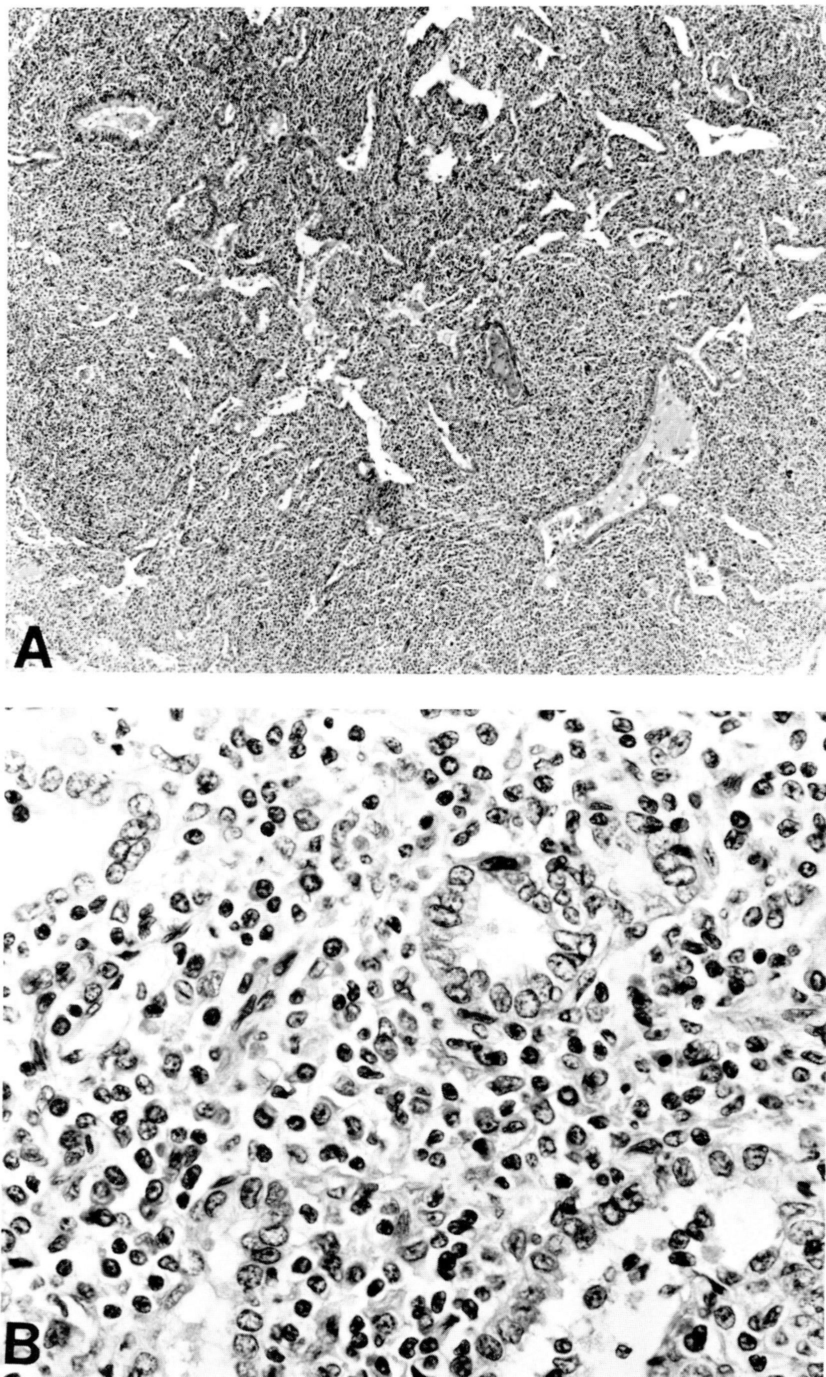

Figure 4 (A).   The extensive interstitial lymphoplasmacytic infiltrate in this lung biopsy from a pediatric AIDS patient is characteristic of lymphocytic interstitial pneumonitis. At this low power view, the process obscures the overall lung architecture (H&E, original magnification ×60). (B) Higher power shows numerous lymphocytes and plasma cells within the interstitium with prominent cuboidal change in the alveolar lining cells (H&E, original magnification ×500).

products that induce an inflammatory response. EBV is known to be a direct polyclonal B-cell activator without the requirement of either T cells or macrophages. Recent evidence also suggests that the lung may be a reservoir for EBV.[141] Considering this evidence, it is possible that EBV becomes activated as a result of the immunosuppression due to HIV infection and induces an "opportunistic lymphoproliferation".[142] EBV is also associated with B-cell lymphoproliferative disorders in other immunosuppressed patients as well as in AIDS patients.[143] A small subset of AIDS patients who present with LIP may develop similar polyclonal lymphoproliferative disorders.[66,71,136]

The most effective treatment for LIP appears to be low doses of steroids.[62,64] Treatment with antiviral agents such as acyclovir has not been successful.[64]

Another form of interstitial pneumonitis in AIDS patients has emerged as a result of the observation that a subgroup of patients who presented with clinical pneumonitis were found to have an interstitial inflammatory process on lung biopsy with no evidence of infection or tumor.[13,144,145] This clinicopathologic condition has been called "nonspecific interstitial pneumonitis" and in one series was found to occur in 12% of 61 AIDS patients with respiratory abnormalities[13] (Figs. 5 and 6).

Desquamative interstitial pneumonitis (DIP) has been described in pediatric AIDS patients,[136] however, these same authors have more recently withdrawn this concept.[66] Follow-up in the original cases revealed associated PCP, *Aspergillus* granulomatous disease, and LIP.[66] DIP-like accumulations of intraalveolar macrophages are known to occur as a nonspecific reaction in a wide variety of pulmonary processes.[146] Therefore, these cases do not appear to represent the fibrotic interstitial lung disease of DIP.

Two cases of alveolar proteinosis have been reported in AIDS patients.[42] One of these patients had associated infection with MTB and the other had combined PCP and CMV pneumonitis.[42] Alveolar proteinosis has also been described in a patient with HIV infection and adult T-cell lymphoma/leukemia.[147]

Alveolar proteinosis is known to occur in association with a variety of infectious agents including *Nocardia asteroides, Histoplasma capsulatum, Cryptococcus neoformans,* MTB, MAI and CMV.[148–151] Although the distinction between the alveolar exudates of PCP and alveolar proteinosis can be very difficult, the association between these two conditions has been reported in at least one other case.[148] It is also known to occur in the context of immune deficiency and a variety of hematologic malignancies.[148,152] The mechanisms for development of alveolar proteinosis in AIDS are not certain. It is possible that alveolar proteinosis in AIDS is related to underlying immune deficiency and that the infections are secondary. Alternately, the infectious agent may provide the inciting injury that leads to development of alveolar proteinosis. Due to the histologic resemblance with the alveolar exudates of PCP, the diagnosis of alveolar proteinosis should be made with caution in AIDS patients.

Eosinophilic pneumonia in association with ketaconazole therapy has also been reported in an AIDS patient.[153] This patient had peripheral eosinophilia and histologic evidence of eosinophilic pneumonia on open lung biopsy. This process probably represented a hypersensitivity drug reaction. A pulmonary hypersensitivity reaction to phenytoin has also been reported in an HIV-infected patient.[154] With the wide variety of medications given to AIDS patients, and the prospects of many new experimental therapies, it is likely that more pulmonary drug reactions will be observed in the coming years.

Intravenous drug abusers may have a foreign body granulomatous reaction to hematogenously spread birefringent crystalline material and associated vascular pulmonary hypertensive changes. However, these are usually incidental findings discovered at autopsy[122] rather than primary causes of inter-

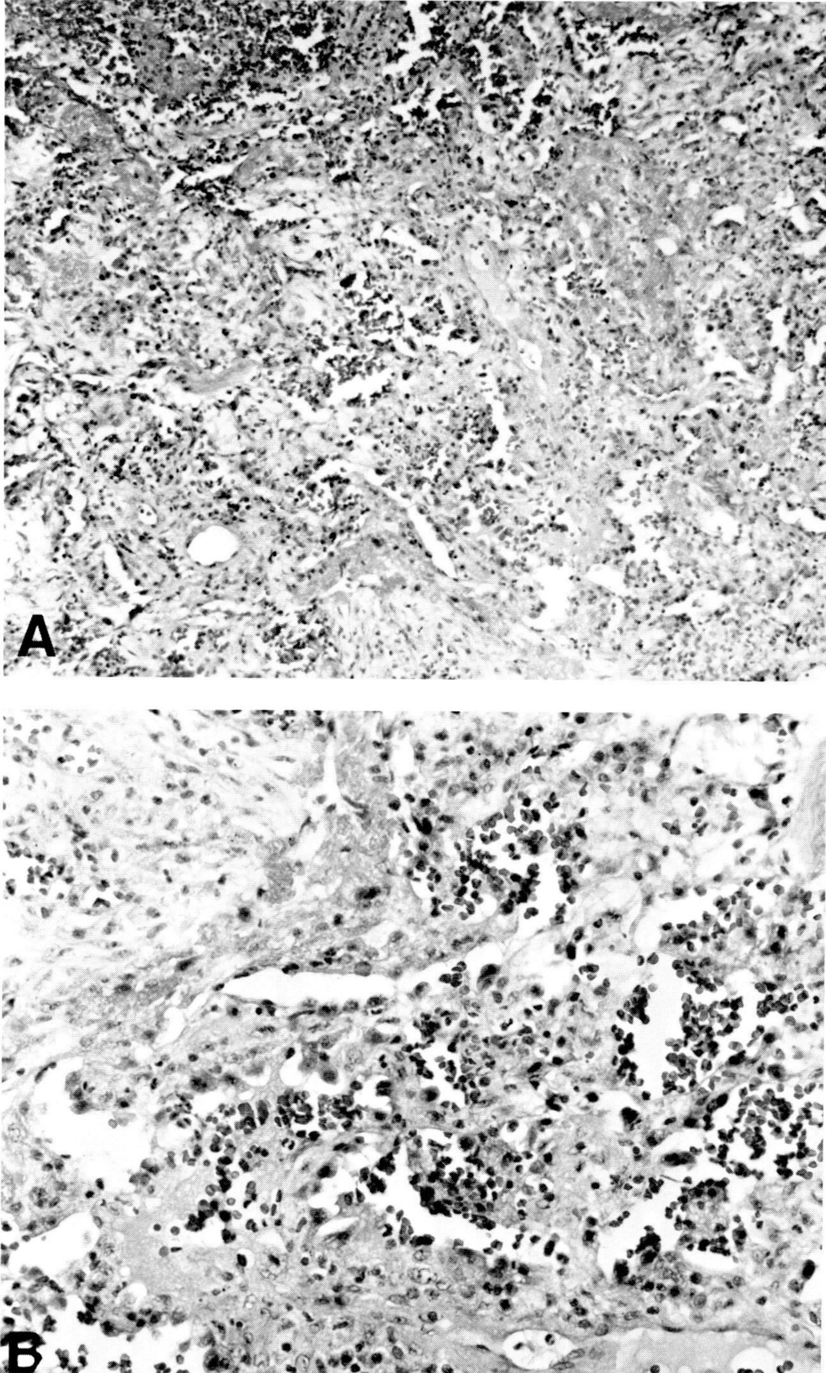

Figure 5 (A).   The acute form of nonspecific interstitial pneumonitis is represented by this transbronchial biopsy, which shows the organizing phase of diffuse alveolar damage with interstitial edema, loose interstitial fibrosis, intraalveolar hemorrhage, and acute and chronic interstitial inflammation. (H&E, original magnification ×125 (B) Higher power shows prominent reactive alveolar lining cells and a closer view of the features of diffuse alveolar damage (H&E, original magnification ×250).

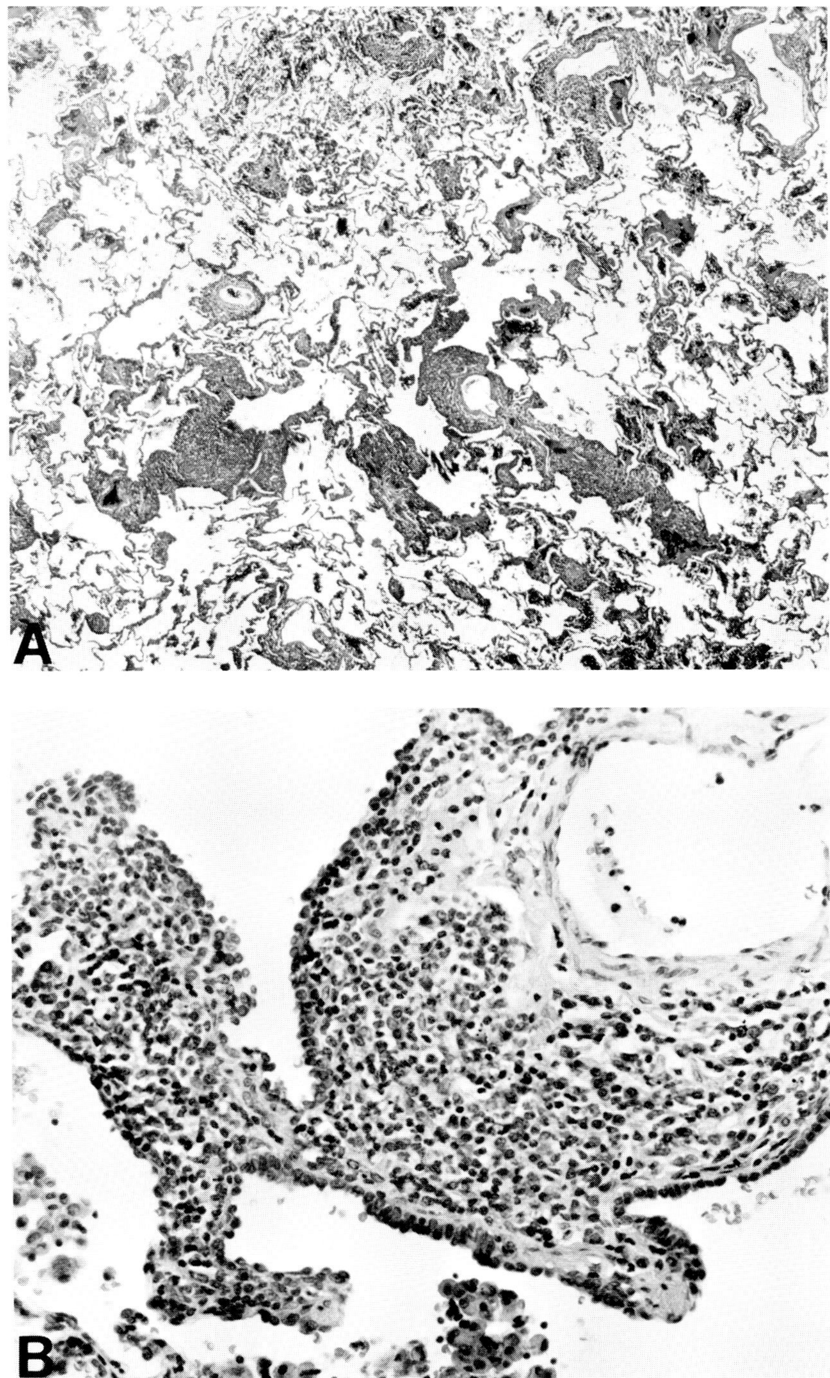

Figure 6 (A). The chronic form of nonspecific interstitial pneumonitis is illustrated by this open lung biopsy, which demonstrates mild to moderate interstitial infiltration by lymphocytes that surround bronchioles and blood vessels and form small nodular aggregates. (H&E, original magnification ×30) (B) A closer view shows peribronchiolar and perivascular infiltration by lymphocytes and plasma cells (H&E, original magnification ×250).

stitial pneumonitis in AIDS.[154a] Plexogenic pulmonary arteriopathy associated with membranoproliferative glomerulonephritis occurred in one AIDS patient who presented with pulmonary hypertension manifested by cardiomegaly and prominent pulmonary arteries without alveolar infiltrates.[155]

PULMONARY KAPOSI'S SARCOMA AND OTHER MALIGNANCIES

Kaposi's Sarcoma

Pulmonary Kaposi's sarcoma (KS) has been reported as a complication of AIDS in 3–20% of cases premortem[8,9,156,157] and 6–35% of patients who come to autopsy.[55,56,57,122,124,158–160] While pulmonary involvement is relatively uncommon in non-African KS without associated HIV infection among AIDS patients who have documented extrapulmonary KS,[160a,161,162] the lung has been reported to be involved in 18–75% of cases.[8,56,57,98,156,159,160,163,163a] The primary presentation of KS in the lung is uncommon, but has been reported both in patients with AIDS[163–166] and without AIDS.[162,167]

The clinical presentation of pulmonary KS may be indistinguishable from that of opportunistic infection.[158] Chest x-rays show nodular or diffuse interstitial pulmonary infiltrates.[158,159] Pleural effusions are common and may be hemorrhagic.[158,159] Complications of pulmonary KS include hemorrhage and airway obstruction. KS is also commonly associated with pulmonary infection.[158,159]

Lung involvement by KS takes the form of parenchymal, pleural, or endobronchial lesions.[159,163a] Kaposi's sarcoma is characterized by the proliferation of spindle-shaped cells forming slit-like spaces containing numerous extravasated erythrocytes (Fig. 7). The spindle-shaped cells of KS are mildly atypical and frequently contain small PAS-positive eosinophilic globules within the cytoplasm. Parenchymal KS infiltrates are distributed along lymphatic routes beneath the pleura, and in relation to bronchioles and blood vessels.[159,163a,168]

There has been little success with the diagnosis of KS by transbronchial biopsy[8,9,12,159,163a] with a few exceptions.[168,169,169a] Since transbronchial biopsies are usually nondiagnostic, in order to establish a histologic diagnosis of KS, an open lung is necessary in most cases. In one study, emphasis was placed on recognition of the inflammatory variant of KS.[168] More recently, the clinical diagnosis of endobronchial KS, by recognition of erythematous papules on bronchoscopy without histologic confirmation, has been advocated due to the difficulty in obtaining diagnostic tissue by transbronchial biopsy.[158,170,171,171a]

The etiology and pathogenesis of KS is not known. Evidence suggests that immunosuppression as well as genetic factors may render individuals susceptible to KS.[172,173] KS is known to occur in renal transplant patients;[172] and patients with KS have been shown to have an increased frequency of HLA-DR5.[173] Several studies have also suggested that viral infection may contribute to the development of KS. Roles of CMV, hepatitis B, and HIV in the pathogenesis of KS have been proposed.[174–178] A recent study, however, demonstrated the lack of HIV and hepatitis B DNA sequences in AIDS-associated KS, and provided evidence suggesting that the presence of CMV DNA in a small percentage of cases is the result of an opportunistic infection rather than a causative agent.[179] In addition, these investigators found that KS cells have a tendency to undergo karyotypic rearrangements.[179] Another recent study using in situ hybridization for CMV DNA similarly indicated no strong association between KS and CMV.[179a]

The histogenesis of KS remains unclear. Ultrastructural studies have demonstrated the presence of endothelial cells, pericytes,

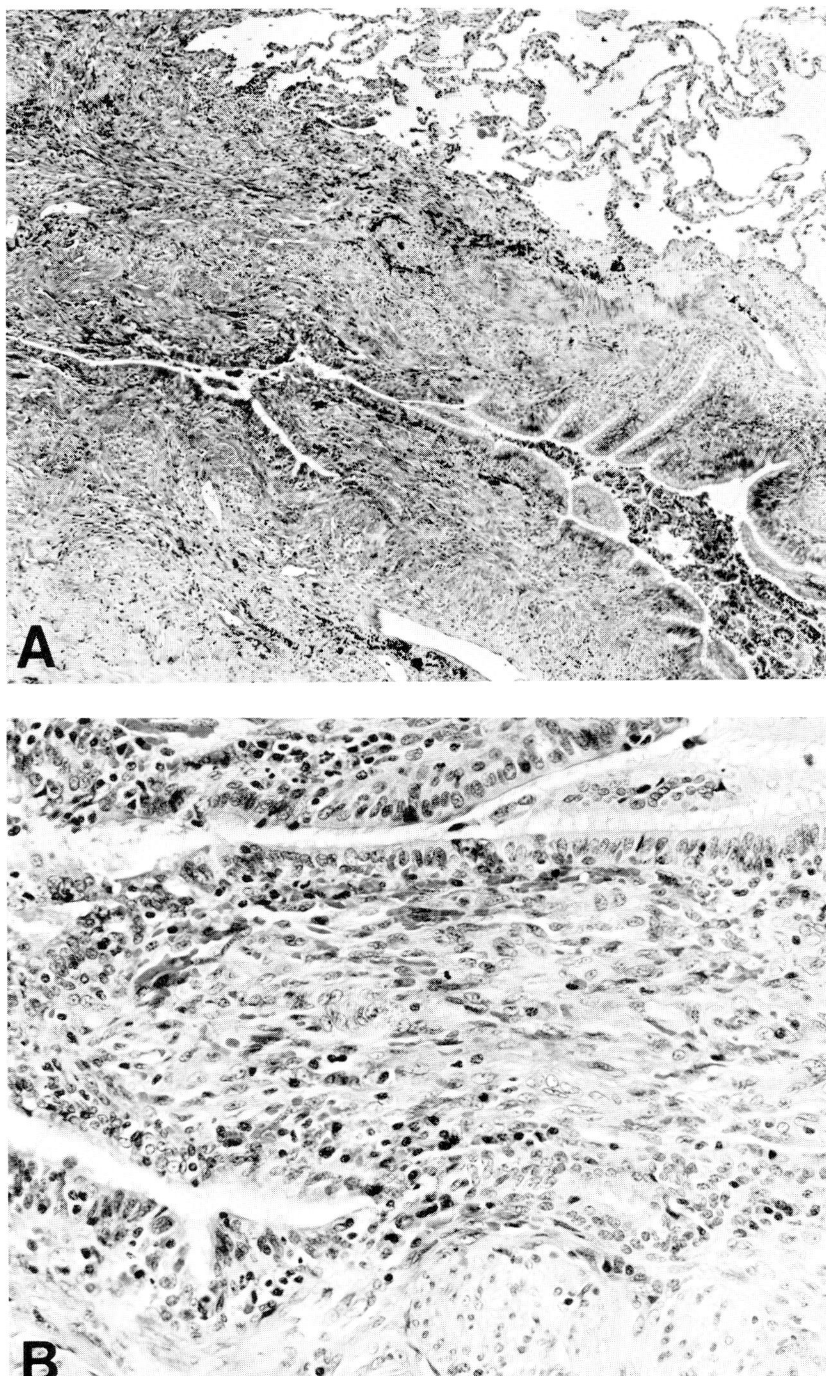

Figure 7 (A). This open lung biopsy shows Kaposi's sarcoma infiltrating around a bronchiole with extension through the wall and into the lamina propria. (B) A high power view shows the characteristic spindle-shaped cells with extravasated erythrocytes diagnostic of KS infiltrating beneath the bronchiolar epithelium (H&E, original magnification ×250).

fibroblasts, and myofibroblasts.[172] Immunohistochemical techniques using monoclonal antibodies to various human sarcoma and connective tissue antigens[180] and antisera to Factor VIII[172,181] have been used to stain KS in tissue sections. Although positive staining for Factor VIII has led some to conclude that KS is of endothelial origin,[181] others have found that Factor VIII stains only endothelial cells rather than the spindle-shaped stromal cells. Consequently, it has been proposed that KS is derived from a primitive vasoformative mesenchyme.[172]

Malignant Lymphoma

Malignant lymphomas arising in AIDS patients are usually extranodal, and most are high grade non-Hodgkin's lymphomas[182,183,183a] (Fig. 8). The lung is involved in 7–9% of cases.[182,183,183a] In addition to the high grade lymphomas, polyclonal B-cell lymphoproliferative disorders have been described.[69-71] The identification of EBV DNA in many of these cases[69-71] suggests that EBV may play an important role in the pathogenesis of these polyclonal lymphoproliferative disorders. This situation has a striking similarity to the EBV associated polyclonal B-cell polyclonal lymphoproliferative disorders described in transplant patients.[184,185] The common finding of EBV in association both with LIP and polyclonal lymphoproliferative disorders in AIDS patients and the reported progression of LIP to a lymphoproliferative disorder in some patients suggests a possible link between these two conditions.

Solid Malignancies

Neoplastic solid tumors of the lung have also been reported in AIDS. Several cases of

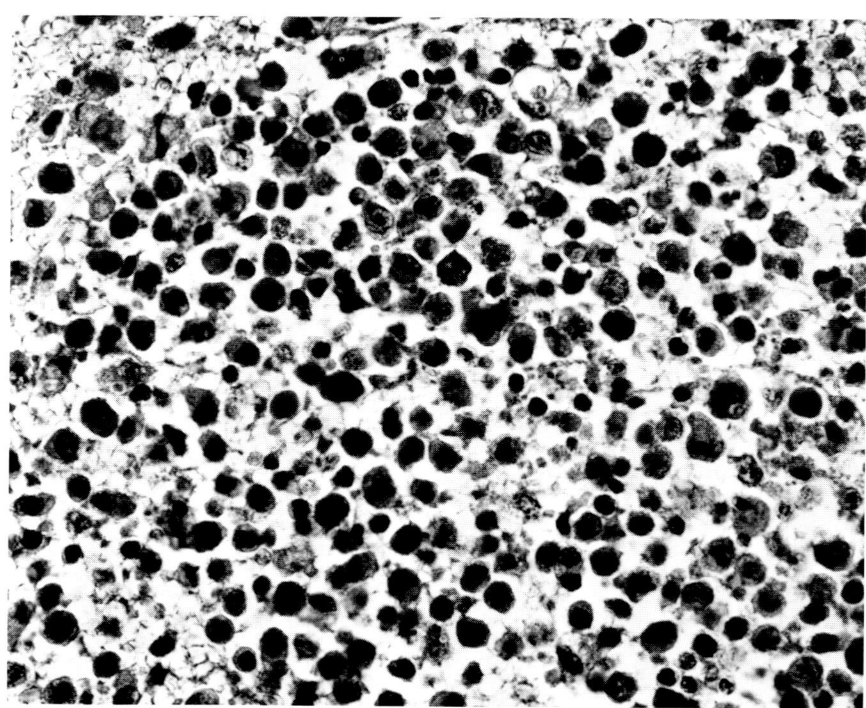

Figure 8. The cytologic preparation of this needle aspirate shows poorly cohesive atypical cells with a high nuclear to cytoplasmic ratio and prominent nucleoli, compatible with malignant lymphoma of the large cell type (H&E, original magnification ×800).

small cell carcinoma have occurred,[186,187] a dysplastic carcinoid tumor reported,[188] and an adenosquamous carcinoma of the lung described.[189] It is possible, however, that the observation of these neoplasms represents the background of naturally occurring neoplasms rather than an association with AIDS.

CASE MATERIAL AND METHODOLOGY

Two hundred thirty-five transbronchial and 26 open lung biopsies were performed on 174 AIDS patients seen at the NIH to evaluate 234 episodes of pneumonitis (Table 2). The various clinical aspects of the pulmonary care of these patients have been published previously.[10,163a,190–195] These AIDS patients were evaluated at the NIH prior to August 1987 for research protocols involving antiretroviral therapy, treatment for an opportunistic infection, or KS. Bronchoalveolar lavage (BAL) was done in conjunction with 191 transbronchial biopsies (TBB) and was the only diagnostic procedure in 32 cases. Open lung biopsies followed TBB in 24 cases and were performed alone in five cases. The majority (58%) of these patients had multiple (up to six) TBB.

Multiple TBB (average 3–4) were obtained in the vast majority of bronchoscopic procedures. These biopsies were routinely processed overnight and given priority for early interpretation. On each biopsy, ten serial sections were cut; three sections were stained with H&E, and one each with the following battery of special stains for microorganisms: Gomori's methenamine silver, toluidine blue, Giemsa, PAS, and the Fite acid-fast stains.

TABLE II

Cause of Pneumonitis in 174 AIDS Patients*

Causes	Episodes N (%)		
	Initial	Subsequent	Total
Pneumocystis	80 (46)	14 (23)	94 (40)
Nonspecific			
Interstitial pneumonitis	58 (33)	17 (28)	75 (32)
Nondiagnostic†	12 (7)	12 (20)	24 (10)
Kaposi's sarcoma ††	11 (6)	3 (5)	14 (6)
Cytomegalovirus	2 (1)	5 (8)	7 (3)
Pneumocystis and Cytomegalovirus	4 (2)	1 (2)	5 (2)
Bacteria	3 (2)	3 (5)	6 (3)
Mycobacteria	3 (2)	2 (3)	5 (2)
Cryptococcus	1 (1)	1 (2)	2 (1)
Pneumocystis and *Cryptococcus*		1 (2)	1 (.5%)
Lymphoma		1 (2)	1 (.5%)
TOTAL	174 (100)	60 (100)	234 (100)

*Ten cases of *Pneumocystis* pneumonia, 2 cases of bacterial pneumonia, and 1 case of cryptococcal pneumonia documented by bronchoalveolar lavage alone; the remaining cases documented by bronchoalveolar lavage and transbronchial biopsy or open lung biopsy.

†Bronchoalveolar lavage performed alone because of biopsy contraindication (24 patients); in 2 patients biopsy specimens were inadequate.

††Concurrent *Pneumocystis* (3 patients), *Cryptococcus* (1 patient), *Legionella* (1 patient), and interstitial pneumonitis (8 patients).

In addition to examination for the presence of infectious organisms, neoplasms, and interstitial abnormalities, lung biopsies were evaluated for the presence and severity of diffuse alveolar damage (DAD). The following features of DAD were looked for: (1) alveolar edema and fibrin deposition, (2) hyaline membrane formation, (3) interstitial inflammation, (4) loose interstitial fibrosis, and (5) dense interstitial fibrosis. In addition, the presence of alveolar macrophages, alveolar hemorrhage, alveolar pneumonitis with neutrophilic infiltration, and interstitial lymphoid aggregates were evaluated. Each of these histologic features was graded on a scale from 0 to 3 with Grade 0 = absent, Grade 1 = mild, Grade 2 = moderate, and Grade 3 = marked.

These histopathologic data were supplemented by the results of BAL, cultures for bacterial, fungal, and mycobacterial organisms, and clinical assessment of the functional status of the patient including physical examination, chest x-ray, arterial blood gases, and pulmonary function studies.

RESULTS AND DISCUSSION

Diagnostic Sensitivity of Transbronchial Biopsy and Bronchoalveolar Lavage

TBB and BAL had the greatest sensitivity in diagnosis of infection (95%), whereas sensitivities for TBB and BAL alone were 86% and 84% respectively. The sensitivity for TBB and BAL in the diagnosis of PCP was 98%. The most common pulmonary abnormalities were PCP followed by nonspecific interstitial pneumonitis, KS, CMV infection, bacterial pneumonia (i.e., *Legionella pneumophilia*), *Cryptococcus,* and malignant lymphoma (Table 2).

In 29 cases, TBB failed to reveal a pathogen. The diagnosis was established by BAL in 15 cases (PCP-13, *Cryptococcus*-1, MAI-1), open lung biopsy in 10 cases (KS-8, PCP-1, MAI-1), and needle aspiration biopsy in one case (lymphoma). Conversely, in 21 episodes of pneumonitis, a specific etiologic agent was not detected by BAL. The organisms not recovered by BAL were found by TBB (CMV-7, PCP-5, Cryptococcosis-1) or open lung biopsy (CMV-3, PCP-1, and MAI-1).

Open Lung Biopsy

Open lung biopsy revealed a diagnosis that had not been detected by TBB in 12 of 18 patients (70%). The added information included: KS (8 cases), infection with CMV (2 cases), and MAI (1 case). Both caseating and noncaseating granulomas were seen in the open lung biopsy that cultured MAI, however, organisms could not be identified histologically in the lung tissue. In two cases, the open lung biopsy revealed CMV in addition to PCP, which had been previously detected on TBB. In eight cases, an open lung biopsy was performed without previous TBB and the following diagnoses were made: NIP (3 cases), KS (3 cases) *Legionella* pneumonia (1 case; also showed KS), and CMV pneumonitis (2 cases). In six cases, the open lung biopsy did not reveal any additional cause for pneumonitis that had not already been found by TBB and BAL: PCP (2 cases) and NIP (4 cases). TBB in combination with BAL detected all cases of PCP in this study except for one where a subsequent open lung biopsy revealed both PCP and CMV.

Transbronchial Biopsy and Clinical Correlations

There is recent evidence that TBB may provide important prognostic information when the severity of PCP is graded.[190] The severity of interstitial edema provides prognostic information in patients with PCP, according to a previous study from the NIH.[190] In this study, decreased long-term survival correlated with severity of interstitial edema on initial TBB (p < 0.05), elevation of alveolar arterial oxygen gradient at the time of diagnosis (p < 0.05), and the persistence of *Pneumocystis* cysts after 3 weeks of therapy (p < 0.05).[190] In addition, longer periods of treatment were required to clear organisms from patients with greater numbers of *Pneumocystis* organisms on initial biopsy.

An attempt to correlate histologic and clinical response to therapy for PCP showed that the histologic response following therapy in AIDS patients differs from that of patients without AIDS.[193] AIDS patients do not clear the *Pneumocystis* cysts or the cellular infiltrate or alveolar exudate as rapidly as patients without AIDS.[193]

Unusual Histology of Pneumocystis Carinii Pneumonia

In one patient we observed an extensive lymphocytic interstitial infiltrate associated with PCP (Fig. 1). This feature was so striking that the diagnosis of PCP was not considered after initial review of an open lung biopsy performed at another hospital, and the patient was referred to the NIH with a diagnosis of a primary interstitial lung disease. Since this was the presenting manifestation of transfusion-acquired AIDS, and the patient was not in any of the known high-risk groups, an opportunistic infection was not considered. *Pneumocystis* cysts were discovered during review of the BAL specimen and the diagnosis was confirmed retrospectively by review of the open lung biopsy with special stains. This case illustrates the importance of considering pulmonary complications of AIDS in the differential diagnosis in patients who appear to have interstitial lung disease.

Nonspecific Interstitial Pneumonitis

Nonspecific interstitial pneumonitis (NIP) was observed in 32% of all episodes of pneumonitis among our series of 174 AIDS patients (Table 2).[195] This diagnosis was made when morphologic evaluation and/or cultures of lung biopsies and BAL did not reveal any specific cause for pneumonitis to account for the patient's episode of respiratory dysfunction. In approximately two thirds of these cases, it was found in association with extrapulmonary KS, experimental therapies, or post-PCP.[195] NIP in the absence of any other detectable cause occurred in 13% of the overall group of AIDS patients.[195] More details about the clinical and radiographic features of AIDS patients with NIP from the NIH have been reported elsewhere.[194,195]

As the name implies, the histology of lung biopsies from these patients is nonspecific and shows features of DAD or interstitial lymphocytic infiltration. The most common histologic feature in this group was interstitial chronic inflammation (77%), followed by alveolar macrophage accumulation (69%), interstitial edema (46%), hemorrhage (31%), and hyaline membranes (15%). The diagnosis is basically one of exclusion, after ruling out the presence of infectious organisms on BAL or biopsy sections.

The pathologic features of the biopsies showing NIP could be categorized into acute and chronic forms: (1) acute: varying degrees of diffuse alveolar damage (Fig. 5); and (2) chronic: mild to moderate patchy chronic inflammatory interstitial infiltrates (Fig. 6). The extent of lymphocytic infiltration in the latter group (Fig. 6) was considerably less than that reported in cases of LIP associated with HIV infection (Fig. 4). Of 13 cases of NIP without any detectable cause, seven (54%) fit into the former category (DAD) and the remaining six (46%) were characterized primarily by interstitial chronic inflammation. Three of the patients in this latter category had autopsies that revealed pulmonary KS in two cases and pneumonia due to CMV and *Candida* in another case.

The relationship between the chronic form of NIP, LIP, and the inflammatory variant of KS is uncertain; however, in some cases the distinction can be difficult. The lymphoid interstitial infiltrate in LIP is much more striking than that usually seen in cases of chronic NIP, however, in several cases the infiltrate was significant enough that LIP was considered. Although some of these cases may represent mild forms of LIP, it may not be possible to resolve this question, since we do not have any specific method to characterize the lymphoid infiltrate in LIP. The significance of the chronic inflammatory interstitial infiltrates seen in the inflammatory variant of KS is not entirely clear for reasons discussed below.

The etiology of NIP in AIDS patients is not known. It is possible that it is caused by an underlying viral infection, such as EBV where viral inclusions are not recognizable by light microscopy. Chronic forms of NIP could represent early manifestations of immune dysfunction similar to the lymphoid abnormalities seen in other organs in AIDS patients or the lymphocytic pulmonary disorders seen in a variety of immunologic conditions.[196-198] Rather than having a single cause, it is likely that the pathogenesis of NIP involves a variety of mechanisms. Perhaps studies using in situ hybridization for viral DNA on pulmonary biopsies will be helpful. Preliminary in situ hybridization studies in ten patients from our institution have failed to show the HIV genome in lung biopsy specimens with NIP.*

Kaposi's Sarcoma and Malignant Lymphoma

Kaposi's sarcoma (KS) involving the parenchyma was identified by TBB in three patients and by open lung biopsy in ten others. The diagnosis of KS was made only when characteristic spindle cells with extravasated red blood cells were seen in areas free of crush artifact, which may give the spurious impression of vascular prolifera-

tion (Fig. 7).[163a,169a] There was often deposition of hemosiderin. Recognition of hypercellular areas around bronchioles and blood vessel walls was helpful in making a diagnosis of KS. A nonspecific interstitial infiltrate was found in the lung parenchyma adjacent to the KS lesions in eight of the ten open lung biopsies.

Our study confirms previous reports that pulmonary KS is frequently associated with lymphoplasmacytic interstitial infiltrates.[160,168] Although it is possible that these lesions are related, our experience suggests that these chronic inflammatory interstitial infiltrates may not necessarily represent an early manifestation of KS. We have seen similar lesions in patients in whom KS was not identified even with follow-up. For this reason, we question the specificity of these infiltrates for KS. As a result, we prefer not to use the term "inflammatory KS"and refer to these infiltrates as interstitial pneumonitis associated with KS.

When chronic inflammatory interstitial infiltrates are seen in lung biopsies, a careful search should be performed for the characteristic spindle-shaped cells of KS. If the spindle-cell infiltrate of KS is identified, a definitive rather than a tentative diagnosis of KS can be established. If the spindle-cell infiltrate of KS is not present, but pulmonary KS is strongly suspected on clinical grounds, we agree that this lesion may be regarded as suspicious for KS.[168] If, however, there is no clinical suspicion for KS and diagnostic KS lesions are not present, the authors believe that chronic NIP should be considered.

One patient with malignant lymphoma had disease restricted to the lung with no evidence of extrapulmonary involvement. The diagnosis was made by needle aspiration cytology (Fig. 8). The tumor was considered high grade with features of a large cell lymphoma. Immunohistochemical staining of the malignant lymphoid cells revealed positive staining for B-cell markers and monotypic staining for the λ-IgG light chains.

---

*Koenig and associates. Unpublished observations.

Although malignant lymphomas are known to be associated with AIDS, and involve the lung in up to 10% of cases, it is not known how many of these present with primary involvement in the lung.[182] The detection of pulmonary lymphoma by fine needle aspiration cytology in the single case from our series illustrates the use of a diagnostic tool rarely used in the approach to pulmonary complications of AIDS.[17] Diagnosis of pulmonary lymphomas by needle aspiration cytology can be difficult if the lymphoma is well differentiated; however, if the lymphoma is of high grade, as in the case reported herein, the diagnosis can be made with confidence.[199,200]

CLINICAL ASPECTS OF THE EVALUATION OF PULMONARY DISEASE IN AIDS PATIENTS

The evaluation of an AIDS patient with pulmonary symptomatology or an abnormal chest roentgenogram requires an understanding of the broad spectrum of pulmonary pathogens and noninfectious pulmonary processes that these patients develop. In general, we feel that an aggressive diagnostic approach towards the pulmonary disease in these patients is warranted. Data have emerged that indicate early detection and therapy of some infectious processes, (*i.e.,* PCP) are likely to improve survival.[190] Patients may present with pulmonary symptoms that are usually cough, dyspenea upon exertion, or sputum production, and/ or they may have an abnormal chest roentgenogram.

Patients with a history of a productive cough or sputum production should have their sputum analyzed by both Gram stain and by routine bacterial and fungal cultures. Patients with pulmonary symptoms such as cough or shortness of breath with or without an abnormal X-ray should be considered for the other more common pulmonary pathogenic processes in AIDS patients. It is im-

portant to realize that up to 5% of AIDS patients with pulmonary symptoms and a normal chest roentgenogram at presentation can still have PCP.[191] The initial workup in these patients should include the use of an ultrasonic nebulizer to inhale 3% saline in an attempt to induce sputum. The material induced by this technique is stained, conventionally with toluidine blue, and experimentally, using monoclonal antibodies[34] in an attempt to identify *Pneumocystis carinii* organisms. Using the sputum induction technique, 50% or more of patients with PCP can be diagnosed in this noninvasive manner without requiring a bronchoscopic procedure.[44] If a sputum induction is negative for *Pneumocystis,* however, then a bronchoscopy is indicated to complete the diagnostic work-up. The bronchoscopic procedure should be thorough and include an anatomic examination to rule out endobronchial abnormalities, a BAL of a bronchial subsegment, and in certain circumstances, multiple TBB done under fluoroscopic guidance. BAL as a diagnostic technique is very sensitive for the diagnosis of PCP, and in most series, sensitivity ranges from 90–100%.[10,12,201] It has been suggested by some clinicians that BAL should be the only technique used to diagnose PCP in a patient with AIDS. Lavage is not as sensitive in identifying other pathogens, however, and the clinician must rely on other diagnostic tools. For example, the presence of CMV or MAI in cultures of BAL fluid is difficult to interpret, in the absence of histologic evidence of either viral or mycobacterial disease.

If the bronchoscopic procedure reveals a pathogen, then therapy should be initiated against that specific pathogen. In a situation where both BAL and TBB are negative, then the patient is either observed or considered for a second diagnostic procedure. A second diagnostic procedure is indicated, especially in a situation where a patient has progressive clinical deterioration such as progressive hypoxemia or deterioration of an already abnormal chest X-ray.The second procedure may either be a repeat bronchoscopy or an open lung biopsy.

The open lung biopsy technique, as a method of diagnosis in AIDS patients is controversial.[8,192,202,203] Its use is currently limited and recommended by most clinicians only under particular circumstances such as: (1) progressive pulmonary dysfunction, and (2) negative BAL in a patient precluded from TBB because of either coagulopathy or refractory hypoxia. In the latter situation, an open lung biopsy is clearly a safer procedure. Controversy still exists as to whether or not an open lung biopsy should be considered in patients for whom a pathogen has been identified by bronchoscopy, but who becomes progressively symptomatic despite therapy. In this situation many have questioned whether an open lung biopsy should be considered in the hope of finding a second, hopefully treatable, process. There are some data suggesting that an open lung biopsy rarely demonstrates a second treatable pathologic process in patients failing to respond to monospecific therapy.[202]

SPECIAL TECHNIQUES IN DIAGNOSIS OF PULMONARY COMPLICATIONS OF AIDS

The AIDS epidemic has provided a tremendous stimulus for the development of new techniques such as in situ hybridization and both monoclonal and polyclonal antibodies for the diagnosis of infectious and neoplastic diseases. The development of monoclonal antibodies for detecting infectious organisms such as cytomegalovirus,[204-208] herpes simplex,[209] and *Pneumocystis carinii*[34,35] may facilitate diagnosis of opportunistic pulmonary infections in AIDS patients. Immunohistochemical techniques have also been developed for the diagnosis of histoplasmosis[123] and aspergillosis.[210] Monoclonal antibodies to *Toxoplasma gondii* have been shown to be useful in the diagnosis of cerebral toxoplasmosis.[211]

Hopefully, this technique can be applied to lung specimens and enhance detection of pulmonary toxoplasmosis.

In situ hybridization has proven to be most useful in detecting viral DNA within infected cells, in tissue sections, when nuclear and/or cytoplasmic inclusions may be difficult or impossible to observe by light microscopy.[212-217] This technique has proven helpful in identifying HIV and other viruses such as CMV and adenovirus in fixed tissue sections.[215-217] Interpretation of in situ hybridization can be difficult, especially in lung biopsy specimens, because of artifactual positive staining.

Several studies have suggested a role for in situ hybridization in the diagnosis of CMV pneumonitis using both tissue biopsy sections and BAL specimens.[215,218-220] It remains to be proven, however, whether detecting CMV pulmonary infection by this method provides any clinically significant additional information compared to other methods.

Another potentially useful method for detecting viral infections involves the isolation of DNA from the paraffin-embedded tissues followed by dot hybridization.[214] Although this method may be simpler to perform and interpret, it needs to be compared more thoroughly with the in situ hybridization technique.

As new methods are developed for detection of the opportunistic infections in AIDS patients, they need to be critically evaluated to determine whether they provide additional clinically relevant information. It is hoped, nevertheless, that these new techniques will lead to more sensitive and specific ways to diagnose pulmonary complications of AIDS.

ACKNOWLEDGEMENTS

The authors gratefully acknowledge Dr. Antonio Perez for providing the case illustrated in Figure 4, and Mr. Larry Ostby for assistance with photography.

REFERENCES

1. Moskowitz L, Hensley GT, Chan JC, Adams K: Immediate causes of death in acquired immunodeficiency syndrome. Arch Pathol Lab Med 1985; 109:735–738

2. Bronnimann DA, Adam RD, Galgiani JN, et al: Coccidioidomycosis in the acquired immunodeficiency syndrome. Ann Intern Med 1987; 106:372–379

3. Wheat LJ, Small CB: Disseminated histoplasmosis in the acquired immunodeficiency syndrome. Arch Intern Med 1984; 144:2147.–2149

4. Maayan S, Wormser GP, Widerhorn J, et al: Strongyloides stercoralis hyperinfection in a patient with the acquired immune deficiency syndrome. Am J Med 1987; 83:945–948

5. Broaddus C, Dake MD, Stulbarg MS, et al: Bronchoalveolar lavage and transbronchial biopsy for the diagnosis of pulmonary infections in the acquired immunodeficiency syndrome. Ann Intern Med 1985; 102:747–752

6. Gal AA, Klatt EC, Koss MN, et al: The effectiveness of bronchoscopy in the diagnosis of *Pneumocystis carinii* and cytomegalovirus pulmonary infections in acquired immunodeficiency syndrome. Arch Pathol Lab Med 1987; 111:238–241

7. Hartman B, Koss M, Hui A, et al: *Pneumocystis carinii* pneumonia in the acquired immunodeficiency syndrome (AIDS). Diagnosis with bronchial brushings, biopsy, and bronchoalveolar lavage. Chest 1985; 87:603–607

8. McKenna RJ, Campbell A, McMurtrey MJ, Mountain CF: Diagnosis for interstitial lung disease in patients with acquired immunodeficiency syndrome (AIDS): a prospective comparison of bronchial washing, alveolar lavage, transbronchial biopsy, and open-lung biopsy. Ann Thorac Surg 1986; 41:318–321

9. Murray JF, Felton CP, Garay SM, et al: Pulmonary complications of the acquired immunodeficiency syndrome, report of a National Heart, Lung, and Blood Institute Workshop. N Engl J Med 1984; 310:1682–1688

10. Ognibene FP, Shelhamer JH, Gil VJ, et al: The diagnosis of *Pneumocystis carinii* pneumonia in patients with the acquired immunodeficiency syndrome using subsegmental bronchoalveolar lavage. Am Rev Resp Dis 1984; 129:929–932

11. Rorat E, Garcia RL, Skolom J: Diagnosis of *Pneumocystis carinii* pneumonia by cytologic examination of bronchial washings. JAMA 1985; 254:1950–1951

12. Stover DE, White DA, Romano PA, Gellene RA: Diagnosis of pulmonary disease in acquired immune deficiency syndrome (AIDS): Role of bronchoscopy and bronchoalveolar lavage. Am Rev Respir Dis 1984; 130:659–662

13. Stover DE, White DA, Romano PA, et al: Spectrum of pulmonary diseases associated with the acquired immune deficiency syndrome. Am J Med 1985; 78:429–437

14. Williams D, Yungbluth M, Adams G, Glassroth J: The role of fiberoptic bronchoscopy in the evaluation of immunocompromised hosts with diffuse pulmonary infiltrates. Am Rev Resp Dis 1985; 131:880–885

15. Wollschlager CM, Khan FA, Chitkara RK, Shivaram U: Pulmonary manifestations of the acquired immunodeficiency syndrome (AIDS). Chest 1984; 85:197–202

16. Caughey G, Wong H, Gamsu G, Golden J: Nonbronchoscopic bronchoalveolar lavage for the diagnosis of *Pneumocystis carinii* pneumonia in the acquired immunodeficiency syndrome. Chest 1985; 88:659–662

17. Wallace JM, Batra P, Gong H, Ovenfors CO: Percutaneous needle aspiration for diagnosing pneumonitis in the patient with acquired immunodeficiency syndrome (AIDS). Am Rev Respir Dis 1985; 131:389–392

18. Gottlieb MS, Schroff R, Schanker HM, et al: *Pneumocystis carinii* pneumonia and mucosal candidiasis in previously healthy homosexual men. Evidence of a new acquired cellular immunodeficiency. N Engl J Med 1981; 305:1425–1431

19. Masur H, Michelis MA, Greene JB, et al: An outbreak of community-acquired *Pneumocystis carinii* pneumonia. Initial manifestation of cellular immune dysfunction. N Engl J Med 1981; 305:1431–1438

20. Centers for Disease Control: Update on acquired immune deficiency syndrome (AIDS)—United States: MMWR 1982; 31:507–514

21. Centers for Disease Control: Revision of the case definition of acquired immunodeficiency syndrome for national reporting—United States. MMWR 1985; 34:373–375

22. Centers for Disease Control: Revision of the CDC surveillance case definition for acquired immunodeficiency syndrome. MMWR (Supplement) 1987; 36:1S–15S

23. Barrio JL, Suarez M, Rodriguez JL, et al: *Pneumocystis carinii* pneumonia presenting as cavitating and noncavitating solitary pulmonary nodules in patients with the acquired immunodeficiency syndrome. Am Rev Respir Dis 1986; 134:1094–1096

24. Milligan SA, Stulbarg MS, Gamsu G, Golden JA: *Pneumocystis carinii* pneumonia radiographically simulating tuberculosis. Am Rev Resp Dis 1985; 132:1124–1126

25. Coulman CU, Greene I, Archibald RWR: Cutaneous pneumocystosis. Ann Intern Med 1987; 106:396–398

26. Unger PD, Rosenblum M, Krown SE: Disseminated *Pneumocystis carinii* infection in a patient with acquired immunodeficiency syndrome. Hum Pathol 1988; 19:113–116

27. Kwok S, O'Donnell J, Wood IS: Retinal cotton-wool spots in a patient with *Pneumocystis carinii* infection (Letter). N Engl J Med 1982; 307:184–185

28. Schinella RA, Breda SD, Hammerschlag PE: Otic infection due to *Pneumocystis carinii* in an apparently healthy man with antibody to the human immunodeficiency virus. Ann Intern Med 1987; 106:399–400

29. Young LS: *Pneumocystis carinii* Pneumonia; Pathogenesis, Diagnosis, Treatment. Lung Biology in Health and Disease, Vol 22, New York, Marcel Dekker, Inc, 1984

30. Domingo J, Waksal HW: Wright's stain in rapid diagnosis of *Pneumocystis carinii*. Am J Clin Pathol 1984; 81:511–514

31. Mones JM, Saldana MJ, Oldham SA: Diagnosis of *Pneumocystis carinii* pneumonia. Roentgeno-graphic-pathologic correlates based on fiberoptic bronchoscopy specimens from patients with the acquired immunodeficiency syndrome. Chest 1986; 89:522–526

32. Shimono LH, Hartman B: A simple and reliable rapid methenamine silver stain for *Pneumocystis carinii* and fungi. Arch Pathol Lab Med 1986; 110:855–856

33. Ghali VS, Garcia RL, Skolom J: Fluorescence of *Pneumocystis carinii* in Papanicolaou smears. Hum Pathol 1984; 15:907–909

34. Kovacs JA, Ng VL, Masur H, et al: Diagnosis of *Pneumocystis carinii* pneumonia: Improved detection in sputum with use of monoclonal antibodies. N Engl J Med 1988; 318:589–593

35. Linder E, Lundin L, Vorma H: Detection of *Pneumocystis carinii* in lung-derived samples using monoclonal antibodies to an 82 kDa parasite component. J Immunol Meth 1987; 98:57–62

36. Case Records of the Massachusetts General Hospital, Case 8-1987, N Engl J Med 1987; 316:466–475

37. Dutz W: *Pneumocystis carinii* pneumonia. Pathol Annu 1970; 5:309–341

38. Askin FB, Katzenstein ALA: *Pneumocystis* infection masquerading as diffuse alveolar damage: A potential source of diagnostic error. Chest 1981; 79:420–422

39. Weber WR, Askin FB, Dehner LP: Lung biopsy in *Pneumocystis carinii* pneumonia. A histopathologic study of typical and atypical features. Am J Clin Pathol 67:11–19

40. Gagliardi AJ, Stover DE, Zaman MK: Endobronchial *Pneumocystis carinii* infection in a patient with the acquired immune deficiency syndrome. Chest, 1987; 911:463–464

41. Hartz JW, Geisinger KR, Scharyji, Muss HB: Granulomatous pneumocystosis presenting as a solitary pulmonary nodule. Arch Pathol Lab Med 1985; 109:466–469

42. Ruben FL, Talamo TS: Secondary pulmonary alveolar proteinosis occurring in two patients with acquired immune deficiency syndrome. Am J Med 1986; 80:1187–1190

43. Watts JC, Chandler FW: *Pneumocystis carinii* pneumonitis. The nature and diagnostic significance of the methenamine silver-positive "intracystic bodies". Am J Surg Pathol 1985; 9:744–751

44. Bigby TD, Margolskee D, Curtis JL, et al: The usefulness of induced sputum in the diagnosis of *Pneumocystis carinii* pneumonia in patients with the acquired immunodeficiency syndrome. Am Rev Respir Dis 1986; 133:515–518

45. Pitchenik AE, Ganjei P, Torres A, et al: Sputum examination for the diagnosis of *Pneumocystis carinii* pneumonia in the acquired immunodeficiency syndrome. Am Rev Respir Dis 1986; 133:226–229

45a. Zaman MK, Wooten OJ, Suprahmanya B, et al: Rapid noninvasive diagnosis of *Pneumocystis carinii* from induced liquified sputum. Ann Intern Med 1988; 109:7–10

46. Schwartz DA, Munger RG, Katz SM: Plastic embedding evaluation of *Pneumocystis carinii* pneumonia in AIDS. Simultaneous demonstration of cyst and sporozoite forms. Am J Surg Pathol 1987; 11:304–309

47. Haque AU, Plattner SB, Cook RT, Hart MN: *Pneumocystis carinii*, taxonomy as viewed by electron microscopy. Am J Clin Pathol 1987; 87:504–510

48. Schulman LL: Cytomegalovirus pneumonitis and lobar consolidation. Chest 1987; 91:558–561

49. Mobley K, Rotterdam HZ, Lerner CW, Tapper ML: Autopsy findings in the acquired immune deficiency syndrome. Pathol Annu 1985; 20, 1:45–65

50. Reichert CM, O'Leary TJ, Levens DL, et al: Autopsy pathology in the acquired immune deficiency syndrome. Am J Pathol 1983; 112:357–382

51. Wallace JM, Hannah J: Cytomegalovirus pneumonitis in patients with AIDS; Findings in an autopsy series. Chest 1987; 92:198–203

51a. Klatt EC, Shibata D: Cytomegalovirus infection in the acquired immunodeficiency syndrome. Clinical and autopsy findings. Arch Pathol Lab Med 1988; 112:540–544

52. Strano AJ: Light microscopy of selected viral diseases (Morphology of viral inclusion bodies). Pathol Annu 1976; 11:53–75

53. Gorelkin L, Chandler FW, Ewing EP: Staining qualities of cytomegalovirus inclusions in the lungs of patients with the acquired immunodeficiency syndrome: A potential source of diagnostic misinterpretation. Hum Pathol 1986; 17:926–929

54. Brodie HR, Broaddus C, Hopewell PC, et al: Is cytomegalovirus (CMV) a cause of lung disease in patients with AIDS? (Abstract) Chest 1985; 131:A227

55. Guarda LA, Luna MA, Smith JL, et al: Acquired immune deficiency syndrome: postmortem findings. Am J Clin Pathol 1984; 81:549–557

56. Niedt GW, Schinella RA: Acquired immunodeficiency syndrome, clinicopathologic study of 56 autopsies. Arch Pathol Lab Med 1985; 109:727–734

57. Welch K, Finkbeiner W, Alpers CE, et al: Autopsy findings in the acquired immunodeficiency syndrome. JAMA 1984; 252:1152–1159

58. Myerson D, Hackman RC, Nelson JA, et al: Widespread presence of histologically occult cytomegalovirus. Hum Pathol 1984; 15:430–439

59. Amberson JB, DiCarlo EF, Metroka CE, et al: Diagnostic pathology in the acquired immunodeficiency syndrome. Surgical pathology and cytology experience with 67 patients. Arch Pathol Lab Med 1985; 109:345–351

60. Quinnan GV, Masur H, Rook AH, et al: Herpesvirus infections in the acquired immune deficiency syndrome. JAMA 1984; 252:72–77

61. Krasinski K, Borkowsky W, Chandwani S, et al: Measles in HIV-infected children, United States. JAMA 1988; 259:2352–2357

62. Chayt KJ, Harper ME, Marselle LM, et al: Detection of HTLV-III RNA in lungs of patients with AIDS and pulmonary involvement. JAMA 1986;256:2356–2359

63. Resnick L, Pitchenik AE, Fisher E, Croney R: Detection of HTLV-III/LAV-specific IgG and antigen in bronchoalveolar lavage fluid from two patients with lymphocytic interstitial pneumonitis associated with AIDS-related complex. Am J Med 1987; 82:553–556

64. Fackler JC, Nagel JE, Adler WH, et al: Epstein-Barr virus infection in a child with acquired immunodeficiency syndrome. AJDC 1985; 139:1000–1004

65. Grieco MH, Chinoy-Acharya P: Lymphocytic interstitial pneumonia associated with the acquired immune deficiency syndrome. Am Rev Resp Dis 1985; 131:952–955

66. Joshi VV, Oleske JM: Pulmonary lesions in children with the acquired immunodeficiency syndrome: A reappraisal based on data in additional cases and follow-up study of previously reported cases. Hum Pathol 1986; 17:641–642

67. Rubenstein A, Morecki R, Silverman B, et al: Pulmonary disease in children with acquired immune deficiency syndrome and AIDS-related complex. J Pediatr 1986; 108:498–503

68. Ziza JM, Brun-Vezinet F, Venet A, et al: Lymphadenopathy-associated virus isolated from bronchoalveolar lavage fluid in AIDS-related complex with lymphoid interstitial pneumonitis (Letter). N Engl J Med 1985; 313:183

69. Beissner RS, Rappaport ES, Diaz JA: Fatal case of Epstein-Barr virus-induced lymphoproliferative disorder associated with a human immunodeficiency virus infection. Arch Pathol Lab Med 1987; 111:250–253

70. Case Records of the Massachusetts General Hospital, Case 9-1986. N Engl J Med 1986; 314:629–640

71. Joshi VV, Kauffman S, Oleske JM, et al: Polyclonal polymorphic B-cell lymphoproliferative disorder with prominent pulmonary involvement in children with acquired immune deficiency syndrome. Cancer 1987; 59:1455–1462

72. Zakowski P, Fligiel S, Berlin GW, Johnson BL: Disseminated *Mycobacterium avium-intracellulare* infection in homosexual men dying of acquired immunodeficiency. JAMA 1982; 248:2980–2982

73. Hawkins CC, Gold JWM, Whimbey E, et al: *Mycobacterium avium* complex infections in patients with the acquired immunodeficiency syndrome. Ann Intern Med 1986; 105:184–188

74. Klatt EC, Jensen DF, Meyer PR: Pathology of *Mycobacterium avium intraceullare* infection in acquired immunodeficiency syndrome. Hum Pathol 1987; 18:709–714

75. Chaisson RE, Schecter GF, Theuer CP, et al: Tuberculosis in patients with the acquired immunodeficiency syndrome. Clinical features, response to therapy, and survival. Am Rev Resp Dis 1987; 136:570–574

76. Louie E, Rice LB, Holzman RS: Tuberculosis in non-Haitian patients with acquired immunodeficiency syndrome. Chest 1986; 90:542–545

77. Centers for Disease Control: Diagnosis and management of mycobacterial infection and disease in persons with human immunodefeiciency virus infection. Ann Intern Med 1987; 106:254–256

78. Murray JF, Garay SM, Hopewell PC, et al: Pulmonary complications of the acquired immunodeficiency syndrome: An update. Am Rev Resp Dis 1987; 135:504–509

79. Stoneburner RL, Ruiz MM, Milberg JA, et al: Tuberculosis and acquired immunodeficiency syndrome—New York City. JAMA 1988; 259:338–345

80. Pitchenik AE, Cole C, Russell BW, et al: Tuberculosis, atypical mycobacteriosis, and the acquired immunodeficiency syndrome among Haitian and non-Haitian patients in south Florida. Ann Intern Med 1984; 101:641–645

81. Pitchenik AE, Rubinson HA: The radiographic appearance of tuberculosis in patients with the acquired immunodeficiency syndrome (AIDS) and pre-AIDS. Am Rev Respir Dis 1985; 131:393–396

82. Sunderam G, McDonald RJ, Maniatis T, et al: Tuberculosis as a manifestation of the acquired immunodeficiency syndrome (AIDS). JAMA 1986; 256:362–366

83. Handwerger S, Mildvan D, Senie R, McKinley FW: Tuberculosis and the acquired immunodeficiency syndrome at a New York City Hospital: 1978–1985. Chest 1987; 91:176–180

84. Syabbalo NC: Pulmonary tuberculosis and acquired immunodeficiency syndrome (Letter). Chest 1987; 92:383–384

85. Shelhamer JH, Ognibene FP, Kovacs J, et al: *Pneumocystis carinii* and *Mycobacterium avium* infections in AIDS patients. Ann N Y Acad Sci 1984; 437:394–399

86. Chester AC, Winn WC: Unusual and newly recognized patterns of nontuberculous mycobacterial infection with emphasis on immunocompromised host. Pathol Annu 1986; 21:251–270

87. Polis MA, Tuazon CU: Clues to the early diagnosis of *Mycobacterium avium-intracellulare* infection in patients with acquired immunodeficiency syndrome. Arch Pathol Lab Med 1985; 109:465–466

88. Sohn CC, Schroff RW, Kliewer KE, et al: Disseminated *Mycobacterium avium-intracellulare* infection in homosexual men with acquired cell-mediated immunodeficiency: A histologic and immunologic study of two cases. Am J Clin Pathol 1983; 79:247–252

89. Urmacher C, Nielsen S: The histopathology of the acquired immune deficiency syndrome. Pathol Annu 1985; 20 1:197–220

90. Polsky B, Gold JWM, Whimbey E, et al: Bacterial pneumonia in patients with the acquired im-

munodeficiency syndrome. Ann Intern Med 1986; 104:38–41

91. Witt DJ, Craven DE, McCabe WR: Bacterial infections in adult patients with the acquired immune deficiency syndrome (AIDS) and AIDS-related complex. Am J Med 1987; 82:900–906

92. Holtz H, Lavery D, Kapila R: Actinomycetales infection in the acquired immunodeficiency syndrome. Ann Intern Med 1985; 102:203–205

93. Rodriguez JL, Barrio JL, Pitchenik AE: Pulmonary nocardiosis in the acquired immunodeficiency syndrome. Chest 1986; 90:912–914

94. Lane HC, Masur H, Edgar LC, et al: Abnormalities of B-cell activation and immunoregulation in patients with the acquired immunodeficiency syndrome. N Engl J Med 1983; 309:453–458

95. Ammann AJ, Schiffman G, Abrams D, et al: B-cell immunodeficiency in acquired immune deficiency syndrome. JAMA 1984; 251:1447–1449

96. Saimies JH, Hathaway BN, Echols RM, et al: Lung abscess due to Corynebacterium equi. Report of the first case in a patient with acquired immune deficiency syndrome. Am J Med 1986; 80:685–688

96a. Weingarten JS, Huang DY, Jackman JD: *Rhodococcus equi* pneumonia. Chest 1988; 94:195–196

97. Holmberg K, Meyer RD: Fungal infections in patients with AIDS and AIDS-related complex. Scand J Infect Dis 1986; 18:179–192

98. Nash G, Fligiel S: Pathologic features of the lung in the acquired immune deficiency syndrome (AIDS): An autopsy study of seventeen homosexual males. Am J Clin Pathol 1984; 81:6–12

99. Wheat LJ, Slama TG, Zeckel ML: Histoplasmosis in the acquired immune deficiency syndrome. Am J Med 1985; 78:203–210

100. Klein RS, Harris CA, Small CB, et al: Oral candidiasis in high-risk patients as the initial manifestation of acquired immunodeficiency syndrome. N Engl J Med 1984; 9:354–357

101. Murray HW, Hillman JK, Rubin BY, et al: Patients at risk for AIDS-related opportunistic infections. Clinical manifestations and impaired gamma interferon production. N Engl J Med 1985; 313:1504–1510

102. Eng RHK, Bishburg E, Smith SM, Kapila R: Cryptococcal infections in patients with acquired immune deficiency syndrome. Am J Med 1986; 81:19–23

103. Gal AA, Koss NM, Hawkins J, et al: The pathology of pulmonary crytococcal infections in the acquired immunodeficiency syndrome. Arch Pathol Lab Med 1986; 110:502–507

103a. Wasser L, Talavera W: Pulmonary cryptococcoccosis in AIDS. Chest 1987; 92:692–695

104. Karaffa CA, Rhem SJ, Keys TF: The acquired immunodeficiency syndrome and cryptococcosis (Letter). Ann Intern Med 1986; 104:891–892

105. Kovacs JA, Kovacs AA, Polis M, et al: Cryptococcosis in the acquired immunodeficiency syndrome. Ann Intern Med 1985; 103:533–538

106. Zuger A, Louie E, Holzman RS, et al: Cryptococcal disease in patients with the acquired immunodeficiency syndrome; diagnostic features and outcome of treatment. Ann Intern Med 1986; 104:234–240

107. Witt D, McKay D, Schwam L, et al: Acquired immune deficiency syndrome presenting as bone marrow and mediastinal cryptococcosis. Am J Med 1987; 82:149–150

108. Newman TG, Soni A, Acaron S, Huang CT: Pleural cryptococcosis in the acquired immune deficiency syndrome. Chest 1987; 91:459–461

109. McDonnell JM, Hutchins GM: Pulmonary cryptococcosis. Hum Pathol 1985; 16:121–128

110. Binford CH, Connor DH: Pathology of tropical and extraordinary diseases. Washington D.C., Armed Forces Institute of Pathology, 1976

111. Sarosi GA, Davies SF: Fungal Diseases of the Lung. Orlando, Grune & Stratton, Inc. 1986

112. Ro JY, Lee SS, Ayala AG: Advantage of Fontana-Masson stain in capsule-deficient cryptococcal infection. Arch Pathol Lab Med 1987; 111:53–57

113. Abrams DI, Robia M, Blumenfeld W, et al: Disseminated coccidioidomycosis in AIDS. N Engl J Med 1984; 310:986–987

114. Ampel NM, Ryan KJ, Carry PJ, et al: Fungemia due to *Coccidioides immitis;* an analysis of 16 episodes in 15 patients and a review of the literature. Medicine 1986; 65:312–321

115. Kovacs A, Forthal DN, Kovacs JA, Overturf GD: Disseminated coccidioidomycosis in a patient with acquired immune deeficiency syndrome. West J Med 1984; 140:447–449

116. Roberts CJ; Coccidioidomycosis in acquired immune deficiency syndrome; depressed humoral as well as cellular immunity. Am J Med 1984; 76:734–736

117. Bonner JR, Alexander J, Dismukes WE, et al: Disseminated histoplasmosis in patients with the acquired immune deficiency syndrome. Arch Intern Med 1984; 144:2178–2181

118. Johnson PC, Sarosi GA, Septimus EJ, Satterwhite TK: Progressive disseminated histoplasmosis in patients with the acquired immune deficiency syndrome: A report of 12 cases and a literature review. Sem Resp Infec 1986; 1:1–8

119. Taylor MN, Baddour LM, Alexander JR: Disseminated histoplasmosis associated with the acquired immune deficiency syndrome. Am J Med 1984; 77:579–580

120. Huang CT, McGarry T, Cooper S, et al: Disseminated histoplasmosis in the acquired immunodeficiency syndrome; report of five cases from a nonendemic area. Arch Intern Med 1987; 147:1181–1184

121. Wheat LJ, Kohler RB, Tewari RP: Diagnosis of disseminated histoplasmosis by detection of *Histoplasma capsulatum* antigen in serum and urine specimens. N Engl J Med 1986; 314:83–88

122. Marchevsky A, Rosen MJ, Chrystal G, Kleinerman J: Pulmonary complications of the acquired immunodeficiency syndrome: A clinico-

pathologic study of 70 cases. Hum Pathol 1985; 16:659–670

123. Klatt EC, Cosgrove M, Meyer PR: Rapid diagnosis of disseminated histoplasmosis in tissues. Arch Pathol Lab Med 1986; 110:1173–1175

124. Hui AN, Koss MN, Meyer PR: Necropsy findings in acquired immunodeficiency syndrome: A comparison of premortem diagnosis with postmortem findings. Hum Pathol 1984; 15:640–676

125. Macher A, Nelson A, DeVinatea M, et al: Disseminated infection by *Histoplasma dubosii* in an African patient with AIDS. (Abstr) Lab Invest 1988; 58:59A

126. Jones PG, Cohen RL, Batts DH, Silva J: Disseminated histoplasmosis, invasive pulmonary aspergillosis, and other opportunistic infections in a homosexual patient with acquired immune deficiency syndrome. Sex Trans Dis 1983; 10:202–204

127. Pervez NK, Kleinerman J, Kattan M, et al: Pseudomembranous necrotizing bronchial aspergillosis; a variant of invasive aspergillosis in a patient with hemophilia and acquired immune deficiency syndrome. Am Rev Resp Dis 1985; 131:961–963

128. Schaffner A: Acquired immune deficiency syndrome: Is disseminated aspergillosis predictive of underlying cellular immune deficiency? J Inf Dis 1984; 149:828–829

129. Brady EM, Margolis ML, Korzeniowski OM: Pulmonry cryptosporidiosis in acquired immune deficiency syndrome. JAMA 1984; 252:89–90

130. Forgacs P, Tashis A, Ma P, et al: Intestinal and bronchial cryptosporidiosis in an immunodeficient homosexual man. Ann Intern Med 1983; 99:793–794

131. Ma P, Villanueva TG, Kaufman D, Gillooley JF: Respiratory cryptosporidiosis in the acquired immune deficiency syndrome. Use of modified cold kinyoun and hemicolor stains for rapid diagnosis. JAMA 1984; 252:1298–1301

132. Catterall JR, Hofflin JM, Remington JS: Pulmonary toxoplasmosis. Am Rev Respir Dis 1986; 133:704–705

133. Tawney S, Masci J, Berger HW, Subietas A: Pulmonary toxoplasmosis: An unusual nodular radiographic pattern in a patient with AIDS. Mt Sinai J Med 1986; 53:683–685

134. Yermakov V, Rashid RK, Vuletin JC et al: Disseminated toxoplasmosis. Case report and review of the literature. Arch Pathol Lab Med 1982; 106:524–528

135. Joshi VV, Oleske JM, Minnefor AB, et al: Pathology of suspected acquired immune deficiency syndrome in children: a study of eight cases Ped Pathol 1984; 2:71–87

136. Joshi VV, Oleske JM, Minnefor AB, et al: Pathologic pulmonary findings in children with the acquired immunodeficiency syndrome: A study of ten cases. Hum Pathol 1985; 16:241–246

137. Scott GB, Buck BE, Leterman JG, et al: Acquired immunodeficiency syndrome in infants. N Engl J Med 1984; 310:76–81

138. Morris JC, Rosen MJ, Marchevsky A, Teirstein AS: Lymphocytic interstitial pneumonia in patients at risk for the acquired immune deficiency syndrome. Chest 1987; 91:63–67

139. Solal-Celigny P, Couderc LJ, et al: Lymphoid interstitial pneumonitis in acquired immunodeficiency syndrome-related complex. Am Rev Repir Dis 1985; 131:956–960

140. Wallace JM, Barbers RG, Oishi JS, Prince H: Cellular and T-lymphocyte subpopulation profiles in bronchoalveolar lavage fluid from patients with acquired immunodeficiency syndrome and pneumonitis. Am Rev Respir Dis 1984; 130:786–790

141. Lung ML, So SY, Chan KH, et al: Evidence that respiratory tract is major reservoir for Epstein-Barr virus. Lancet 1985; 1:889–892

142. Andiman WA, Martin K, Rubinstein A, et al: Opportunistic lymphoproliferations associated with Epstein-Barr viral DNA in infants and children with AIDS. Lancet 1985; 2:1390–1393

143. Hanto DW, Frizzera G, Gajl-Peczalska KJ, et al: Epstein-Barr virus-induced B-cell lymphoma after renal transplantation. Acyclovir therapy and transition from polyclonal to monoclonal B-cell proliferation. N Engl J Med 1982; 306:913–918

144. Ramaswamy G, Jagadha V, Tchertkoff V: Diffuse alveolar damage and interstitial fibrosis in acquired immunodeficiency syndrome patients without concurrent pulmonary infection. Arch Pathol Lab Med 1985; 109:408–412

145. Ettensohn DB, Mayer KH, Kessimian N, et al: Lymphocytic bronchiolitis associated with HIV infection. Chest 1988; 93:201–202

146. Bedrossian CWM, Kuhn C, Luna MA: Desquamative interstitial pneumonia-like reaction accompanying pulmonary lesions. Chest 1977; 72:166

147. Case Records of the Massachusetts General Hospital, Case 14-1984. N Engl J Med 1984; 310:906–916

148. Prakash UBS, Barham SS, Carpenter HA, et al: Pulmonary alveolar phospholipoproteinosis: Experience with 34 cases and a review. Mayo Clin Proc 1987; 62:499–518

149. Ranchod M, Bissell M: Pulmonary alveolar proteinosis and cytomegalovirus infection. Arch Pathol Lab Med 1979; 103:139–142

150. Steer A: Focal pulmonary alveolar proteinosis in pulmonary tuberculosis. Arch Pathol 1969; 87:347–352

151. Sunderland WA, Campbell RA, Edwards MD: Pulmonary alveolar proteinosis and pulmonary cryptococcosis in an adolescent boy. J Pediatr 1972; 80:450–456

152. Aymard J-P, Gyger M, Lavalee R, et al: A case of pulmonary alveolar proteinosis complicating chronic myelogenous leukemia; a peculiar pathologic aspect of busulfan lung? Cancer 1984; 53:954–956

153. Abrahams C, DeChristopher P, Williams W, Morales F: Unusual pulmonary manifestations in AIDS. (Abstract) Lab Invest 1987; 56:1

154. Hostettler C, Amundson D, O'Connor S: Phe-

nytoin hypersensitivity with pulmonary involvement in a hemophiliac patient with human immunodeficiency virus infection. Drug Intell Clin Pharm 1987; 21:875–876

154a. Lewis JH, Sundeen JT, Simon GL, et al: Disseminated talc granulomatosis. Arch Pathol Lab Med 1985; 109:147–150

155. Kim KK, Factor SM: Membranoproliferative glomerulonephritis and plexogenic pulmonary arteriopathy in a homosexual man with acquired immunodeficiency syndrome. Hum Pathol 1987; 18:1293–1296

156. Cohn DL, O'Brien RF, Arnall MF: Pleural pulmonary Kaposi's sarcoma in AIDS: Clinical, radiographic, and pathologic manifestations. (Abstract) Am Rev Resp Dis 1985; 131:A82

157. Zibrak JD, Costello P, Legg M, et al: Manifestations of Kaposi's sarcoma (KS) in the respiratory tract. (Abstract) Chest 1985; 88:49S

158. Garay S, Belenko M, Fazzini E, Schinella R: Pulmonary manifestations of Kaposi's sarcoma. Chest 1987; 91:39–43

159. Meduri GU, Stover DE, Lee M, et al: Pulmonary Kaposi's sarcoma in the acquired immunodeficiency syndrome, clinical, radiographic and pathologic manifestations. Am J Med 1986; 81:11–18

160. Moskowitz LB, Hensley GT, Gould EW, Weiss SD: Frequency and anatomic distribution of lymphadenopathic Kaposi's sarcoma in the acquired immunodeficiency syndrome: An autopsy series. Hum Pathol 1985; 16:447–456

160a. Dantzig PI, Richardson D, Rayhanzadeh S, et al: Thoracic involvement of non-African Kaposi's sarcoma. Chest 1974; 66:522–525

161. Hanno R, Owen LG, Callen JP: Kaposi's sarcoma with extensive silent internal involvement. Int J Dermatol 1979; 18:718–721

162. Misra DP, Sunderrajan EV, Hurst DJ, et al: Kaposi's sarcoma of the lung: Radiography and pathology. Thorax 1982; 37:155–156

163. Epstein DM, Gefter WB, Conrad K, et al: Lung disease in homosexual men. Radiology 1982; 143:7–10

163a. Ognibene FP, Steis RG, Macher AM, et al: Kaposi's sarcoma causing pulmonary infiltrates and respiratory failure in the acquired immunodeficiency syndrome. Ann Intern Med 1985; 102:471–475

164. Kornfeld H, Axelrod JL: Pulmonary presentation of Kaposi's sarcoma in a homosexual patient. Am Rev Resp Dis 1983; 127:248–249

165. Nash G, Fligiel S: Kaposi's sarcoma presenting as pulmonary disease in the acquired immunodeficiency syndrome: Diagnosis by lung biopsy. Hum Pathol 1984; 15:999–1001

166. Rucker L, Meador J: Kaposi's sarcoma presenting as homogeneous pulmonary infiltrates in a patient with acquired immunodeficiency syndrome. West J Med 1985; 142:831–833

167. Antman KH, Nadler L, Mark EJ, et al: Primary Kaposi's sarcoma of the lung in an immunocompetent 32-year-old heterosexual white man. Cancer 1984; 54:1696–1698

168. Purdy LJ, Colby TV, Yousem SA, Battifora H: Pulmonary Kaposi's sarcoma, premortem histologic diagnosis. Am J Surg Pathol 1986; 10:301–311

169. Hamm PG, Judson MA, Aranda CP: Diagnosis of pulmonary Kaposi's sarcoma with fiberoptic bronchoscopy and endobronchial biopsy, a report of five cases. Cancer 1987; 59:807–810

169a. Fouret PJ, Touboul JL, Mayaud CM, et al: Pulmonary Kaposi's sarcoma in patients with acquired immune deficiency syndrome: a clinicopathological study. Thorax 1987; 42:262–268

170. Lau K-Y, Av J, Rubin A, et al: Kaposi's sarcoma of the tracheobronchial tree. Chest 1986; 89:158–159

171. Pitchenik AE, Fischl MA, Saldana MJ: Kaposi's sarcoma of the tracheobronchial tree. Chest 1985; 87:122–124

171a. Kaplan LD, Hopewell PC, Jaffe H, et al: Kaposi's sarcoma involving the lung in patients with the acquired immunodeficiency syndrome. J Acquired Imm Def Syndr 1988; 1:23–30

172. Akhtar M, Bunuan H, Ali MA, Godwin JT: Kaposi's sarcoma in renal transplant recipients, ultrastructural and immunoperoxidase study of four cases. Cancer 1984; 53:258–266

173. Friedman-Kien AE, Laubenstein LJ, Rubinstein P, et al: Disseminated Kaposi's sarcoma in homosexual men. Radiology 1982; 96:693–700

174. Boldogh I, Beth E, Huang ES, et al: Kaposi's sarcoma. IV Detection of CMV DNA, CMV RNA, and CMNA in tumor biopsies. Int J Cancer 1981; 28:469–474

175. Drew WL, Conant MA, Miner RC, et al: Cytomegalovirus and Kaposi's sarcoma in young homosexual men. Lancet 1982; 2:125–127

176. Fenoglio CM, Oster MW, Gerfo PL, et al: Kaposi's sarcoma following chemotherapy for testicular cancer in a homosexual man: Demonstration of cytomegalovirus RNA in sarcoma cells. Hum Pathol 1982; 13:955–959

177. Giraldo G, Beth E, Huang ES: Kaposi's sarcoma and its relationship to cytomegalovirus (CMV). III CMV DNA and CMV early antigens in Kaposi's sarcoma. Int J Cancer 1980; 26:23–39

178. Siddiqui A: Hepatitis B virus DNA in Kaposi's sarcoma. Proc Natl Acad Sci USA 1983; 80:4861–4864

179. Delli Bovi P, Donti E, Knowles DM, et al: Presence of chromosomal abnormalities and lack of AIDS retrovirus DNA sequences in AIDS-associated Kaposi's sarcoma. Cancer Res 1986; 46:6333–6338

179a. Grody WW, Lewin KJ, Naeim F: Detection of cytomegalovirus DNA in classic and epidemic Kaposi's sarcoma by in situ hybridization. Hum Pathol 1988; 19:524–528

180. Bartal AH, Lichtig C, Friedman-Birnbaum R, et al: The interaction of Kaposi's sarcoma with monoclonal antibodies to human sarcoma and connective tissue differentiation antigens. Cancer 1985; 56:1071–1074

181. Guarda LG, Silva EG, Ordonez NG, Smith JL: Factor VIII in Kaposi's sarcoma. Am J Clin Pathol 1981; 76:197–200

182. DiCarlo EF, Amberson JB, Metroka CE, et al:

Malignant lymphomas and the acquired immunodeficiency syndrome. Evaluation of 30 cases using a working formulation. Arch Pathol Lab Med 1986; 110:1012–1016

183. Ziegler JL, Beckstead JA, Volberding PA, et al: Non-Hodgkin's lymphoma in 90 homosexual men, relation to generalized lymphadenopathy and the acquired immunodeficiency syndrome. N Engl J Med 1984; 311:565–70

183a. Lowenthal DA, Straus DJ, Campbell SW, et al: AIDS-related lymphoid neoplasia. The Memorial Hospital experience. Cancer 1988; 61: 2325–2337

184. Frizzera G, Hanto DW, Gajl-Peczalska KJ, et al: Polymorphic diffuse B-cell hyperplasias and lymphomas in renal transplant recipients. Cancer Res 1981; 41:4262–4279

185. Shearer WT, Ritz J, Finegold MJ, et al: Epstein-Barr virus-associated B-cell proliferations of diverse clonal origins after bone marrow transplantation in a 12-year-old patient with severe combined immunodeficiency. N Engl J Med 1985; 312:1151–1159

186. Moser RJ, Tenholder MF, Ridenour R: Oat-cell carcinoma in transfusion-associated acquired immunodeficiency syndrome. Ann Intern Med (Letter) 1985; 105:478

187. Nusbaum NJ: Metastatic small-cell carcinoma of the lung in a patient with AIDS. (Letter) N Engl J Med 1985; 312:1706

188. Weitberg AB, Mayer K, Miller ME, Mikolich DJ: Dysplastic carcinoid tumor and AIDS-related complex (Letter). N Engl J Med 1986; 314:1455

189. Irwin LE, Begandy MK, Moore TM: Adenosquamous carcinoma of the lung and the acquired immunodeficiency syndrome. Ann Intern Med (Letter) 1984; 100:158

190. Brenner M, Ognibene FP, Lack EE, et al: Prognostic factors and life expectancy of acquired immunodeficiency syndrome patients with *pneumocystis* pneumonia. Am Rev Resp Dis 1987; 136:1199–1206

191. Kovacs J, Hiemenez J, Macher A, et al: *Pneumocystis carinii* pneumonia: A comparison of the clinical features in patients with the acquired immunodeficiency syndrome and patients with other immune diseases. Ann Intern Med 1984; 100:663–671

192. Pass HI, Potter D, Shelhamer J, et al: Indications for and diagnostic efficacy of open-lung biopsy in the patient with acquired immunodeficiency syndrome (AIDS). Ann Thorac Surg 1986; 41:307–312

193. Shelhamer JH, Ognibene FP, Macher AM, et al: Persistence of *Pneumocystis carinii* in lung tissue of acquired immunodeficiency syndrome patients treated for *pneumocystis* pneumonia. Am Rev Respir Dis 1984; 130:1161–1165

194. Simmons JT, Suffredini AF, Lack EE, et al: Nonspecific interstitial pneumonitis in AIDS: Radiologic features. AJR 1987; 149:265–268

195. Suffredini AF, Ognibene FP, Lack EE, Nonspecific interstitial pneumonitis: A common cause of pneumonia in the acquired immuno-deficiency syndrome. Ann Intern Med 1987; 172:7–13

196. Benisch B, Peison B: The association of lymphocytic interstitial pneumonia and systemic lupus erythematosus. Mt Sinai J Med 1979; 46: 398–401

197. Greenberg SD, Haley MD, Jenkins DE, Fischer SP: Lymphoplasmacytic pneumonia with accompanying dysproteinemia. Arch Pathol Lab Med 1973; 96:73–80

198. Strimlan CV, Rosenow EC, Weiland LH, Brown LR: Lymphocytic interstitial pneumonitis. Review of 13 cases. Ann Intern Med 1978; 88:616–621

199. Erwin BC, Brynes RK, Chan WC, et al: Percutaneous needle biopsy in the diagnosis and classification of lymphoma. Cancer 1986; 57: 1074–1078

200. Kern WH: Exfoliative and aspiration cytology of malignant lymphomas. Sem Diag Pathol 1986; 3:211–218

201. Golden JA, Hollander H, Stulbarg MS, Gamsu G: Bronchoalveolar lavage as the exclusive diagnostic modality for *Pneumocystis carinii* pneumonia; a prospective study among patients with acquired immunodeficiency syndrome. Chest 1986; 90:18–22

202. Fitzgerald W, Bevelaqua F, Garay S, Aranda C: The role of open lung biopsy in patients with the acquired immunodeficiency syndrome. Chest 1987; 91:659–666

203. Hopewell PC, Luce JM: Pulmonary involvement in the acquired immunodeficiency syndrome. Chest 1985; 87:104–112

204. Emanuel D, Peppard J, Stover D, et al: Rapid immunodiagnosis of cytomegalovirus pneumonia by bronchoalveolar lavage using human and murine monoclonal antibodies. Ann Intern Med 1986; 104:476–481

205. Gleaves CA, Smith TF, Wold AD, Wilson WR: Detection of viral and chlamydial antigens in open lung biopsy specimens. Am J Clin Pathol 1985; 83:371–374

206. Hackman RC, Myerson D, Meyers JD, et al: Rapid diagnosis of cytomegaloviral pneumonia by tissue immunofluorescence with a murine monoclonal antibody. J Infect Dis 1985; 151:325–329

207. Shuster EA, Beneke JS, Tegtmeier GE, et al: Monoclonal antibody for rapid laboratory detection of cytomegalovirus infections: characterization and diagnostic application. Mayo Clin Proc 1985; 60:577–585

208. Volpi A, Whitley RJ, Ceballos R, Stagno S: Rapid diagnosis of pneumonia due to cytomegalovirus with specific monoclonal antibodies. J Infect Dis 1983; 147:1119–1120

209. Goldstein LC, Corey L, McDougall JK, et al: Monoclonal antibodies to herpes simplex viruses: Use in antigenic typing and rapid diagnosis. J Infect Dis 1983; 147:829–837

210. Phillips P, Weiner MH: Invasive aspergillosis diagnosed by immunohistochemistry with monoclonal and polyclonal reagents. Hum Pathol 1987; 18:1015–1024

211. Sun T, Greenspan J, Tenenbaum M, et al: Diagnosis of cerebral toxoplasmosis using fluorescein-labeled antitoxoplasma monoclonal antibodies. Am J Surg Pathol 1986; 10:312–316

212. Grody WW, Cheng L, Lewin KJ: In situ viral DNA hybridization in diagnostic surgical pathology. Hum Pathol 1987; 18:535–543

213. Robey SS, Gage WR, Kuhajda FP: Comparison of immunoperoxidase and DNA in situ hybridization techniques in the diagnosis of cytomegalovirus colitis. Am J Clin Pathol 1988; 89:666–671

214. Wolber RA, Lloyd RV: Cytomegalovirus detection by nonisotopic in situ DNA hybridization and viral antigen immunostaining using a two color technique. Hum Pathol 1988; 19:736–741

215. Myerson D, Hackman RC, Myers JD: Diagnosis of cytomegaloviral pneumonitis by in situ hybridization. J Infect Dis 1984; 150:272

216. Unger ER, Budgeon LR, Myerson D, Brigati DJ: Viral diagnosis by in situ hybridization, description of a rapid simplified colorimetric method. Am J Surg Pathol 1986; 10:1–8

217. Ward JM, O'Leary TJ, Baskin GB, et al: Immunohistochemical localization of human and simian immunodeficiency viral antigens in fixed tissue sections. Am J Pathol 1987; 127:199–205

218. Hilborne LH, Nieberg RK, Cheng L, Lewin K: Direct in situ hybridization for rapid detection of cytomegalovirus in bronchoalveolar lavage. Am J Clin Pathol 1987; 87:766–769

219. Keh W, Gerber MA: In situ hybridization for cytomegalovirus DNA in AIDS patients. Am J Clin Pathol 1987; 86:405A

220. Seto E, Benedict TS: Detection of cytomegalovirus infection by means of DNA isolated from paraffin-embedded tissues and dot hybridization. Am J Pathol 1987; 127:409–413

5

The Expanding Spectrum of *Pneumocystis carinii* Infection in the Acquired Immunodeficiency Syndrome

Edwin P. Ewing, Jr.
Francis W. Chandler

PNEUMOCYSTIS CARINII, a protozoan parasite of humans and many animals,[1] causes disease almost exclusively in immunosuppressed hosts. As the organism proliferates, it constantly cycles between cyst and trophozoite forms. Thus, two forms are always present when the protozoan is viable and multiplying. Both forms are extracellular and usually inhabit the lung.

The cyst forms have a pathognomonic morphology, and the accepted standard staining procedure for cysts is the Gomori methenamine silver (GMS) stain.[2] In positive tissue sections or cytologic preparations, cysts appear as black 4–6 μm round, oval, or cup-shaped structures with a dot-like focal cyst wall thickening[3] (Fig. 1). Cysts are usually associated with frothy or honeycombed material that represents numerous thin-walled trophozoites seen by electron microscopy.[4] Rapid modifications of the GMS procedure, such as that described by Shimono and Hartman,[5] enhance the value of this stain.

Other stains have been described for *P. carinii* in cytologic preparations. Cyst walls will stain with periodic acid-Schiff, cresyl violet,[6] and toluidine blue[7-9] and will fluoresce with the orange G of a Papanicolaou stain.[8,10] Within individual cysts, up to eight sporozoites can be seen by Papanicolaou stain fluorescence,[10] Giemsa,[11] and Gram stain.[9,12] Trophozoites are stained by Giemsa[11,13] and Wright[14] stains; they measure 2–5 μm in diameter and contain a single eccentric nucleus. The usefulness of these alternative stains is limited to varying degrees by their inability to discriminate *P. carinii* from background staining of host components and from other microorganisms with similar staining characteristics.

P. carinii pneumonia is the most common opportunistic infectious disease in patients with the acquired immunodeficiency

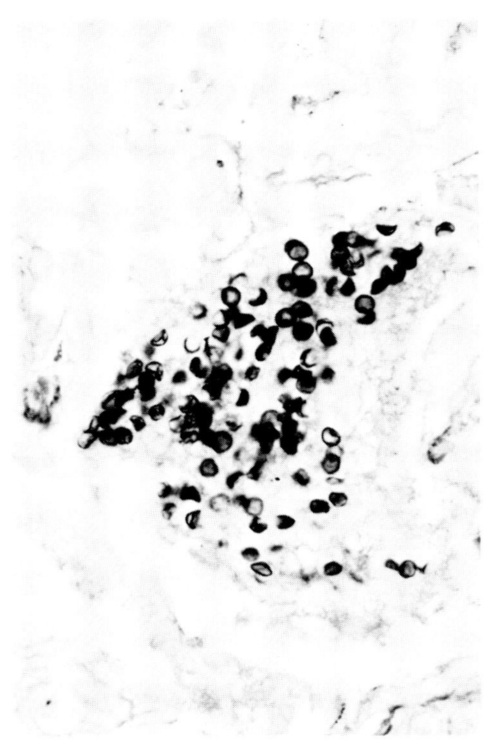

Figure 1. Cyst forms of *P. carinii.* Nonstaining trophozoites appear as numerous clear "holes" in exudate (GMS, original magnification X 567).

PULMONARY PNEUMOCYSTOSIS

Classical Form

In its familiar form, pneumocystosis occurs as a diffuse infection of the lungs. The organisms multiply extracellularly in, and are largely confined to, alveolar spaces. Cysts and trophozoites are embedded in frothy fibrinous exudates. A GMS stain readily demonstrates cyst forms in the exudates, and in AIDS, these forms are often very numerous. Exudates contain few cells of host origin and often appear retracted from alveolar walls in histologic sections (Fig. 2). The exudate may occasionally contain macrophages, and rarely, multinu-

syndrome (AIDS), eventually occurring in 80–85% of these patients.[15] This disease is encountered more and more often by pathologists as the AIDS epidemic grows. Pneumocystosis represents the emergence of a latent infection acquired early in childhood[16,17] and is almost exclusively a complication of AIDS or other immune deficiency conditions. As the incidence of AIDS-associated pneumocystosis increases, new or previously rare manifestations of this disease are reported more frequently. While most pathologists are familiar with the histopathologic features of classical *P. carinii* pneumonia, atypical presentations are not as well known. In this brief review of pneumocystosis associated with AIDS, we describe classical and variant histologic patterns of pulmonary involvement, then consider some unusual extrapulmonary forms.

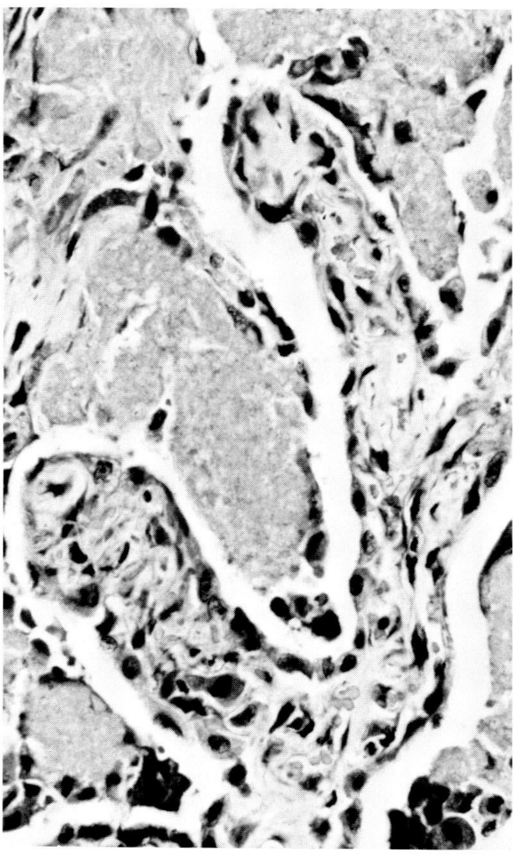

Figure 2. Lung with retracted exudates and widened septa (H&E, original magnification X 360).

cleated giant cells. Septa are intact but contain scattered lymphocytes and sometimes plasma cells, and they may be widened by fibrosis in chronic infections. After treatment with appropriate antibiotics, cysts may be phagocytosed and degraded by macrophages, at which time they appear as GMS-positive granular material (Fig. 3).

Minimal Pathology

Also described as grade 1 infection,[18] this presentation may represent a variant or an early stage of infection, which can be overlooked because of its subtlety. Few or no exudates are seen, and the interstitium is unremarkable except for a mild diffuse lymphocytic infiltrate. A GMS stain, which should be performed routinely on all lung biopsies from patients with known or suspected AIDS, may reveal small groups or rows of cysts adjacent to alveolar walls. The number of cysts does not always correlate with severity of disease. A few cysts may be seen in major respiratory impairment,[19] while many cysts are sometimes found in patients with good respiratory function.[19,20]

Noncavitating Pulmonary Nodules

Pneumocystosis has presented in AIDS as a solitary pulmonary nodule on chest roentgenogram in well documented cases.[21,22] The nodules may occur in any lobe of either lung and are typically about 3 cm in diameter. Histopathologically, there are abundant cysts of *P. carinii* in the absence of other infectious agents. Necrosis may be present, and in one report, organisms were surrounded by atypical granulomas.[22] Nodules may be multiple as well as solitary.[23]

Cavitating Pulmonary Nodules

Evolution of a pulmonary nodule from noncavitating to cavitating has been observed in sequential roentgenograms.[21] Necrosis of pulmonary parenchyma is a dominant feature in the development of this lesion, and alveolar septa appear as ghostlike remnants or are absent (Fig. 4). Large expanses of exudate contain numerous organisms but few intact host cells. Cavitating lesions may be seen in patients with normal arterial blood gases and later progress to diffuse disease with deteriorating pulmonary function.[24]

Diffuse Interstitial Involvement

Pneumocystosis with a predominantly interstitial location of exudate and organisms has been observed in a bronchoscopic biopsy.[25] The exudate also involved the walls of blood vessels. Dissemination of *P. carinii* to multiple organs occurred in this patient.

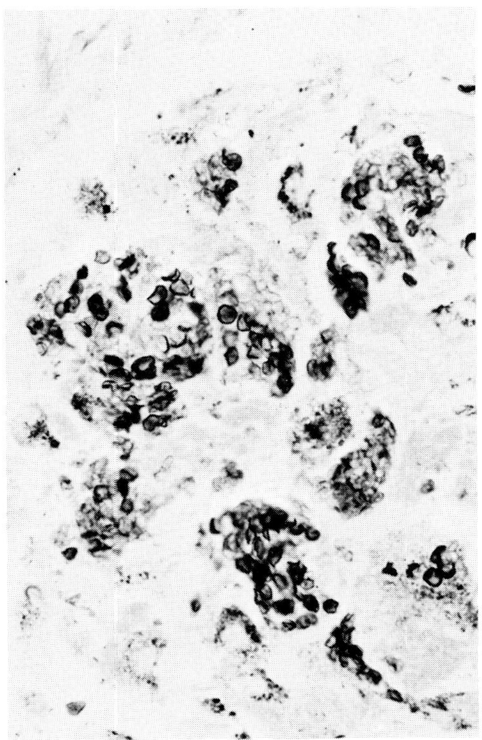

Figure 3. Cysts and granular remnants of cysts in lung (GMS, original magnification X 567).

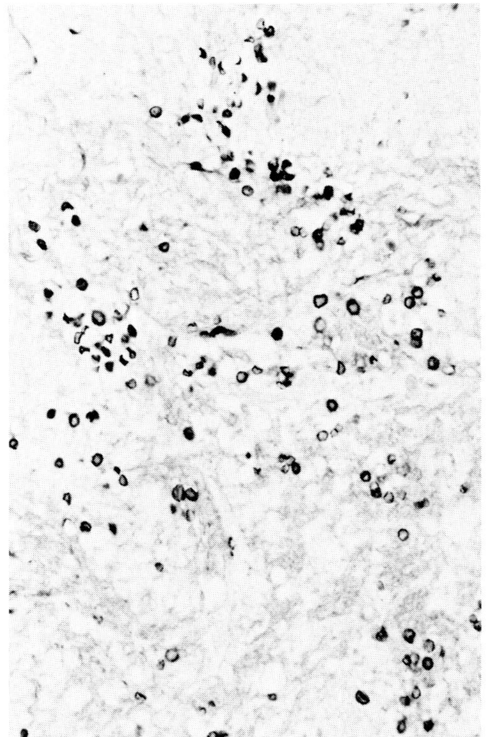

Figure 4. Cysts in an area of necrosis in lung (GMS, original magnification X 360).

Endobronchial Nodule

An obstructing endobronchial mass as the sole manifestation of *P. carinii* infection has been reported.[26] Biopsy of the mass revealed sheets of *P. carinii* cysts. Sections were negative for neoplasm, granuloma, or other organisms including acid-fast bacilli.

EXTRAPULMONARY PNEUMOCYSTOSIS

Lymphoreticular

Multiple lesions have been reported in lymph nodes from many sites[23,25] and in the liver,[23,25] spleen,[25,27,28] and bone marrow.[23,25,27] In all but bone marrow, lesions were visible grossly as gray or yellow foci of necrosis. Microscopically, foci of eosinophilic exudate described as "amorphous," "frothy," or "foamy" were observed alone or within necrotic areas. Lesions typically contained large numbers of organisms and were accompanied by few or no inflammatory cells.

Alimentary Tract

Lesions similar to those described above have occurred in the submucosa of the esophagus.[25] They have also been seen in stomach,[25] small intestine,[23,25] appendix,[25] and large intestine,[23] where both the mucosa and serosa were involved. In addition, lesions have been observed in the mesentery, appendices epiploicae, and omentum.[23]

Other Sites

Lesions have been documented in pancreas,[23,25] thyroid,[23] adrenal,[23,25] kidney,[23,25] ureter,[23] heart,[23,25] eye,[23,29] and external auditory canal.[30,31] Heart involvement has included endocardium and epicardium,[23] and in the eye, both retina[29] and choroid[23] have been affected. The auditory canal lesions presented as polypoid masses of the skin; microscopically, "foamy" material with many organisms was demonstrated in the dermis with essentially no directly related inflammatory response. In one case, the lesions were conspicuously angiocentric, and abundant fibrin deposition was noted in the surrounding intervascular dermis.[30]

CONCLUSION

P. carinii is acquired by virtually everyone early in childhood, and the infection persists latently for a lifetime. When host defenses, especially cell-mediated immunity, are severely impaired as they are with AIDS, this organism can proliferate out of control and damage Type I pneumocytes.[25,32] Pneumonia with desquamation of pneumocytes and filling of alveolar spaces with organisms and exudate can lead to respiratory failure and death.

For unknown reasons, damage in a few cases of pneumocystosis is not limited to pneumocytes, and the destruction becomes more extensive. Interstitial involvement may lead to cavitating pulmonary nodules or recurrent pneumothorax.[24] Extension of lesions to the interstitium undoubtedly facilitates extrapulmonary dissemination of organisms. The finding of organisms in diaphragmatic lymphatics[23] and in a wide variety of other tissues suggests that dissemination can take place by both lymphatic and hematogenous routes.

The large numbers of organisms usually encountered in extrapulmonary lesions indicates that *P. carinii* can flourish in many kinds of tissue when immune defenses are sufficiently impaired. Thus, its usual confinement to the lungs is perhaps as much a reflection of its presumed airborne route of infection as it is a fundamental tissue preference. Both immunologic and anatomic barriers probably act to prevent dissemination in most cases of *P. carinii* pneumonia. However, the organism clearly can disseminate to cause pathology in many other organs, and pathologists confronted with biopsy specimens from AIDS patients must consider this possibility when necrotic or exudative lesions are present.

REFERENCES

1. Chandler FW, McClure HM, Campbell WG Jr, et al: Pulmonary pneumocystosis in nonhuman primates. Arch Pathol Lab Med 1976; 100:163–167
2. Grocott RG: A stain for fungi in tissue sections and smears using Gomori's methenamine-silver nitrate technic. Am J Clin Pathol 1955; 25:975–979
3. Watts JC, Chandler FW: *Pneumocystis carinii* pneumonitis. The nature and diagnostic significance of the methenamine silver-positive "intracystic bodies". Am J Surg Pathol 1985; 9:744–751
4. Sueishi K, Hisano S, Sumiyoshi A, et al: Scanning and transmission electron microscopic study of human pulmonary pneumocystosis. Chest 1977; 72:213–216
5. Shimono LH, Hartman B: A simple and reliable rapid methenamine silver stain for *Pneumocystis carinii* and fungi. Arch Pathol Lab Med 1986; 110:855–856
6. Moas CM, Evans DA, Stein-Streilein J, et al: Cresyl violet: A rapid and sensitive stain for diagnosing *Pneumocystis carinii* by sputum examination. Abstract from the III International Conference on AIDS, June 1–5, 1987:187
7. Blumenfeld W, Hadley WK, Griffiss J: Identification of *Pneumocystis carinii* (PC) in sputum; underestimation of cyst number with Giemsa. Abstract from the III International Conference on AIDS, June 1–5, 1987: 190
8. Flint A, Beckwith AL, Naylor B: *Pneumocystis carinii* pneumonia. Cytologic manifestations and rapid diagnosis in routinely prepared Papanicolaou-stained preparations. Am J Med 1986; 81:1009–1011
9. Macher AM, Shelhamer J, Maclowry J, et al: *Pneumocystis carinii* identified by Gram stain of lung imprints. Ann Intern Med 1983; 99: 484–485
10. Ghalli VS, Garcia RL, Skolom J: Fluorescence of *Pneumocystis carinii* in Papanicolaou smears. Hum Pathol 1984; 15:907–909
11. Blumenfeld W, Wagar E, Hadley WK: Use of the transbronchial biopsy for diagnosis of opportunistic pulmonary infections in acquired immunodeficiency syndrome (AIDS). Am J Clin Pathol 1984; 81:1–5
12. Rankin JA, Young KR Jr: Gram staining of *Pneumocystis* sporozoites (Letter). Ann Intern Med 1984; 100:919
13. Bigby TD, Margolskee D, Curtis JL, et al: The usefulness of induced sputum in the diagnosis of *Pneumocystis carinii* pneumonia in patients with the acquired immunodeficiency syndrome. Am Rev Respir Dis 1986; 133:515–518
14. Domingo J, Waksal HW: Wright's stain in rapid diagnosis of *Pneumocystis carinii*. Am J Clin Pathol 1984; 81:511–514
15. Mills J: *Pneumocystis carinii* and *Toxoplasma gondii* infections in patients with AIDS. Rev Infect Dis 1986; 8:1001–1011
16. Meuwissen JHET, Tauber I, Leeuwenberg ADEM, et al: Parasitologic and serologic observations of infection with *Pneumocystis* in humans. J Infect Dis 1977; 136:43–49
17. Pifer LL, Hughes WT, Stagno S, et al: *Pneumocystis carinii* infection: evidence for high prevalence in normal and immunosuppressed children. Pediatrics 1978; 61:35–41
18. Mones JM, Saldana MJ, Oldham SA: Diagnosis of *Pneumocystis* pneumonia. Roentgenographic-pathologic correlates based on fiberoptic bronchoscopy specimens from patients with the acquired immunodeficiency syndrome. Chest 1986; 89:522–526
19. Kovacs JA, Hiemenz JW, Macher AM, et al: *Pneumocystis carinii* pneumonia: A comparison between patients with the acquired immunodeficiency syndrome and patients with other

immunodeficiencies. Ann Intern Med 1984; 100:663–671

20. Kelly AR, Sutker WL: Pneumocystis pneumonia in a patient with normal chest roentgenograms and normal arterial blood gas values. South Med J 1986; 79:1315–1316

21. Barrio JL, Suarez M, Rodriquez JL, et al: *Pneumocystis carinii* pneumonia presenting as cavitating and noncavitating solitary pulmonary nodules in patients with the acquired immunodeficiency syndrome. Am Rev Respir Dis 1986; 134:1094–1096

22. Masur H, Michelis MA, Greene JB, et al: An outbreak of community-acquired *Pneumocystis carinii* pneumonia. Initial manifestation of cellular immune dysfunction. N Engl J Med 1981; 305:1431–1438

23. Macher AM, Bardenstein DS, Zimmerman LE, et al: *Pneumocystis carinii* choroiditis in a male homosexual with AIDS and disseminated pulmonary and extrapulmonary *P. carinii* infection (Letter). N Engl J Med 1987; 316:1092

24. Eng RHK, Bishburg E, Smith SM: Evidence for destruction of lung tissues during *Pneumocystis carinii* infection. Arch Intern Med 1987; 147: 746–749

25. Grimes MM, LaPook JD, Bar MH, et al: Disseminated *Pneumocystis carinii* infection in a patient with acquired immunodeficiency syndrome. Hum Pathol 1987; 18:307–308

26. Gagliardi AJ, Stover DE, Zaman MK: Endobronchial *Pneumocystis carinii* infection in a patient with the acquired immune deficiency syndrome. Chest 1987; 91:463–464

27. Heyman MR, Rasmussen P: *Pneumocystis carinii* involvement of the bone marrow in acquired immunodeficiency syndrome. Am J Clin Pathol 1987; 87:780–783

28. Pilon VA, Echols RM, Celo JS, et al: Disseminated *Pneumocystis* pneumonia infection in AIDS. N Engl J Med 1987; 316:1410–1411

29. Kwok S, O'Donnell J, Wood IS: Retinal cotton-wool spots in a patient with *Pneumocystis carinii* infection (letter). N Engl J Med 1982; 307: 184–185

30. Coulman CU, Greene I, Archibald RWR: Cutaneous pneumocystosis. Ann Intern Med 1987; 106:396–398

31. Schinella RA, Breda SD, Hammerschlag PE: Otic infection due to *Pneumocystis carinii* in an apparently healthy man with antibody to the human immunodeficiency virus. Ann Intern Med 1987; 106:399–400

32. Walzer PD: Attachment of microbes to host cells: Relevance of *Pneumocystis carinii*. Lab Invest 1986; 54:589–592

33. Long EG, Smith JS, Meier JL: Attachment of *Pneumocystis carinii* to rat pneumocytes. Lab Invest 1986; 54:609–615

6

Diagnosis of Cytomegalovirus Infection of the Lung in the Acquired Immune Deficiency Syndrome (AIDS): By In Situ DNA Hybridization

Cheryl P. Frydman
Ira J. Bleiweiss
Ok H. Yoo
Jaishree Jagirdar

HUMAN CYTOMEGALOVIRUS (CMV) is a frequent cause of life threatening opportunistic pulmonary infection in the acquired immune deficiency syndrome (AIDS) population. The rapid diagnosis of CMV in these patients is essential with the advent of therapeutic trials for effective antiviral agents,[1-5] as well as for diagnostic purposes, prognosis,[6,7] and prevention of nosocomial outbreaks. CMV infection is readily detected serologically by a rise in antibody titer to CMV antigen. Specific IgM antibodies can be detected by radioimmunossay (RIA) or enzyme linked immunosorbent assay (ELISA) and may persist 3–4 months following primary infection, but have little diagnostic significance in profoundly immunosuppressed patients. To date, the only reliable method for detecting active CMV infection in AIDS patients is by demonstrating the virus itself. Human lung fibroblast cultures are conventionally used for the identification of CMV and have been considered the most sensitive procedure.[8] Viral growth is slow, however, and there may be no evidence of cytopathic effect for up to 2–6 weeks following specimen inoculation.[9] Despite sensitive culture techniques, the virus may remain undetected due to a sampling error.[10]

Pulmonary CMV infection can be demonstrated upon routine examination by the presence of distinctive intranuclear and intracytoplasmic inclusions, cellular enlargement, and perinuclear halo formation in the endothelium, pneumocytes, and alveolar macrophages. However, the sensitivity of this technique is low, since cytomegalic cells are usually only observed in tissues containing large amounts of virus, and examination of routine histologic sections may give no indication that infection is present.[11-13] Cy-

"

tomegalic alterations may also be confused with hyperplastic Type II pneumocytes due to other causes.

Several methods have been evaluated for their ability to provide sensitive and more rapid diagnosis of CMV infection in body fluids and tissues from immunocompromised hosts. These include: electron microscopy, the use of monoclonal antibodies directed against nuclear and cytoplasmic viral antigens, and DNA in situ hybridization using biotinylated and ^{32}P labeled cloned fragments of human CMV DNA.[10,14-23] CMV in situ hybridization has been found to approach or exceed the diagnostic sensitivity of viral cultures, far surpassing that of routine histologic examination.[10,23-25] In situ hybridization has, in fact, revealed the presence of CMV DNA in cells that did not appear to be infected by standard histologic criteria, and such occult CMV infection may account for a large number of the infected cells in disseminated CMV infection.[21,26] This study demonstrates the usefulness of human CMV DNA probes for detecting occult CMV infection in lung biopsy specimens from AIDS patients treated at our institution.

MATERIALS AND METHODS

Tissue

Histologic sections of lung tissue obtained from patients treated at the Bronx Veterans Administration Medical Center between 1983 and 1987 were reviewed. We studied 50 biopsy specimens from 40 AIDS patients with *Pneumocystis carinii* pneumonia (PCP). Twelve of these patients had several biopsies performed. In addition, five specimens from AIDS patients without histologic evidence of PCP infection were also included.

Bronchoscopic biopsy and open lung biopsy specimens were fixed in neutral buffered formalin for approximately 24

hours, embedded in paraffin, and sectioned onto poly-L-lysine (M.W. > 300,000) coated glass slides for hybridization. Tissue for early nuclear antigen studies was frozen and stored at $-70°C$. In addition, all tissue sections were routinely stained with hematoxylin-eosin, Grocott's methenamine silver (GMS) and by the Ziehl-Neelsen method for acid-fast bacilli.

In Situ Hybridization

In situ hybridization was performed according to the method of Brigati et al[27] with the following modifications: histologic sections were deparaffinized in xylene, rehydrated in graded ethanols, and washed with phosphate buffered saline (PBS). The sections were immersed in 0.01% hydrogen peroxide in methanol to inhibit endogenous peroxidase activity followed by treatment with 0.1 mg/ml Proteinase K (Sigma Chem. Co., St. Louis, MO) in PBS for 15 minutes at $37°C$. Proteolytic activity was terminated by washing in 2 mg/ml glycine in PBS. For hybridization, tissue sections were covered with 20 μL of biotinylated CMV DNA (Cytomegalovirus deoxy Bio-Probe™, labeled probe, Enzo Biochem., Inc., New York), or in the control experiments, 20 μL of biotinylated Epstein-Barr virus (EBV) DNA (Epstein-Barr virus deoxy Bio-Probe™, labeled probe, Enzo Biochem., Inc., New York). The CMV DNA probe consists of a mixture of plasmid pBR 322. The insert sizes are 17.2 kb and 25.2 kb. The EBV DNA probe consists of a single 3.1 kb sequence from the BAM H1 "V" (internal repeat 1) region of the EBV genome cloned into pBR 322. Denaturation was performed in a moist chamber at $90°C$, for 15 minutes followed by hybridization at $37°C$ for two hours. The sections were washed at room temperature in 50% formamide followed by wash buffer (Triton X-100 in PBS) for two minutes each. The slides were then incubated with streptavidin-horseradish peroxidase (Enzo Biochem., Inc., New York) for 15 minutes at room temperature. The tissue sections were washed in buffer followed by incubation with a solution of aminoethylcarbazole in acetate buffer and hydrogen peroxide (Enzo Biochem., Inc., New York) for five minutes at room temperature. Some sections were counterstained with fast green for one minute. Coverslips were mounted with water, and the slides were examined by light microscopy. Positive control slides consisted of lung tissue with known CMV infection demonstrating typical cytomegalic changes. Negative controls included tissue infected with varicella zoster virus and EBV. Control slides for nonspecific staining were included with each case by performing the procedure substituting PBS for the biotinylated probe during the hybridization step.

Two cases were rehybridized after pretreatment with DNAase (0.5 mg/ml in 0.1 M MgCl$_2$) in PBS buffer at a concentration of 0.1 ul/ml. Slides were incubated with DNAase at 37°C for 1 hour, washed in PBS four times, and then hybridized.

Detection of CMV Early Nuclear Antigen

Detection of the early nuclear antigen of CMV was performed on frozen tissue sections fixed in cold acetone and air dried. The specimens were incubated with a 1:10 dilution of mouse monoclonal anti-CMV early nuclear protein IG2A (New England Nuclear Products, Boston) in 3% bovine serum albumin for 30 minutes at 37°C followed by 30 minutes at room temperature. Specimens were washed four times in PBS and air dried. Tissue sections were incubated with a detection complex consisting of a 1:50 dilution of horseradish peroxidase labeled goat anti-mouse IgG (DAKO Immunoglobulins, Denmark) in 3% bovine serum albumin for 30 minutes at 37°C followed by room temperature for 30 minutes. The sections were then washed four times in PBS followed by incubation with a solution of aminoethylcarbazole in hydrogen peroxide

for five minutes. Coverslips were mounted with water, and the sections were examined by ight microscopy. Positive control slides consisted of human diploid fibroblast (MRC-5) monolayer cell cultures (Earl-Clay Lab., Inc., Norcross, Ga.) infected with CMV ATCC strain AD169, and negative control slides consisted of uninfected fibroblast monolayers.

Electron Microscopy

Lung biopsy and pulmonary lavage specimens were fixed in a mixture of glutaraldehyde and paraformaldehyde, impregnated with 2% osmium tetroxide, and dehydrated and embedded in epoxy resin. Thick sections (1–2u) were stained with toluidine blue and examined by light microscopy. Thin sections (60–100 mu) were stained with uranyl acetate, lead citrate and examined for viral particles using a Phillips 400 electron microscope.

Viral Cultures

Bronchial washings, urine, blood, or sputum were inoculated in 0.2 ml aliquots into duplicate human diploid fibroblast (MRC-5) monolayer cell culture tubes (Earl Clay Lab., Inc., Norcross, Ga.). Cultures were incubated at 37°C and were observed for cytopathic effect twice weekly for 6 weeks.

Results

Fifty-five biopsy specimens were obtained from 41 AIDS patients undergoing evaluation for suspected pneumonitis. Clinical data were available on 28 of the patients (Table 1). The patients ranged in age from 29–59 years (mean 39.4 years). All patients were male. OK T4:T8 ratios ranged from 0.2–1.24. CMV antibody titers ranged from 1:4–1:256. Currently, 18 of the patients

TABLE I
Summary of Clinical Data

Risk Factors	Number of Patients
Homosexuality	5/28 (17%)
Intravenous drug abuse	21/28 (75%)
Homosexuality and drug abuse	1/28 (4%)
Unknown risk factor	1/28 (4%)
Associated Infections and Disease	
Candidiasis	20/28 (71%)
Toxoplasmosis	3/28 (11%)
Mycobacterium avium complex	4/28 (14%)
Cryptococcosis	1/28 (4%)
Herpes simplex virus	3/28 (11%)
Kaposi's sarcoma	1/28 (4%)

with available records have expired. The specimens included 54 transbronchial biopsies obtained by fiberoptic bronchoscopy and one open lung biopsy. Twelve of the patients underwent two or more biopsies.

PATHOLOGIC FINDINGS

Light Microscopy

Fifty of 55 lung biopsy specimens contained foamy eosinophilic intraalveolar exudate, chronic inflammatory cells, and cell debris within alveoli. GMS stain revealed characteristic *Pneumocystis carinii* cysts within the exudate. Three lung biopsies contained acid fast bacilli (one in addition to *Pneumocystis carinii*), and the presence of *Mycobacterium avium intracellulare* complex was confirmed by bacteriologic cultures. One lung biopsy contained cryptococcal blastoconidia in addition to *Pneumocystis carinii*. One biopsy did not show any histologic abnormality. Many of the specimens showed varying degrees of interstitial fibrosis and inflammation as well as hyperplastic Type II pneumocytes. A minimum of three hematoxylin-eosin stained tissue sections were examined from each

case both prior to and following hybridization; however, none of the cells demonstrated any cytomegalic changes. Three of the cases later had typical CMV inclusions on second biopsy.

In Situ Hybridization

In situ human CMV DNA hybridization detected the presence of CMV DNA in the nucleus, cytoplasm, and/or on bronchial epithelial surfaces of pneumocytes in 19 of 55 (35%) lung biopsy specimens. Positive cells were readily visualized by light microscopy under medium power (20×) and high power (40×) objectives as finely granular brick red staining (Fig. 1A&B). Nonspecific background staining and environmental pigment were distinguished from true staining by their quality (coarse and angulated), location (out of tissue plane), and color (brown). Each section contained between one and greater than 50 hybridizing cells. Both the location of the viral DNA and the number of hybridizing cells were found to be reproducible, as seen on serial sections.

CMV DNA was detected in 35 out of 50 PCP cases (70%) (Table 2). In 15 of 50 cases (30%) staining was confined to pneumocyte cytoplasm, nucleus, or bronchial epithelial surface. In 31 of 50 cases (62%) there was staining in the alveolar exudate, either in the form of granular staining on the surfaces of the pneumocystis or within the exudate (Figs. 2A&B). The number of organisms staining varied from case to case; in some cases only a few of the organisms contained CMV DNA, while in other specimens many of the organisms were positive. Eleven of 50 (22%) cases of PCP had both positive staining on the organisms and the cells.

On sequential biopsies, eight out of 12 (67%) of the cases were probe-positive for CMV DNA either simultaneously on the *Pneumocystis* and in the pneumocytes or sequentially in the same order (Table 3). Seven cases contained CMV DNA in the pneumocytes on the second serial biopsy.

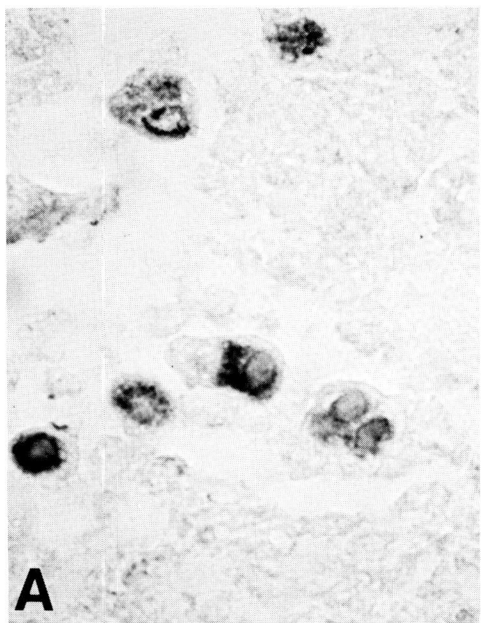 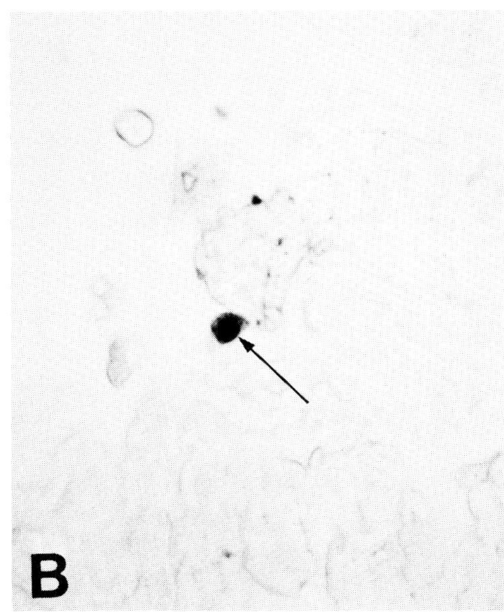

Figure 1. In situ hybridization for CMV DNA. (A) Nuclear and cytoplasmic staining in pneumocytes (control). (B) Positive staining of non cytomegalic alveolar lining cell (arrow).

TABLE II
In Situ Hybridization for CMV
in *Pneumocystis carinii* Pneumonia

Location of Positive Staining	Percentage
A. Pneumocyte cytoplasm, nucleus, or bronchial epithelial surface	30%
B. *Pneumocystis carinii* in alveolar exudate	62%
C. Pneumocytes and *Pneumocystis carinii* in alveolar exudate	22%
D. No staining	30%

Previous biopsies in six out of seven (86%) of these cases contained probe-positive *Pneumocystis* with two of the cases showing concurrent positivity in the pneumocytes.

Four PCP-negative cases contained CMV DNA in pneumocytes on second biopsy. Previous biopsies in all four patients contained probe-positive *Pneumocystis* with one also showing probe-positive pneumocytes. The fifth PCP-negative case (no.1) also showed CMV DNA in pneumocytes; however, this patient did not have a previous PCP infection documented. The presence of probe-positive *Pneumocystis* (nos. 5 and 10) may not necessarily lead to the presence of CMA DNA in the pneumocytes on subsequent biopsy. In two cases (nos. 1 and 6), probe-positive pneumocytes were seen in the first biopsy; however, the second biopsy did not show probe-positive pneumocytes.

The specificity of the CMV DNA probe was evaluated by hybridization with normal paraffin embedded lung tissue and with tissue infected with varicella zoster virus and EBV. In addition, a DNA probe directed against EBV DNA was hybridized with tissue containing CMV DNA. Hybridization did not occur in any of these tissue specimens.

Two cases were rehybridized after pretreatment with DNAase. DNA specific hybridization was demonstrated as no positive staining was observed in the slides pretreated with DNAase.

TABLE III
In Situ Hybridization for CMV on Sequential Lung Biopsy Specimens

Case #	First Biopsy in PCP	in Cells	Second Biopsy in PCP	in Cells	Time Interval Between Biopsies
1	*	+	+	−	7 months
2	−	−	+	+	9 months
3	+	+	*	+	5 months
4	+	−	+	+	8 months
5	+	−	−	−	5 months
6	+	+	−	−	1 month
7	+	+rare	+	+	17 months
8	−	−	−	−	6 months
9	+	−	*	+	19 months
10	+	−	+	−	9 months
11	+	−	*	+	18 months
12	+	−	*	+	9 months

*Specimens were negative for PCP

Note: 67% of cases showed positivity for CMV DNA either simultaneously on the *Pneumocystis* and in the pneumocytes or sequentially in the same order.

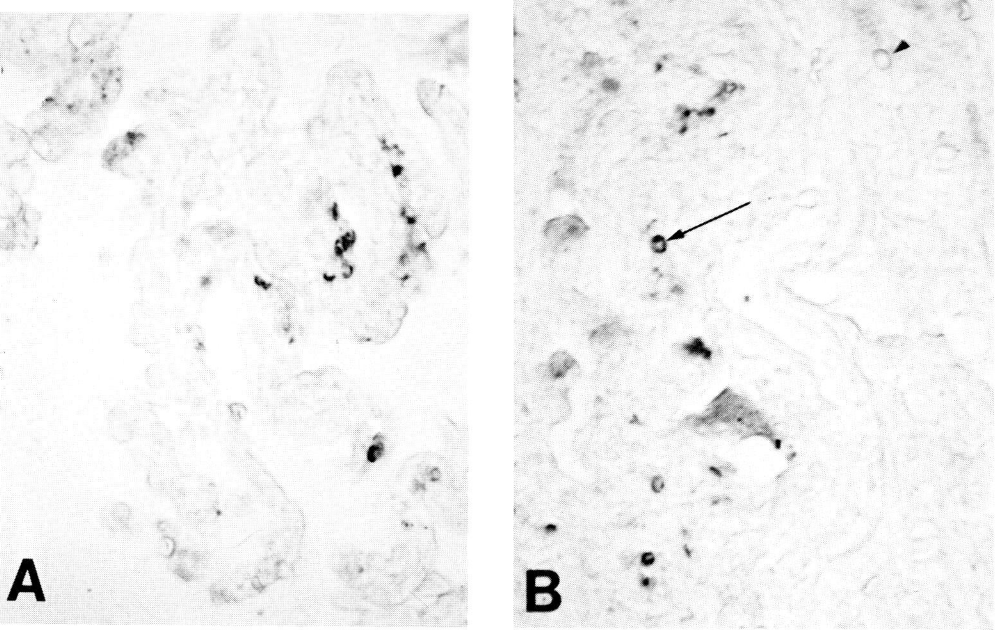

Figure 2. In situ hybridization for CMV DNA. (A,B) Positive staining of discrete *Pneumocystis carinii* cysts for CMV DNA (long arrow). Note: absence of staining on erythrocytes (short arrow).

Monoclonal Antibodies

Fresh frozen tissue for the detection of the early antigen of CMV was available on one case, which contained probe positive pneumocytes and *Pneumocystis*. The early nuclear antigen was readily visualized in positive cells as coarse red intranuclear staining by light microscopy (Fig. 3A). CMV antigen was also detected on the pneumocytes and *Pneumocystis* of the case studied (Fig. 3B).

Viral Cultures

Viral culture results were available on 22 of the patients studied. Various specimens were cultured including: blood, urine, bronchial washings, and sputum. Specimens were obtained at various time intervals before or after biopsy. Ten of 16 (63%) probe-positive cases were negative by viral culture (Table 4). All of the probe-negative cases had negative viral cultures.

Electron Microscopy

Six lung biopsy specimens containing hybridizing pneumocytes and/or *Pneumocystis* and pulmonary lavage specimens from patients with corresponding biopsy specimens containing CMV DNA were evaluated extensively by electron microscopy for the presence of viral particles; however, none were found.

TABLE IV
In Situ Hybridization for CMV in Lung Biopsy Specimens Compared with Routine Viral Cultures

In Situ Hybridization	Viral Cultures		
	Positive	Negative	Total
Positive	6	10	16
Negative	0	6	6

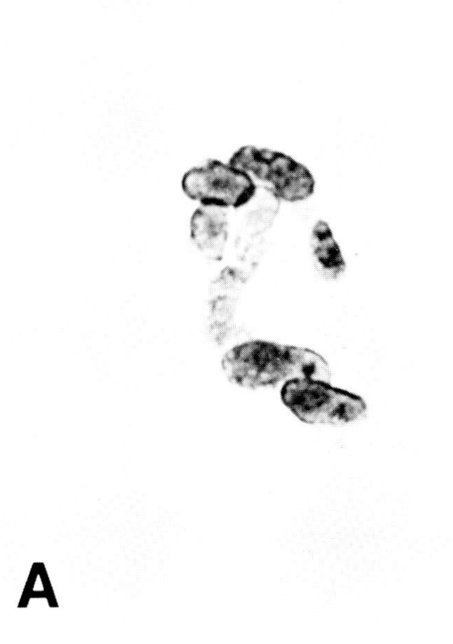
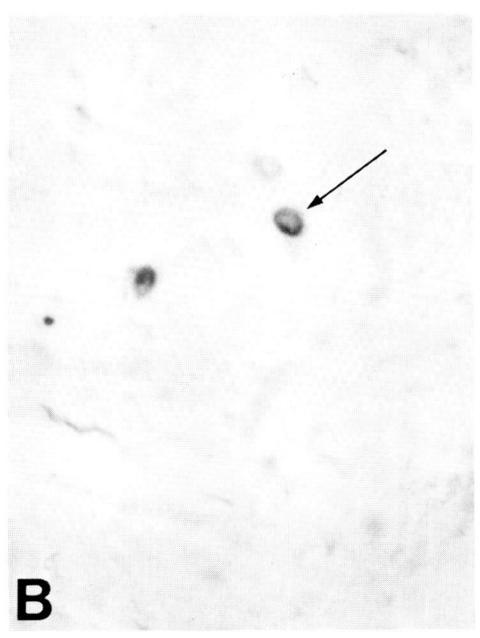

Figure 3. Staining of CMV early nuclear antigen. (A) Control. (B) Positive staining of *Pneumocystis carinii* cysts (arrow).

Discussion

In situ hybridization is a specific and reproducible diagnostic method for detecting CMV DNA in routine biopsy specimens. The use of biotinylated DNA probes is highly advantageous for several reasons. They are stable for up to 2 years and do not necessitate the use of radioactive isotopes. Results are available within 24–36 hours following biopsy, while visible cytopathic effect in tissue culture can take up to 6 weeks and may yield false negative results due to cytotoxic substances inoculated with the specimen. In addition, CMV is a labile virus, and the infective virus titer may be below the sensitivity of routine viral cultures.

Examination of routine histologic lung biopsy specimens in this institution between 1983 and 1987 failed to reveal CMV as the etiologic agent of AIDS related pneumonitis. There was no correlation between the clinical characteristics of the patients and the presence or absence of CMV DNA in any of the biopsy specimens. Previous studies have shown that up to 67% of pneumonitis in AIDS patients is due to CMV, and between 14% and 83% of these cases were detected by routine examination of bronchoscopic and open lung biopsy specimens.[6,28,29] In this study, CMV infection was detected by in situ hybridization in approximately 33% of patients with suspected pneumonitis; however, typical cytomegalic inclusions were not seen on routine hematoxylin-eosin stained tissue sections. Cytomegalic alterations are usually not seen unless a large amount of virus is present, and the patients reported in these previous studies often had more advanced disease (50% with Kaposi's sarcoma) than patients in our population, possibly harboring larger amounts of virus, and thus allowing for more ready detection of CMV infection.[6]

A review of viral culture results showed that 63% of probe-positive cases had negative viral cultures, so in situ hybridization may be a more sensitive technique for detecting CMV DNA than routine culture. In situ hybridization may detect defective or incomplete occult viral particles that are unable to grow in tissue culture. In addition, many of the body fluids cultured were obtained from disparate body sites, were not always obtained coincidentally with the biopsy, and therefore, may not truly have reflected a pulmonary process. Rabah and Jaffe,[30] however, studying allograft liver biopsies, found in situ hybridization to be no more sensitive than routine histologic examination. The reason for this discrepancy is unclear.

The presence of occult CMV infection has been suspected in the past.[12,28,31-33] Myerson et al.[26] studied autopsy tissue from patients with disseminated CMV infection by in situ hybridization and found the majority of CMV DNA to be localized in normal appearing cells. Therefore, the presence of cytomegaly may be the exception rather than the rule. The percentage of infected biopsies and the number of cells in biopsy specimens containing viral DNA may, in fact, be much higher than suspected since the size of the specimen is usually very small and the tissue may contain very few or no viral particles. There are three histologic patterns of CMV pneumonia: (1) miliary, (2) diffuse, and (3) the category of scattered infected cells recently added by Myerson et al.[26,34] Tissue studies have shown that the distribution of CMV in the lungs is highly variable with only 50% of the tissue sections sampled containing hybridizing cells. Thus, a single negative biopsy specimen may only reflect sampling variation.[7,10,21]

Concurrent PCP and CMV infection is a frequent occurrence.[28,35-38] In this study, 22% of the patients with PCP also had CMV probe positivity, and, in one case, this finding was complimented by monoclonal antibody directed against CMV early antigen. Symbiosis of CMV and *Pneumocystis carinii* has been reported.[39,40] *Pneumocystis carinii* in lung tissue from patients with known PCP and CMV infection has been shown to contain viral particles by electron microscopy.[39,40] These particles had a similar appearance to the dense core of CMV found in alveolar epithelial cells and macrophages from the same specimens.[39] We, however, studied six cases of PCP by EM and were not able to find any viral particles. It is possible that the complete virion may not be present. Protozoa and fungi have been shown to be infected by viruses.[41]

Sequential biopsies showed that 67% of the probe-positive cases did have previous or simultaneous *Pneumocystis carinii* infections. It is, therefore, not unlikely that *Pneumocystis carinii* may serve as an intermediate host or reservoir for CMV. This would explain the frequent coexistence of the two infections. Furthermore, *Pneumocystis carinii* is relatively more common than CMV in lung biopsy specimens from patients with AIDS[6,29,42]; however, at autopsy, CMV pneumonitis is more common than PCP.[7,29] As in this study, it has been found that many of these patients with CMV pneumonitis had been treated for PCP in the past.[7] The prevalence of CMV at autopsy may be explained by the more immunocompromised state of the patient immediately prior to the demise, as well as previous *Pneumocystis carinii* infection serving as a route of entry for CMV. It is speculated that when PCP is treated, CMV remains waiting to manifest itself clinically with further immunocompromise. PCP, though, should not be regarded as an absolute prerequisite for CMV infection, and, indeed, it has been suggested that CMV infection may predispose to PCP.[35] Therefore, specimens from immunocompromised patients with PCP should also be suspected to harbor CMV regardless of the clinical response to antibiotic therapy. Lung biopsies from such patients should undergo in situ hybridization for the presence of CMV DNA, so that prophylactic antiviral therapy for CMV can be instituted.[1,5]

REFERENCES

1. Collaborative DHPG Treatment Study Group: Treatment of serious cytomegalovirus infections with 9-(1,3-Dihydroxy-2-propoxymethyl) guanine in patients with AIDS and other immunodeficiencies. N Engl J Med 1986; 314:801–806
2. Blacklock HA, Griffiths PD, Stirk PR, Prentice HG: Specific hyperimmune globulin for cytomegalovirus pneumonitis. Lancet 1985; 2:152–153
3. Cheng YC, Huang ES, Lin JC, et al: Unique spectrum of activity of 9-(1,3-dihydroxy-2-propoxy methyl) guanine against herpesviruses in vitro and its mode of action against Herpes Simplex virus type I. Proc Natl Acad Sci USA 1983; 80:2767–2770
4. Ringden O, Wilczek H, Lonnquist B, et al: Foscarnet for cytomegalovirus infections. Lancet 1985; 2:1503–1504
5. Erice A, Jordan MC, Chace BA, et al: Ganciclovir treatment of cytomegalovirus disease in transplant recipients and other immunocompromised hosts. JAMA 1987; 257:3082–3087
6. Stover DE, White DA, Romano PA, Gellene RA: Diagnosis of pulmonary disease in acquired immune deficiency syndrome (AIDS). Am Rev Resp Dis 1984; 130:659–662
7. Reichert CM, O'Leary TJ, Levens DL, et al: Autopsy pathology in the Acquired Immune Deficiency Syndrome. Am J Pathol 1983; 112:357–382
8. Smith TF, Holley KE, Keys TF, Macasalt FF: Cytomegalovirus studies of autopsy tissue I. Virus isolation. Am J Clin Pathol 1975; 63:854–858
9. Stagno S, Pass RF, Reynolds DW, Alford CA: Diagnosis of cytomegalovirus infections. In: Nahmias AJ, Dowdle WR, Schinazi RF, eds. The Human Herpesviruses. New York, Elsevier, 1981; 363–373
10. Myerson D, Hackman RC, Meyers JD: Diagnosis of cytomegaloviral pneumonia by in situ hybridization. J Infect Dis 1984; 150:272–277
11. Schulman HM, Hackman RC, Sale GE, Meyers JD: Rapid cytologic diagnosis of cytomegalovirus interstitial pneumonia on touch imprints from open lung biopsy. Am J Clin Pathol 1982; 77:90–94
12. Craighead JE: Cytomegalovirus pulmonary disease. Pathobiol Annu 1975; 5:197–220
13. Kanich RE, Craighead JE: Cytomegalovirus infection and cytomegalic inclusion disease in renal homotransplant recipients. Am J Med 1966; 40:874–882
14. Lee FK, Nahmais AJ, Stagno S: Rapid diagnosis of cytomegalovirus infection in infants by electron microscopy. N Engl J Med 1978; 299:1266–1270
15. Goldstein LC, McDougall J, Hackman R, Myers JO, et al: Monoclonal antibodies to cytomegalovirus: rapid identification of clinical isolates and preliminary use in diagnosis of cytomegalovirus pneumonia. Infect Immun 1982; 38:273–281
16. Griffiths PD, Panjwani DD, Stirk PR, et al: Rapid diagnosis of cytomegalovirus infection in immu-

nocompromised patients by detection of early antigen fluorescent foci. Lancet 1984; 2:1242–1245

17. Gleaves CA, Smith TF, Shuster EA, Pearson GR: Rapid detection of cytomegalovirus in MRC-5 cells inoculated with urine specimens by using low-speed centrifugation and monoclonal antibody to early antigen. J Clin Microbiol 1984; 19:917–919

18. Volpi A, Whitley RJ, Ceballos R, et al: Rapid diagnosis of pneumonia due to cytomegalovirus with specific monoclonal antibodies. J Infect Dis 1983; 147:1119–1120

19. Martin WJ, Smith TF: Rapid detection of cytomegalovirus in bronchoalveolar lavage specimens by a monoclonal antibody method. J Clin Microbiol 1986; 23:1006–1008

20. Chou S, Merigan TC: Rapid detection and quantitation of human cytomegalovirus in urine through DNA hybridization. N Engl J Med 1983; 308:921–925

21. Loning T, Milde K, Foss HD: In situ hybridization for the detection of cytomegalovirus (CMV) infection. Virch Arch (Pathol Anat) 1986; 409:777–790

22. Spector SA, Spector DH. The use of DNA probes in studies of human cytomegalovirus. Clin Chem 1985; 31:1514–1520

23. Spector SA, Rua JA, Spector DH, Mcmillan R: Detection of cytomegalovirus in clinical specimens by DNA-DNA hybridization. J Infect Dis 1984; 150:121–126

24. Hilborne LH, Nieberg RK, Cheng L, Lewin KJ. Direct in situ hybridization for rapid detection of cytomegalovirus in brochoalveolar lavage. Am J Clin Pathol 1987; 87:766–769

25. Masih AS, Linder J, Shaw BW, et al: A comparison of in situ hybridization (IH), routine light microscopy, and viral culture in post-transplant liver biopsies with suspected cytomegalovirus (CMV) hepatitis. (Abstract) Lab Invest 1987; 56:48A

26. Myerson D, Hackman RC, Nelson JA, et al: Widespread presence of histologically occult cytomegalovirus. Hum Pathol 1984; 15:430–439

27. Brigati DJ, Myerson D, Leary JJ, et al: Detection of viral genomes in cultured cells and paraffin-embedded tissue sections using biotin-labeled hybridization probes. Virology 1983; 126:32–50

28. McKenna RJ, Campbell A, McMurtrey MJ, Mountain CF: Diagnosis for interstitial lung disease in patients with acquired immune deficiency syndrome (AIDS); A prospective comparison of bronchial washing, alveolar lavage, transbronchial lung biopsy, and open lung biopsy. Ann Thorac Surg 1986; 41:318–321

29. Gal AA, Klatt EC, Koss MW, et al: The effectiveness of bronchoscopy in the diagnosis of *Pneumocystis carinii* and cytomegalovirus pulmonary infections in the acquired immune deficiency syndrome. Arch Pathol Lab Med 1987; 111:238–241

30. Rabah R, Jaffe R. Early detection of CMV in allograft liver biopsy. (Abstract). Lab Invest 1987; 56:5P

31. Naraqi S, Jackson GG, Jansson O, et al: Search for cytomegalovirus in renal allografts. Infect Immun 1978; 19:699–703

32. Fioretti A, Furukawa T, Santoli D, et al: Nonproductive infection of guinea pig cells in the human cytomegalovirus. J Virol 1973; 11:998–1003

33. Mocarski ES, Stinski MF: Persistence of cytomegalovirus in human cells. J Virol 1978; 31:761–775

34. Bescharner WE, Hutchins GM, Burns WH, et al: Cytomegalovirus pneumonia in bone marrow transplant recipients: miliary and diffuse patterns. Am Rev Resp Dis 1980; 122:107–114

35. Follansbee SE, Busch DF, Wufsby CB, et al: An outbreak of *Pneumocystis carinii* pneumonia in homosexual men. Ann Intern Med 1982; 96:705–713

36. Rifkind D, Starzl TE, Marchioro TL, et al: Transplantation pneumonia. JAMA 1964; 189:808–812

37. Kaposi's sarcoma and *Pneumocystis* pneumonia among homosexual men—New York City and California. MMWR 1981; 30:3054–3058

38. Le Clair RA: Descriptive epidemiology of interstitial pneumocystic pneumonia. An analysis of 107 cases from the United States, 1955–1967. Am Rev Resp Dis 1969; 99:542–547

39. Wang NS, Huang SN, Thurlbeck WM: Combined *Pneumocystis carinii* and cytomegalovirus infection. Arch Pathol 1970; 90:529–535

40. Ernst P, Chem MF, Wang NS, Cosio M: Symbiosis of *Pneumocystis carinii* and cytomegalovirus in a case of fatal pneumonia. Can Med Assoc J 1983; 128:1089–1092

41. Schuster FL: Intranuclear virus-like bodies in the amoebo-flagellate *Naegleria gruberi.* J Protozool 1969; 16:724–727

42. Marchevsky A, Rosen MJ, Chrystal G, Kleinerman J: Pulmonary complications of the Acquired Immune Deficiency Syndrome. Hum Pathol 1985; 16:659–670

7

Neuropathologic Complications of Infection with the Human Immunodeficiency Virus (HIV)

Harry V. Vinters
Uwamie Tomiyasu
Karl H. Anders

THE PRIMARY GOALS of this chapter will be to: (1) review and illustrate the neuropathologic complications of acquired immune deficiency syndrome (AIDS) and AIDS related complex (ARC) involving both the central and peripheral nervous systems, using the UCLA experience as a basis for this; (2) place the pathologic observations in a clinical context, (i.e., attempt to establish a clinicopathologic correlation whenever this is possible); (3) assess the relative importance of different types of neuropathology (e.g., opportunistic infection, tumor, human immunodeficiency virus [HIV] infection of the central nervous system [CNS]) in the production of neurologic syndromes in AIDS patients; and (4) briefly discuss recent virologic and molecular findings relevant to direct HIV infection of the brain. Of necessity, this chapter builds on previous work in our laboratory[1,2] and that of others, much of which has been reviewed in previous published comprehensive articles.[3-13] The bibliography will, therefore, emphasize papers that have been published since the completion of our earlier reviews,

though the findings described in certain early key articles will warrant reemphasis.

There is a substantial discrepancy in most series between the percentage of AIDS patients who have significant neurologic signs and symptoms during life, and the percentage in whom neuropathology is discovered at autopsy. The former figure is usually given as 25–30%, the latter as 50–85%. Between 10 and 30% of patients have neurologic dysfunction as the initial manifestation of AIDS or infection with HIV. Recent sporadic case reports and small series attest to the fact that a defined subset of patients presents with exclusively neurologic manifestations of AIDS (usually reflecting direct HIV infection of the brain) with none of the usual visceral or peripheral sequelae of the syndrome.[14] We do not yet know what long-term effects of HIV infection of the CNS are likely to appear, although given the apparently severe abnormalities (particularly of white matter) induced by acute infection, they might be expected to be devastating. Specific therapies for AIDS might also be anticipated to induce neuropathology, depending on the ability of agents to penetrate the blood-brain barrier (BBB). We have recently reported an example of Wernicke's encephalopathy that occurred in close temporal proximity to treatment with azidothymidine (Zidovudine, Burroughs Welcome, Research Triangle, North Carolina).[15]

Correlation between neuropathologic abnormalities and neurologic syndromes is poor in many cases. It appears that different types of CNS abnormality can induce similar neurologic syndromes. Even neuroradiologic techniques, refined as they are, are often ineffective in predicting the types of lesions to be expected when tissue is examined.[16-18] MRI (magnetic resonance image) scans appear to be more sensitive than CT (computerized tomographic) scans in detecting intracranial disease in AIDS patients. This makes the job of the neuropathologist the more important in providing feedback to clinicians on the histopathology of autopsy or biopsy material. The difficulty in establishing clinicopathologic correlations is probably multifactorial: Patients who are terminally ill, often with respiratory embarrassment, are unlikely to have a detailed neurologic examination or work-up; clinicians often seek a single etiology to explain neurologic signs and symptoms, whereas it is a common experience to find several types of lesion in the nervous system of AIDS patients, often encompassing both infectious and neoplastic disease.

The best established clinical syndrome specific to AIDS patients is the AIDS dementia complex (ADC) or AIDS encephalopathy, which results from direct HIV infection of the brain.[19-21] Even in this condition, there are frequently discrepancies between the clinical degree of dementia in a given patient and the evidence of cerebral injury when such individuals come to autopsy.[20] Rare and unusual neurologic syndromes are now sometimes attributed to HIV infection of the nervous system, and psychiatric sequelae of AIDS have been described.[22-24] Biochemical and serologic studies of cerebrospinal fluid (CSF) in neurologically ill patients frequently show non-

specific results, often precisely because of the patients' immunosuppressed state.[25] CSF antibodies to HIV are frequently detectable, indicating local synthesis, and can be present at an early stage of disease before clinical features of AIDS or ARC are apparent.[26-28]

The importance of meticulous autopsy examination of neural tissues in an effort to arrive at neuropathologic diagnoses cannot be overemphasized. There is often a discrepancy between gross findings (even at the time of brain cutting) and final microscopic diagnoses. We have frequently found significant microscopic lesions in grossly normal or minimally abnormal brains. Some of the data to be presented are the result of extensive systematic sampling of all AIDS brain and spinal cord tissues in our laboratory. In the case of unusual clinical syndromes, the neuropathologist is also wise to fix appropriate material for electron microscopy and snap freeze a portion of the tissue for possible DNA analysis and other investigations, depending on the interests of AIDS research personnel at the respective institution.

THE UCLA EXPERIENCE

The CNS was examined in 158 AIDS patients, including the spinal cord in over half of the cases. All autopsies were performed at the UCLA Center for the Health Sciences or the Wadsworth Veterans Administration Hospital, except for three brains referred to UCLA from primary care hospitals. Brains were fixed in 10% neutral buffered formalin for 1–2 weeks, cut under the supervision of a neuropathologist, and routinely sampled for microscopic evaluation (with extra sections submitted for grossly suspicious lesions). The patient's clinical chart (when available) and autopsy reports were reviewed for clinical and systemic manifestations of AIDS.

Only four patients in this series were female. Risk factors for AIDS included: homosexuality-109 (69%), bisexuality-18 (11%), intravenous drug abuse-15 (9%), blood transfusion therapy-5 (3%), heterosexual partner at risk for AIDS-5 (3%), and emigration from Haiti-1 (1%). The risk factors for AIDS were not known in 15 (9%) patients, while 14 (9%) individuals had multiple risk factors. The ages ranged from 24 to 65 years, with a mean of 41 years. Most patients were Caucasian (98), with 45 Blacks, 13 Hispanics, 1 Asian, and one patient of unknown racial origin. Patients survived from 1 to 35 months after AIDS was diagnosed (mean 7 months).

Signs and symptoms related to neurologic manifestations were uncommon at the time of the AIDS diagnosis, being noted in only 14 patients. However, 101 patients had clinical CNS manifestations prior to their death, including 62 patients in whom the process was severe (e.g., producing seizures, encephalopathy, meningitis, blindness, hemiparesis).

Table 1 summarizes important systemic manifestations of AIDS discovered clinically or at autopsy. In addition, 42 patients had a documented history of hepatitis, 37 had prior gonorrhea, and 36 had previous syphilis. Pneumonic infection due primarily to *Pneumocystis,* cytomegalovirus, or interstitial pneumonia was the immediate cause of death in the majority of patients.

Sixty-two brains had gross abnormalities. In 20 of these, the changes were relatively minimal (mild edema or atrophy, focal hemorrhage). However, the remaining brains showed more significant pathology, including 31 cases with abscesses, infarction or necrosis, 9 cases with diffuse meningeal opacification, and one case each with widespread parenchymal hemorrhages or bilateral subdural hematomas.

Table 2 summarizes the abnormalities seen in the central nervous system of AIDS

TABLE I
Systemic (Non-CNS) Manifestations Found Clinically or at Autopsy in 158 AIDS Patients

	Patients	
Pathologic Process	Number	Percentage
I: Infections		
Pneumocystis carinii	105	66
Cytomegalovirus	90	57
Candidiasis	84	53
Herpex simplex virus	37	23
Mycobacterium avium-intracellulare	36	23
Gram-positive bacterial pneumonia/sepsis	20	13
Cryptococcosis	19	12
Amebiasis	15	9
Hepatitis B	14	9
Cryptosporidiosis	13	8
Giardiasis	13	8
Herpes zoster	11	7
Gram-negative bacterial pneumonia/sepsis	7	4
Mycobacterium tuberculosis	5	3
Aspergillosis	4	3
Histoplasmosis	4	3
Mycoplasma pneumonia	3	2
II: Other		
Kaposi's sarcoma	64	41
Lymphoma	7	4
Nonbacterial thrombotic endocarditis	3	2

TABLE II
Summary of CNS Histopathologic Abnormalities in AIDS Patients at UCLA (n = 158)

| | Patients | |
Pathologic Process	Number	Percentage
I: *Microglial nodule encephalitis*	99	63
few, scattered	(63)	(40)
diffuse, marked	(36)	(23)
II: *Viral infections*		
Cytomegalovirus	27	17
Multinucleate HIV-type giant cells	16	10
Progressive multifocal leukoencephalopathy	8	5
III: *Fungal infections*		
Cryptococcus	13	8
Histoplasma	1	1
Aspergillus	1	1
IV: *Protozoal-Parasitic*		
Toxoplasma	12	8
V: *Bacterial*		
Mycobacterium avium-intracellulare	4	3
VI: *Neoplasms*		
Primary lymphoma	5	3
Secondary lymphoma	2	1
Primary lymphoma associated with lymphomatoid granulomatosis	2	1
Lymphomatoid granulomatosis	1	1
VII: *Vascular complications*		
Infarcts	18	11
Hemorrhage		
subdural	1	1
subarachnoid	8	5
intraparenchymal	6	4
Siderocalcinosis (calcific vasculopathy)	19	12
VIII: *White matter abnormalities*		
Central pontine myelinolysis	2	1
Focal pontine leukoencephalopathy	3	2
Vacuolar myelopathy	6	4
Miscellaneous	23	15
IX: *Other lesions*		
Anoxic-ischemic changes	9	6
Granular ependymitis	13	8
Bergmann gliosis, cerebellum	2	1
Parenchymal microcalcification	3	2
Alzheimer II astrocytes	12	8
Mild lymphoid infiltrate around vessels/within leptomeninges	18	11

patients in this series. The details of these findings and associated disease processes are subsequently discussed.

OPPORTUNISTIC VIRAL INFECTIONS

Two main groups of viruses dwarf all others in their importance as opportunistic pathogens within the nervous system of AIDS patients: The herpesviruses, especially cytomegalovirus (CMV) but also varicella or herpes zoster (HZV) and herpes simplex (HSV); and papovaviruses. The latter produce a single well defined syndrome — progressive multifocal leukoencephalopathy (PML), whereas the former viruses induce highly variable neuropathology in different patients; and different herpesviruses can be found in a single brain.[29]

CMV can cause a variety of morphologic CNS and peripheral nervous system (PNS) lesions.[2,29-34] Historically, it was the first pathogen to be associated with the microglial nodules (MGNs), commonly observed in brains from AIDS patients.[1,35] MGN encephalitis (Fig. 1) is still a controversial entity, though it appears that at least some examples (or some MGN's even within brains infected by CMV) result from HIV infection. In addition to MGNs, CMV can cause one or more of the following histologic lesions: (1) isolated inclusions within single cells, often in the middle of an MGN, (2) focal parenchymal necrosis with or without surrounding demyelination, (3) necrotizing ventriculo-encephalitis, (4) necrotizing radiculomyelitis, (5) meningo-encephalitis, and (6) choroid plexitis.[31] In the 28 cases we have encountered,[36] as in other series, the extent of neuropathology has been highly variable, ranging from scattered occasional inclusion-bearing cells that probably have not contributed to neurologic signs and symptoms to severe necrotizing

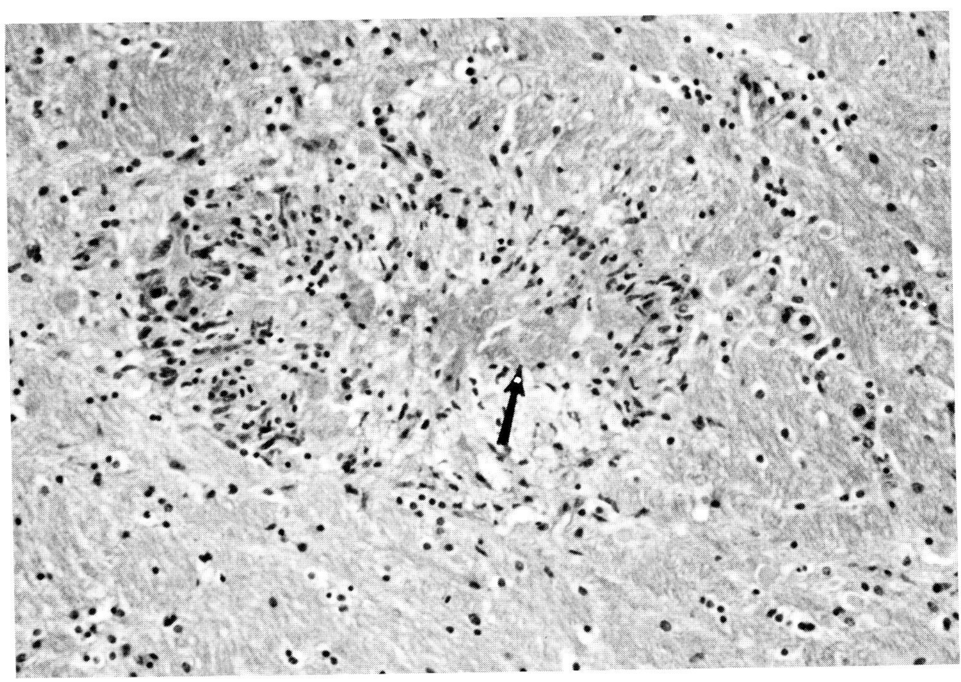

Figure 1. Microglial nodule (MGN) encephalitis. MGN in brainstem shows central region of necrosis (arrow) (H&E, original magnification ×180).

multifocal ventriculitis, encephalitis, and choroid plexitis that was the major cause of neurologic morbidity. A severe case of the latter is illustrated in Figure 2.

The affinity of CMV for ependymal surfaces and the tendency for the virus to spread in a ventriculofugal fashion have been documented by immunocytochemical and hybridization techniques,[37] and are particularly well illustrated by this example. There is moderate dilatation of the lateral ventricles, which may in part represent an ex vacuo phenomenon. However, the ependymal lining of the cerebral aqueduct in the midbrain was absent, the periaqueductal tissues were very hemorrhagic, and microscopically, heavily involved by necrotizing CMV encephalitis (Fig. 3), suggesting that an element of obstructive hydrocephalus may have been operative in this patient. CSF secretion, flow, and dynamics would also be hampered by the presence of CMV within epithelial cells of the choroid plexus. This component of the overall CMV infection was, however, minimal and we have consistently found this — the choroid plexus showing focal CMV inclusions surrounded by a mononuclear cell inflammatory infiltrate, which is never overwhelming. CMV probably enters the brain via the blood and then is disseminated by the CSF before further movement into brain parenchyma.[31]

The extent to which CMV can cause CNS demyelination in the absence of overt tissue necrosis has not been quantitatively assessed, though the association has been suggested.[38] It is clear, however, that CMV can produce a syndrome clinically identical to the Guillain-Barré polyneuropathy (GBP), a rapidly ascending polyradiculoneuropathy. The pathologic correlate of this is a severe radiculomyelitis and predominantly spinal meningitis; CMV inclusions are readily identified within the resultant inflammatory infiltrate.[31,39,40] In one such case we encountered, the radiculomyelitis had produced necrosis of the spinal nerve roots (Fig. 4), and partly or totally occluded blood vessels with inflamed walls could be identi-

fied within the subarachnoid space near foci of tissue injury, reflecting the previously described affinity of CMV for endothelium.[41,42] The role, if any, that CMV has in the induction of peripheral neuropathy in AIDS is not yet known, but the association between CMV infection and polyneuritis has been made in other clinical settings.[43]

Occasionally, reports describe neurologic syndromes caused by HSV and HZV, including radiculitis caused by the latter.[7,44] HSV Type II has been cultured from brain biopsies of affected patients, and an appropriate immunofluorescent antibody technique has demonstrated viral antigen within the CNS.[45] HSV Type II has also been shown to cause a progressive necrotizing myelopathy.[46] A well documented case of HZV encephalomyelitis showed multifocal areas of necrosis and demyelination in the brain — lesions initially suggestive of PML.[47] Such cases demonstrate the significance of careful histologic examination of such autopsy material and the valuable contributions in arriving at a final diagnosis of ancillary diagnostic techniques (e.g., Southern blot analysis of extracted cerebral DNA). No specific disorder resulting from Epstein-Barr virus (EBV) infection of nervous tissue has been found, though it has been implicated in the pathogenesis of CNS lymphoma, either in the presence or absence of AIDS.[48,49]

PML, caused by papovaviruses, commonly occurs in AIDS patients, though it is seen less often than CMV infection of the brain. Gross and microscopic appearances of the brain are similar to those of brains affected by PML in other clinical settings,[1,2,50-52] except that a particularly severe, widespread, and necrotizing type of pathology is often observed (Fig. 5). Microscopically, no unique features are encountered, and there is no evidence that systemic HIV infection induces a more profound or widespread infection by papovavirus (e.g., JC virus) without a pathologic correlate in AIDS brains.[53] Papovavirus is demonstrated in oligodendrocytes and transformed astro-

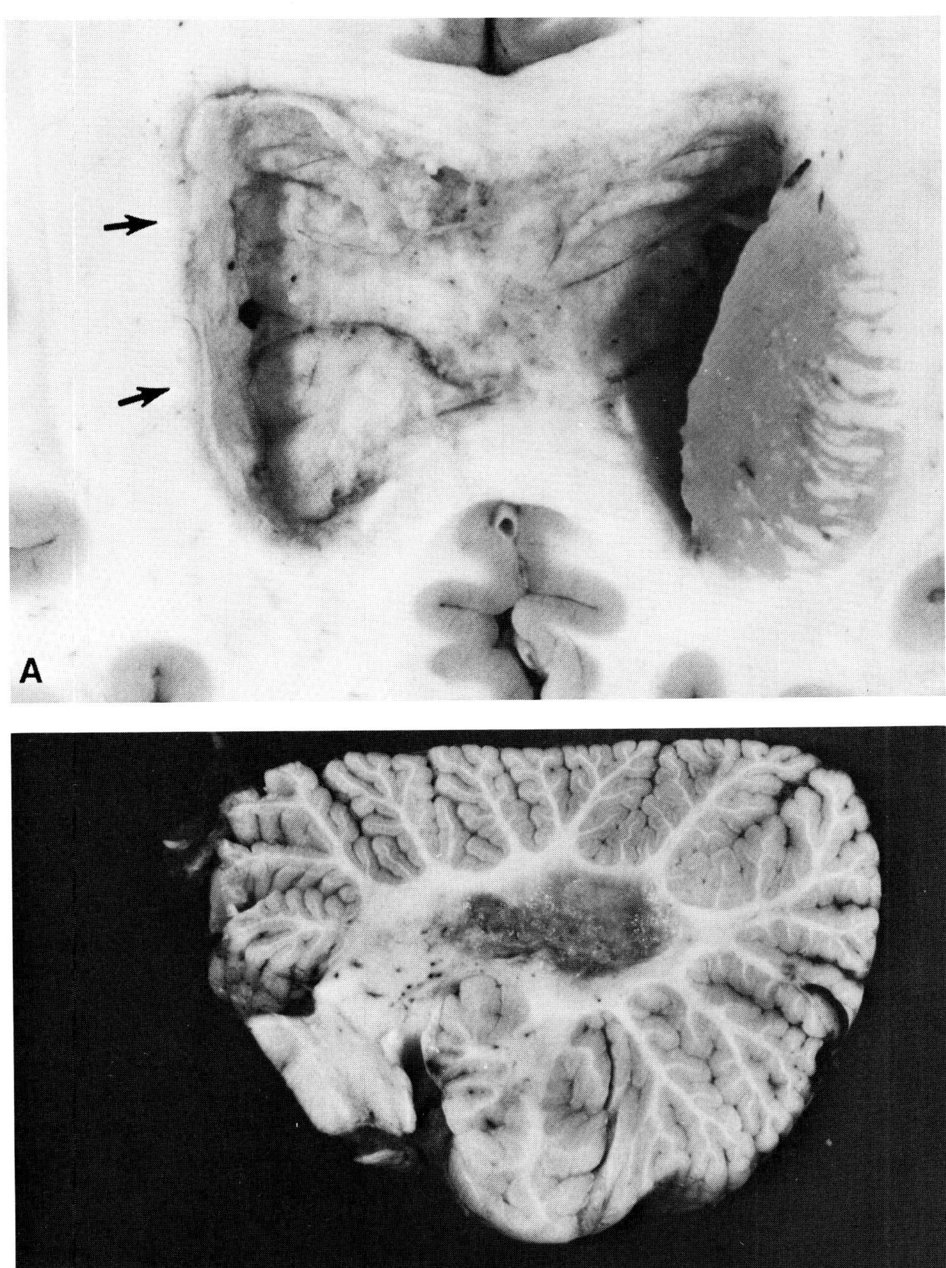

Figure 2. (A) CMV ventriculitis. Coronal section through frontal lobes of fixed brain. Note ventricular dilatation and shaggy irregular material that lines ependymal surface and extends into periventricular white matter (arrows). (B) CMV encephalitis. Parasagittal section of cerebellar hemisphere. Dentate nucleus and central white matter show poorly demarcated gelatinous lesion resulting from necrotizing CMV encephalitis. Other cerebellar hemisphere contained a similar lesion identically located.

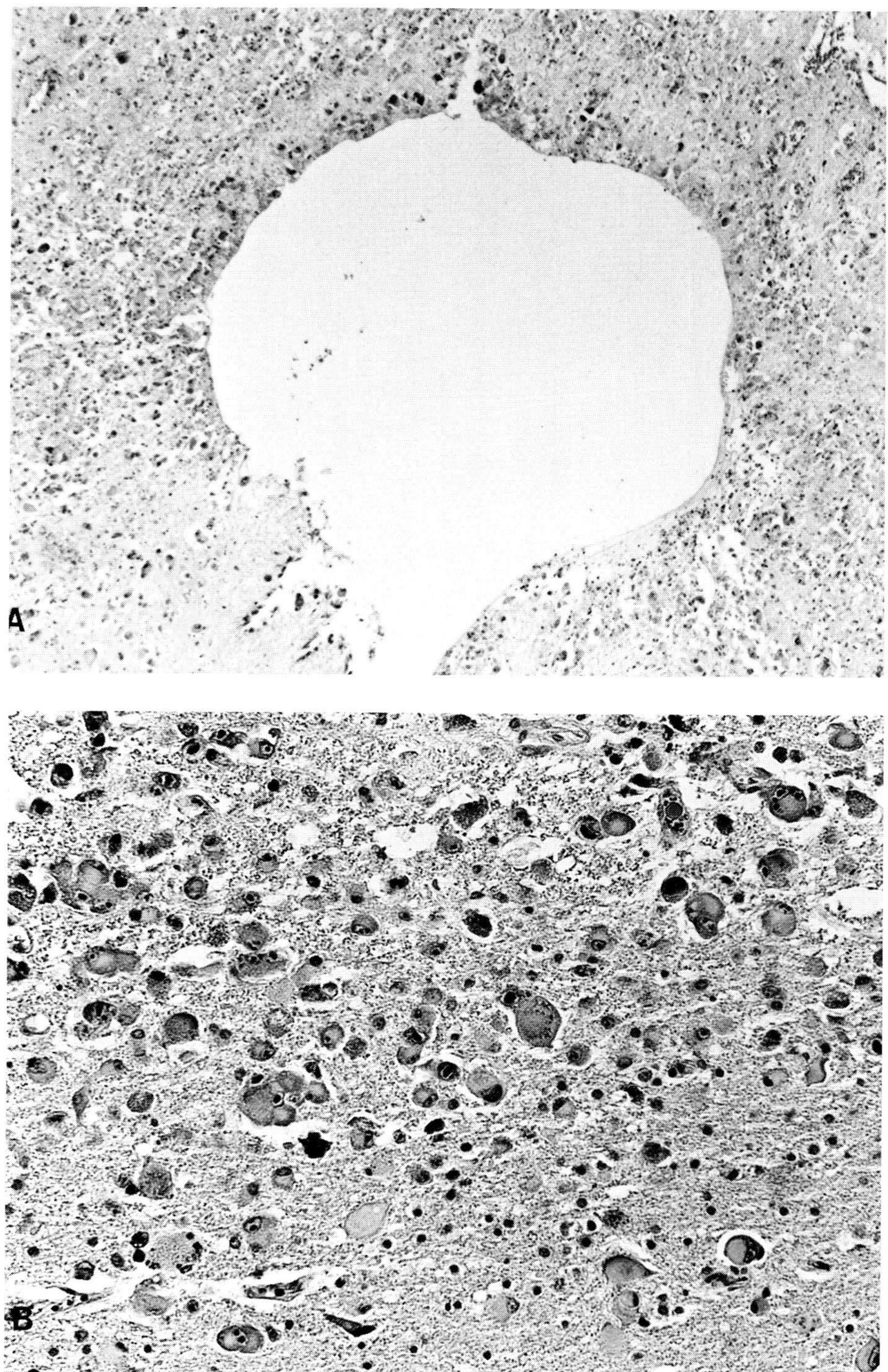

Figure 3. (A) CMV ependymitis and periaqueductal encephalitis. Low power view of cerebral aqueduct from same patient as illustrated in Figure 2A. There is total loss of ependyma with surrounding necrosis and slight inflammatory infiltrate, within which typical CMV inclusions were identified (H&E, original magnification ×75). (B) CMV encephalitis. Typical field shows numerous cytomegalic cells with intranuclear and cytoplasmic inclusions (H&E, original magnification ×190).

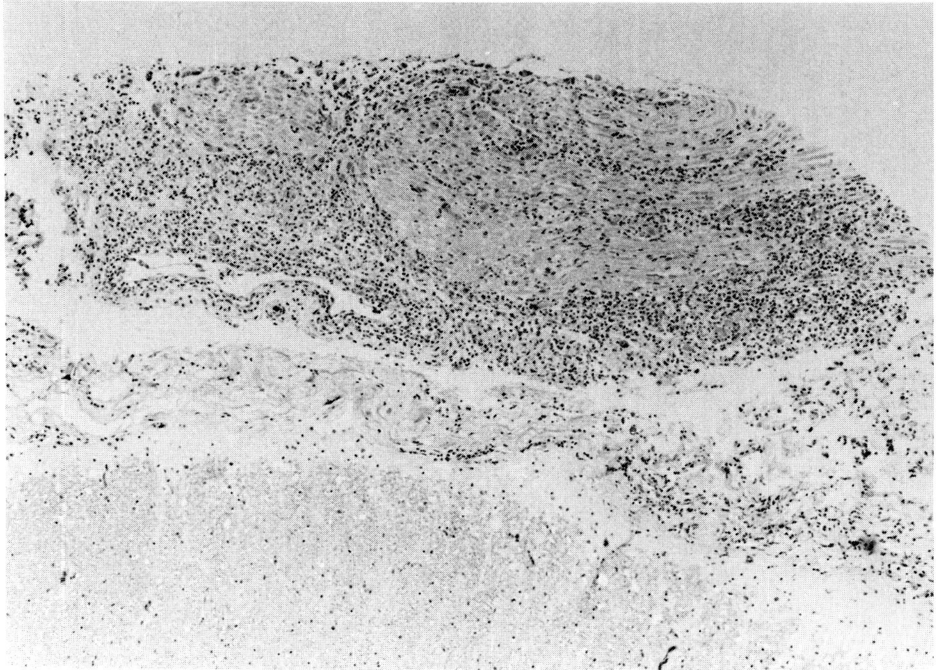

Figure 4. CMV radiculitis in a patient with a history of ascending polyradiculoneuropathy. Spinal nerve root shows acute and chronic inflammation enveloping the root. CMV inclusions were easily identified within and around roots, portions of which demonstrated frank necrosis. Spinal cord is seen in lower portion of micrograph (H&E, original magnification ×80).

cytes only.[54] The affected white matter shows demyelination or necrosis with abundant lipid-laden histiocytes, atypical astrocytes, and amphophilic intranuclear inclusions (Fig. 6); the cortex is usually spared. The diagnosis can be made from an adequate brain biopsy.[55,56] Papovavirus virions can usually be demonstrated ultrastructurally and by immunocytochemical and in situ hybridization techniques[53,57] that allow for more definitive assignment of etiology of the white matter lesions.

As is the situation with most other neurologic syndromes observed in AIDS patients, PML has been noted in the absence of other clinical manifestations of immunodeficiency in HIV seropositive patients.[58] In the largest reported series,[59] death occurred 10 days to 18 months after symptom onset, but occasional patients were alive as long as 23 months after clinical presentation and, re-markably, two patients had experienced significant clinical improvement without therapy. Various therapies were felt to be ineffective in amelioration of neurologic symptoms.

FUNGAL INFECTIONS

Fungal organisms are among the most common opportunistic agents identified in AIDS patients at neuropathologic examination. The fungal infection encountered most frequently in published series,[60,61] including our own,[2] is due to *Cryptococcus neoformans*. Infection by *Cryptococcus* may be limited to the central nervous system, or it can be part of a disseminated systemic infection. The lung is the usual site of primary infestation.

Grossly, brains infected with *Crypto-*

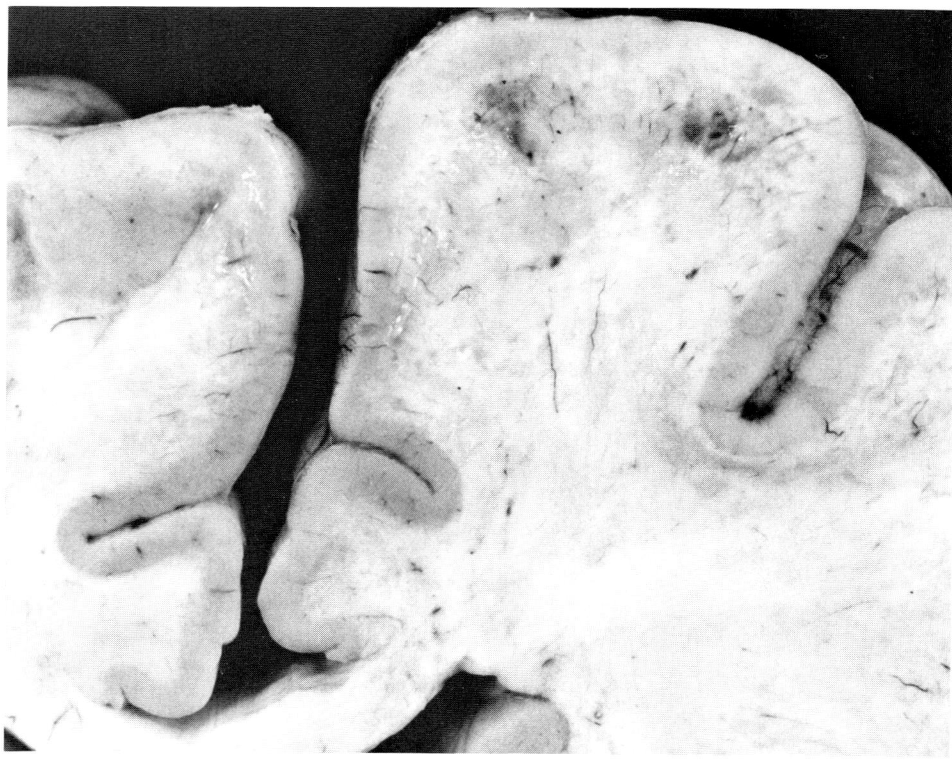

Figure 5. Progressive multifocal leukoencephalopathy (PML). Coronal section of cerebral hemispheres shows focally gelatinous, discolored white matter within centrum semiovale bilaterally. Virtually no normal white matter remains, but cortex is relatively preserved.

coccus show thickened, somewhat opacified meninges, having a slimy quality on cut section. Histologically, the meninges are usually diffusely involved, with extension of the organisms along (and expansion of) perivascular (Virchow-Robin) spaces into the brain parenchyma. Proliferation of the organism within the brain results in a grossly spongy or cribriform appearance (Fig. 7). Though sometimes referred to as cryptococcomas, these lesions are not surrounded by a capsule. The organisms are of variable sizes, from 3–15 μm, and have a thick mucicarmine-positive mucopolysaccharide capsule. They are characterized by a budding form with a thin tapered neck. A variable inflammatory reaction to cryptococcus is seen. In most patients the inflammation is minimal to absent, however, occasionally, a marked

histiocytic response is seen with formation of multinucleate histiocytic giant cells bearing a superficial resemblance to HIV giant cells (see below), but phagocytosis of fungi is easily seen (Fig. 8). Despite an intermittent response to antifungal chemotherapy, relapsing infection is common and patients frequently die of their cryptococcal infection.

We have encountered a single case of meningoencephalitis secondary to *Histoplasma capsulatum*.[2] Numerous poorly formed granulomata were noted throughout the central nervous system of this patient. The organisms are characteristically small (1–5 μm) and round to oval in shape. A methenamine silver stain greatly aids in their visualization. While histoplasma infection appears to be rather uncommon in

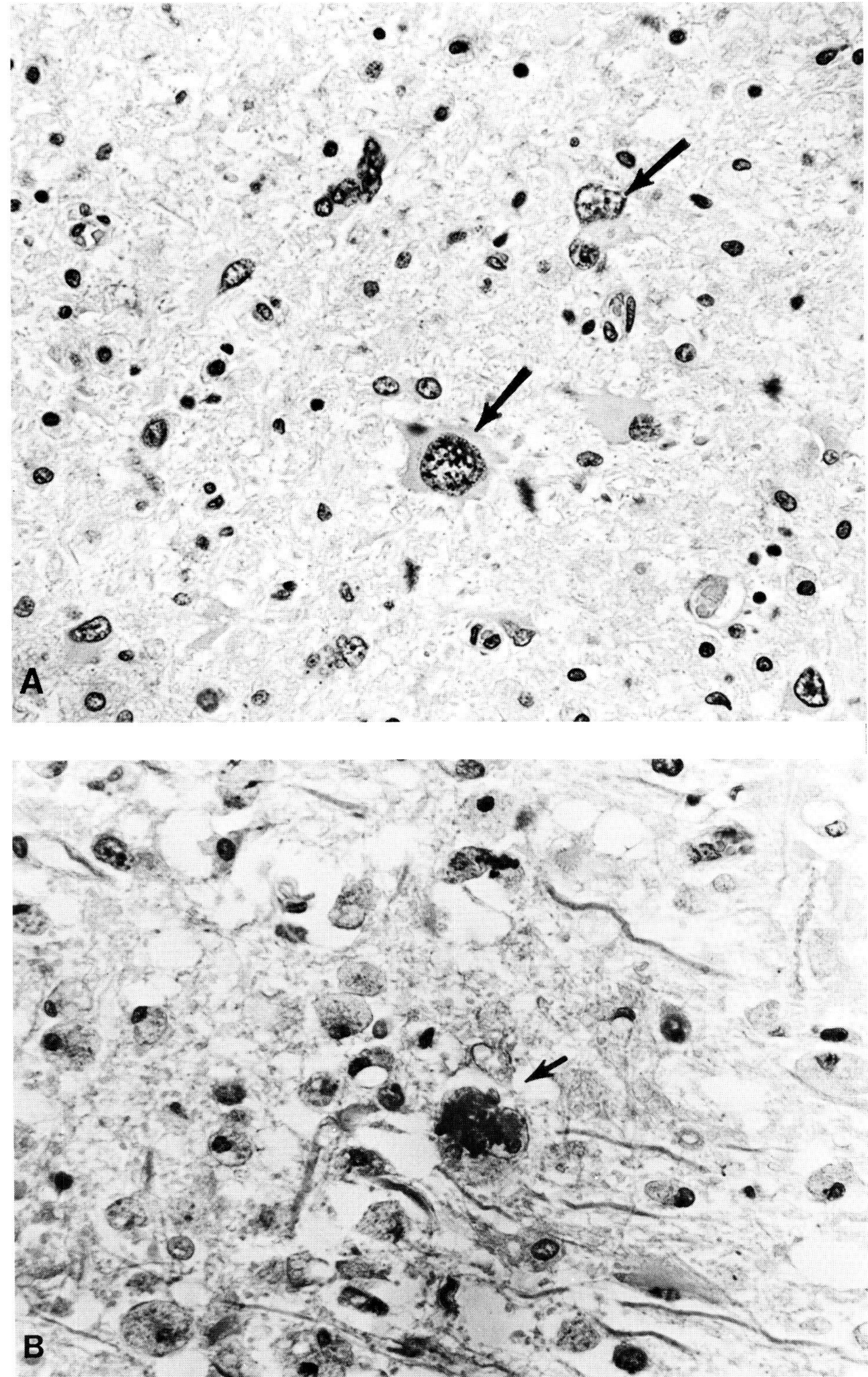

Figure 6. Histologic features of PML (amphophilic oligodendroglial inclusions not illustrated). (A) Spongy change and astrogliosis within white matter, with atypical astrocytes with bizarre nuclei (arrows) (H&E, original magnification ×325). (B) Extensive tissue destruction with foamy histiocytes. A single atypical mitotic figure (arrow) is present (H&E, original magnification ×300).

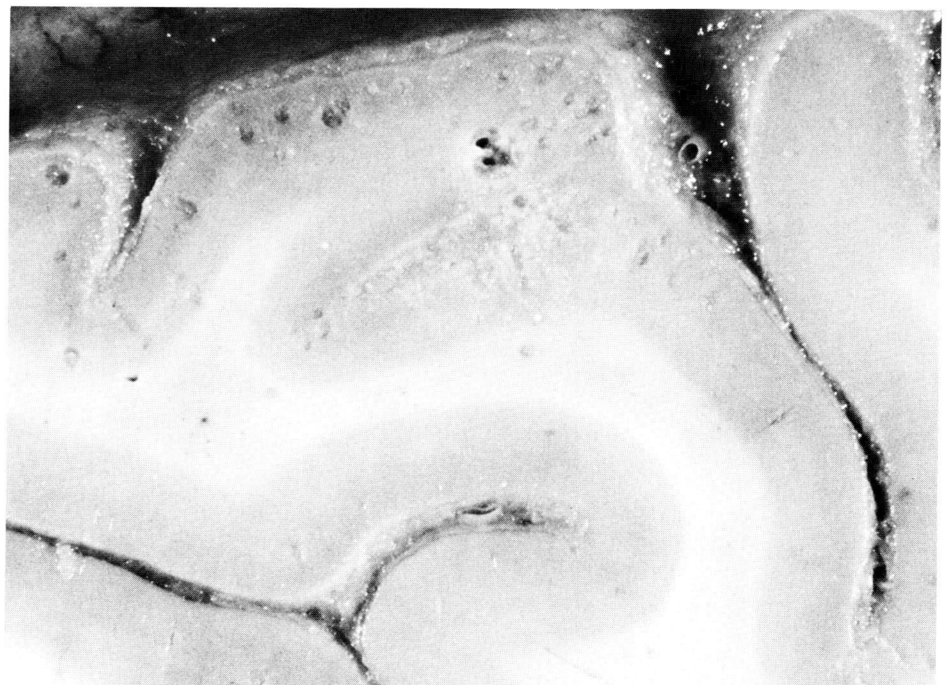

Figure 7. Cryptococcosis. Magnified view of coronal section of cerebral hemisphere shows cyst-like lesions (primarily in cortex, but a few in white matter). Subarachnoid space is thickened with gelatinous material.

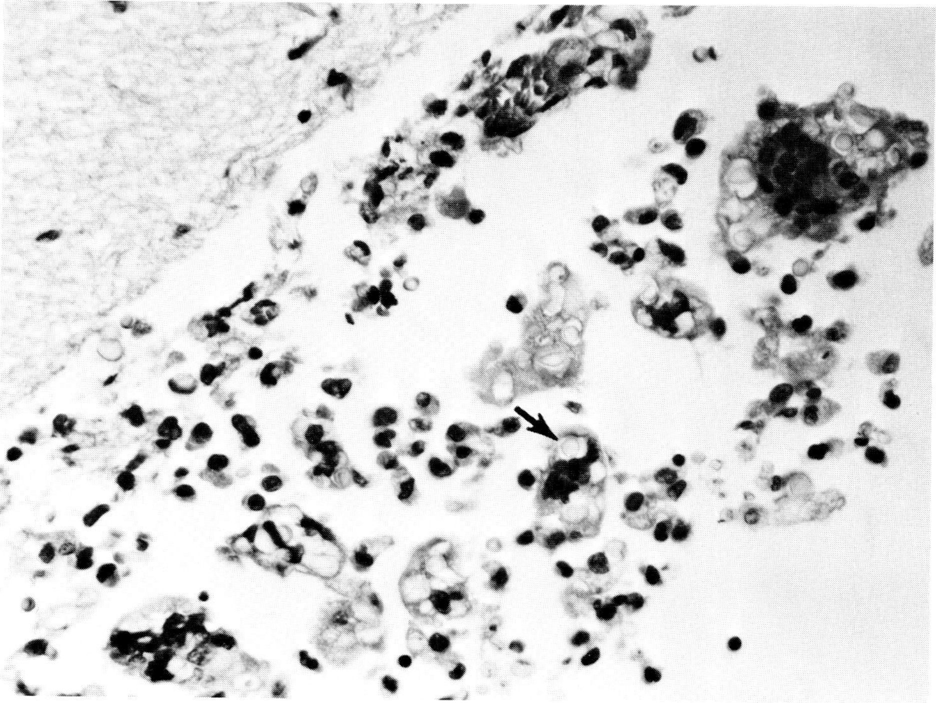

Figure 8. Encapsulated cryptococcal organisms in subarachnoid space may be recognized as single units or within clusters. Multinucleate giant cells (e.g. arrow) show organisms within their cytoplasm (H&E, original magnification ×300).

AIDS patients, reports of progressive disseminated histoplasmosis in the southeastern United States may result in more frequently encountered cases in the near future.[62,63]

Despite the prevalence of *Coccidioides immitis* in the southwestern United States, this infection has not significantly increased within the central nervous system of AIDS patients, and very few cases have been reported.[2,64] The large spherules are easily identified in routine sections.

Infections with *Candida* or *Aspergillus* species may result in a meningoencephalitis or abscess formation, but are fairly uncommon in AIDS patients. Only one of our patients had an *Aspergillus* infection, a meningeal aspergilloma. Likewise, *Blastomyces dermatitidis* infections are also uncommon.

PARASITIC AND BACTERIAL INFECTIONS

The most important parasitic infection of the nervous system in AIDS patients is caused by *Toxoplasma gondii*.[2,65,66] It is often associated with considerable tissue necrosis (Fig. 9), localized vasculitis or periarteritis, and a variable, but sometimes prominent, inflammatory reaction (Fig. 10)—one often out of proportion to the number of organisms identified.[67] In CNS infection in AIDS patients, bradyzoites are often encountered without any tissue reaction.

In general, brain lesions can be identified as necrotizing, organizing, or chronic.[65] Scattered free tachyzoites in the parenchyma indicate active infection, whereas encysted organisms are seen in the quiescent state. Clinically, the diagnosis can be suspected on the basis of imaging studies. However, serologic results on blood and CSF can be misleading; *Toxoplasma* is rarely cultured from CSF, and since the treatment for cerebral toxoplasmosis is not risk-free, brain biopsy is often performed to confirm the diagnosis. The neuropathologist must then search diligently for toxoplasma cysts, which

can be identified on hematoxylin and eosin or Giemsa stained sections. An immunocytochemical technique is available to confirm the presence of toxoplasma bradyzoites[68] and electron microscopy of tissue has been advocated as a precise and rapid method of diagnosis.[69] Not surprisingly, cerebral toxoplasmosis occurs concurrently with other CNS infections in some AIDS patients.[70,71]

Other parasitic infections of the CNS or PNS are rare in AIDS. *Pneumocystis carinii* has never been definitely identified in either locus to our knowledge. *Acanthamoeba castellanii* infection of muscle[72] has been found in one patient with disseminated infection, and an example of fatal suppurative hemorrhagic meningoencephalitis produced by *Acanthamoeba culbertsoni* has been documented.[73] In the latter case, typical trophozoites (approximately 20 μm in diameter) were found throughout necrotic foci and were stained with periodic acid-Schiff and silver methenamine stains. The presence of organisms was also confirmed by culture and inoculation of appropriate tissue culture material (derived from necropsy CNS tissue) into the brains of mice. An example of meningoencephalitis caused by achloric algae *(Prototheca)* has recently been presented.[74,75]

Bacterial infections of the nervous system (e.g., causing meningitis) do not constitute a major clinical problem in patients with systemic HIV infection.[2,76] In a study of 200 AIDS patients, Eng et al.[77] found that several subjects had fever without known sites of infection. Identifiable pathogens isolated from blood cultures included a variety of microorganisms, most notably coagulase negative *Staphylococcus*, *Salmonella* species, and *Cryptococcus neoformans*. *Mycobacterium avium-intracellulare* (MAI) was cultured from the blood of one patient and has been detected in a similar fashion from several AIDS patients at UCLA. Normally, when tissues are injured a polymorphonuclear leukocytic reaction is evoked by chemotaxic signals. In AIDS, tissue damage is often associated with a dampened seg-

Vinters et al.

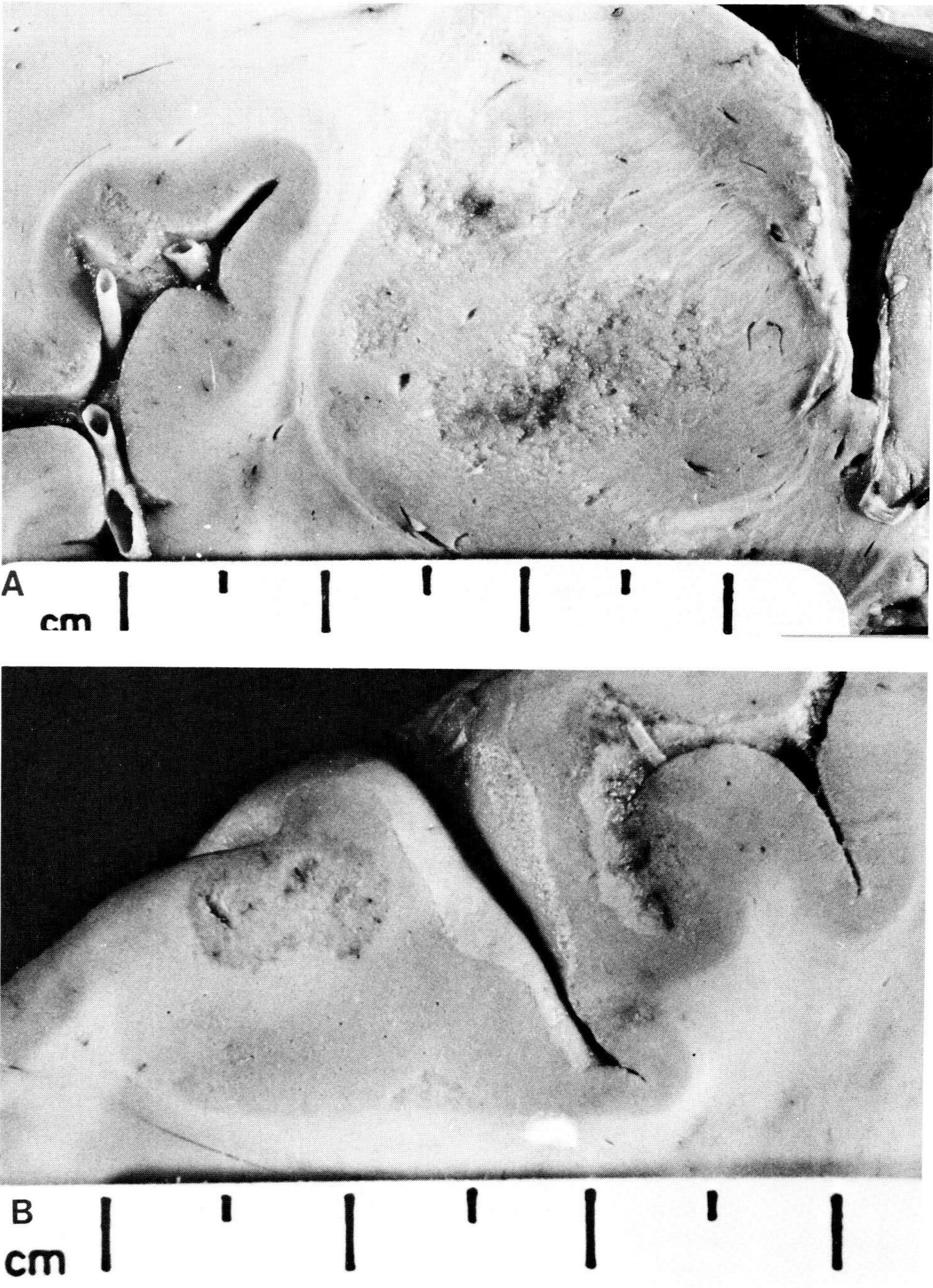

Figure 9. Toxoplasma encephalitis. (A) Extensive patchy ill-defined necrosis of putamen encroaches on the lateral margin of anterior limb of internal capsule. (B) Abscesses involve cerebral cortex and extend into subarachnoid space.

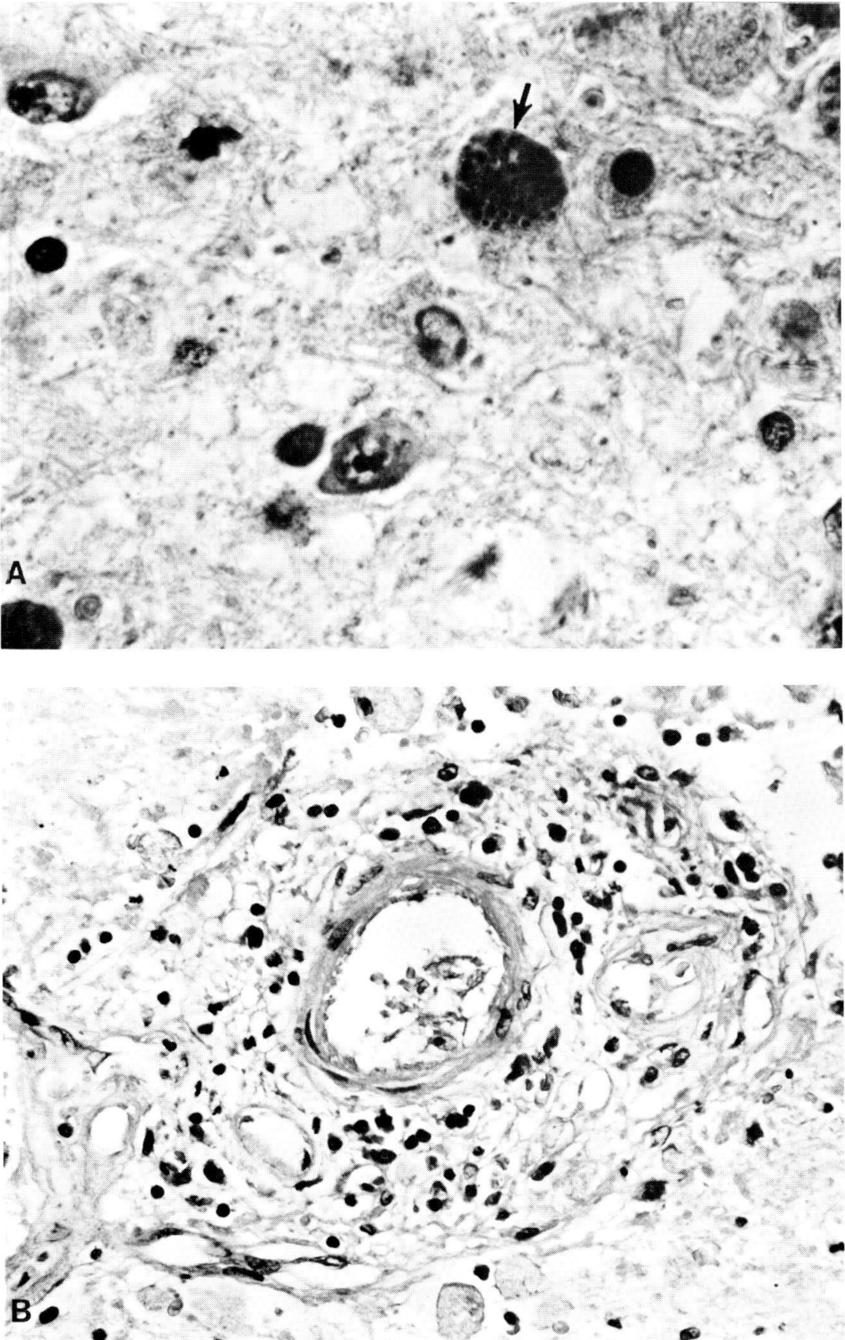

Figure 10. Toxoplasma encephalitis. (A) Toxoplasma bradyzoite (arrow) has sparse surrounding reaction (H&E, original magnification ×750). (B) Subarachnoid space adjacent to cerebellum severely involved by toxoplasmosis. No microorganisms seen in this field. Perivascular mononuclear cell infiltrate, mild fibrosis and occasional histiocytes within necrotic material are present (H&E, original magnification ×300).

mented leukocytic reaction. This seems curious since the AIDS literature infrequently mentions neutropenia as a feature, although cytopenias are often seen. Neutrophil counts in AIDS appear to be at least 500/ mm^3 and often range between 1000–2000/ mm^3, which may be sufficient to successfully counter bacteremia.[77]

Mycobacteria are occasionally present in the CNS, and include MAI and *Mycobacterium tuberculosis* (TB). MAI occurs less commonly in the CNS than in other organs,[78] and, when present, numerous MAI organisms are packed into collections of macrophages, resembling the reaction seen in lepromatous leprosy. The lesions lack giant cells or inflammation, which would provide a clue to the presence of acid-fast bacteria. The examples we have previously described were all discovered by essentially random staining of brain sections with an acid-fast technique, especially at sites of disruption of the BBB. MAI has been isolated at post mortem examination from numerous body sites, including (in decreasing order of frequency), the brain, muscle, peripheral nerve, and eye.[79] The associated histopathology would suggest that MAI infection of neural tissues is not a significant cause of morbidity. AIDS patients with MAI complex infection show poor response when treated with two or more antimycobacterial drugs.[79] Tuberculosis in the brains of AIDS or ARC patients is relatively rare but has presented as leptomeningitis, multiple cerebral abscesses, and tuberculomas.[80]

Listeria monocytogenes behaves like an intracellular parasite and is infectious primarily in individuals whose cell-mediated immunity is impaired. Why then is an infection with this organism infrequently seen in AIDS patients, where all aspects of cell-mediated immunity are severely compromised?[81,82] Very rare examples of *Listeria* meningitis have been described.[83] An example of Whipple's disease of the brain in an AIDS patient has been documented.[84] Considering the large number of AIDS patients

with a past history of venereal disease (including syphillis), manifestations of treponemal infection of the nervous system are surprisingly rare.[85]

CENTRAL NERVOUS SYSTEM NEOPLASMS

A markedly increased incidence of non-Hodgkin's lymphoma in AIDS patients has been identified.[2,86–91] Extranodal involvement is common, with lymphomatous lesions frequently affecting the central nervous system. Many lymphomas involve only the central nervous system, and while occasionally symptomatic, they are often incidental autopsy findings (i.e. they are clinically unsuspected). These lesions are primarily intraparenchymal, although they may extend to, and involve, the leptomeninges. Occasionally, the CNS is secondarily involved by a systemic lymphoma. These usually present as diffuse subarachnoid lesions with associated invasion of the parenchyma.[2]

While brains with primary CNS lymphoma are often grossly normal, occasionally, large destructive tumorous masses are noted (Fig. 11). These lesions are soft and fleshy tan, and frequently associated with extensive necrosis. The neoplastic lymphoid cells are primarily angiocentric in location, with prominent infiltration of the brain parenchyma seen in larger tumors (Fig. 12). In AIDS patients, lymphomas are primarily of B-cell lineage, and mainly intermediate to high grade lesions (frequently immunoblastic or Burkitt-like).[88,90] Immune phenotyping has shown cells to have monoclonal lambda or kappa light chains, IgG heavy chain, and other B-cell surface antigens (e.g. LN-1).[89]

Kaposi's sarcoma is an extremely common neoplasm among AIDS patients, afflicting approximately 30% of the population at risk (especially homosexual men).[2] The disease is frequently of multifocal pre-

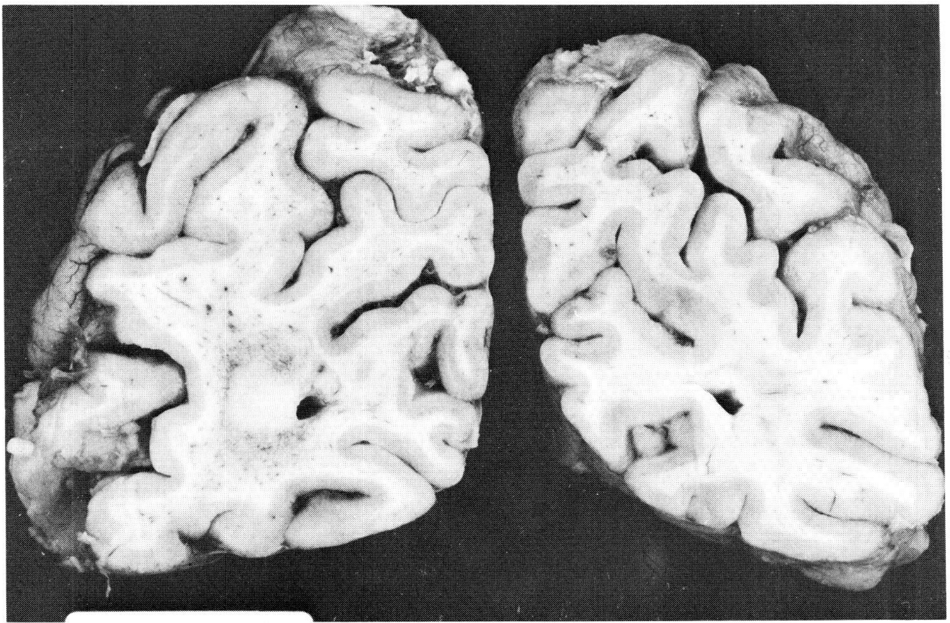

Figure 11. Cerebral lymphoma. Discolored region of white matter with hyperemic margin is seen adjacent to left lateral ventricle within parietal lobe.

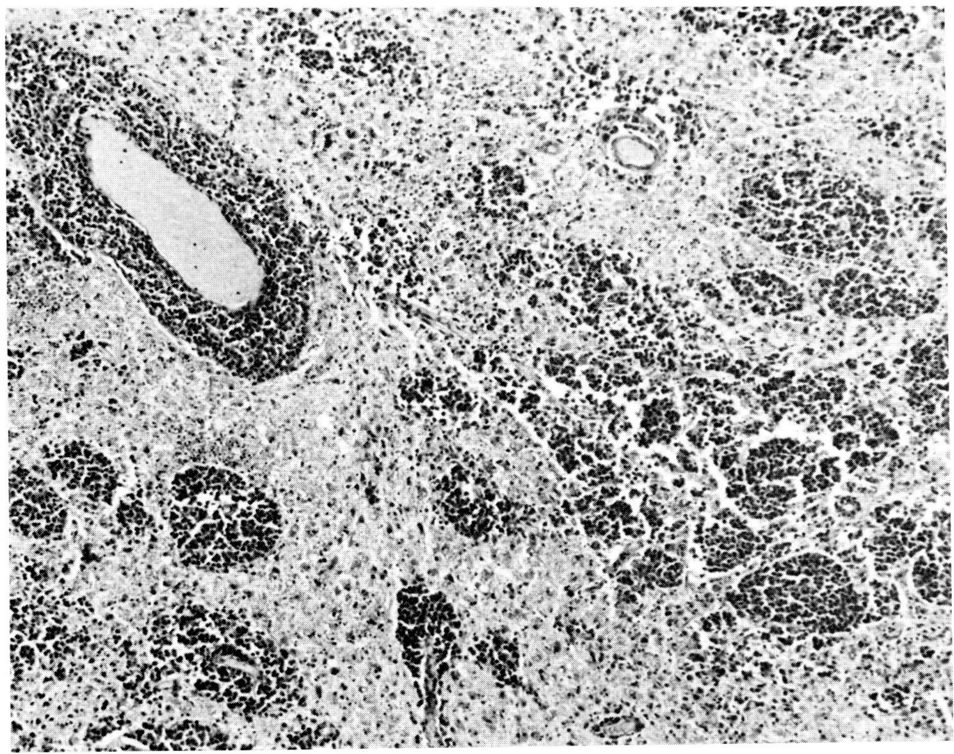

Figure 12. Cerebral lymphoma. Characteristic atypical mononuclear (lymphoid) infiltrate is angiocentric but extends into surrounding parenchyma, which shows reactive change, including astrocytic gliosis (H&E, original magnification ×76).

sentation, involving numerous sites in the skin, lymph nodes, gastrointestinal tract, and lungs. Despite this very high incidence, intracranial Kaposi's sarcoma is an extremely uncommon lesion in AIDS, and we have not yet encountered a case. The rarity of CNS metastasis, some postulate, is perhaps due to the hypothesized origin of this neoplasm. Many believe the stem cell is endothelial (possibly lymphatic endothelium); since the brain lacks lymphatic drainage, one would not expect this multifocal neoplasm to afflict this organ. Hence, the paucity of CNS Kaposi's sarcoma is perhaps not unexpected. The few reported cases of Kaposi's sarcoma involving the brain likely represent metastatic lesions from aggressive primary neoplasms elsewhere.[2]

Lymphomatoid granulomatosis is a disease of unknown etiology. While multiple organ involvement is usual, and the lung is generally involved, the process may occasionally affect only the central nervous system.[92,93] Lymphomatoid granulomatosis is characterized by a mixed atypical lymphoreticular infiltrate comprised of histiocytes, lymphocytes, atypical mononuclear cells and plasma cells. Like malignant lymphoma, the process is angiocentric, with significant thickening of blood vessel walls. The process is, however, also angiodestructive, with characteristic fibrinoid necrosis, and thrombosis of the lumen, a feature required for absolute characterization of the process. Many patients with lymphomatoid granulomatosis will ultimately develop malignant lymphoma before death. We have encountered three patients who had lymphomatoid granulomatosis confined to the central nervous system. In one patient, the process was very focal and involved only the deep grey matter.[1] In the two additional patients, the process was much more generalized involving large portions of the cerebral hemispheres. The necrotizing lesions of lymphomatoid granulomatosis gradually merged with high grade (immunoblastic) non-Hodgkin's lymphomas in both individuals.

VASCULAR COMPLICATIONS

Vascular complications that affect the nervous system in AIDS patients constitute a heterogeneous group and have been thus perhaps the most difficult to study systematically. Hemorrhages into one or another intracranial compartment are common, often reflecting disseminated intravascular coagulation or thrombocytopenia.[2] Anoxic-ischemic lesions or small bland infarcts are frequently encountered because respiratory compromise and hypotensive episodes are such common clinical problems in this critically ill patient population. Larger infarcts may be caused by emboli from nonbacterial thrombotic endocarditis, and these are sometimes fatal.[2,94]

Rare instances of vasculitis, not always clearly affecting the nervous system, are seen in AIDS patients. One example of leukocytoclastic vasculitis has been presented.[95] Cerebral granulomatous angiitis affecting large arteries was found in one patient from whose CNS and CSF HIV was isolated.[96] An AIDS patient with amaurosis fugax was found to have a severe eosinophilic vasculitis on temporal artery biopsy.[97] We have encountered a patient with ARC who developed a rapidly ascending polyradiculoneuropathy, died within 48 hours of clinical presentation, and at necropsy was shown to have necrotizing (small vessel) vasculitis (with resultant hemorrhagic necrosis) involving primarily the spinal cord and cauda equina, although there was no obvious etiology for the angiitis.[98] Since HIV has been localized to microvascular endothelium within the CNS,[99] one might postulate that the retrovirus itself, or a peculiar host response to its presence within the blood vessel wall, results in the inflammation, though this is speculative. As mentioned above, herpes viruses, especially CMV and HZV, are observed to cause severe, large or small vessel angiitis with resultant extensive brain necrosis in non-AIDS patients.[100,101] There is reason to expect that this might also occur in AIDS. Well documented examples of this phenomenon have been rare, however.

Pronounced intimal proliferation (by smooth muscle cells and fibroblasts), without inflammation within leptomeningeal arteries has been described in a few AIDS patients.[102] All of the brains had associated cerebral parenchymal infarcts of varying ages. The affected vessels showed no evidence of inflammation or HIV type giant cells, and stains for microorganisms were negative, but the possibility that the vascular change might be related to primary HIV infection of the brain was raised.

One must also keep in mind that a significant proportion of patients with AIDS have a history of intravenous abuse of recreational drugs, and thus are also prone to the vasculitides that can complicate drug abuse.[103,104]

A microvascular lesion often noted in the brains of AIDS patients is described as siderocalcinosis or ferruginization. Microscopically, it consists of metal deposition within the walls of capillaries and small arteries (usually branches of the lenticulostriate arteries) in the basal ganglia and is less often seen in the deep cerebellar nuclei.[2] The microvascular change does not seem to affect integrity of the surrounding brain parenchyma. Although anecdotal evidence suggests that this vascular calcification occurs with greater frequency in AIDS patients than in age-matched controls, a systematic study to confirm this has not been carried out. An identical lesion is seen in several other clinical settings.[105,106] The vascular calcification or calcific vasculopathy tends to be particularly prominent, and often associated with parenchymal calcium deposits in the basal ganglia of infants and children with AIDS.[107]

ABNORMALITIES OF WHITE MATTER (INCLUDING SPINAL CORD)

In a previous paper,[2] we made a rudimentary attempt to classify the various lesions of white matter tracts that are found within the CNS of AIDS patients. A subset of these various leukoencephalopathies is clearly related to opportunistic viral infections, most commonly by papovaviruses, CMV, or HZV. One very rare entity, described as progressive diffuse leukoencephalopathy (PDL) has been tentatively linked to infection of the brain by either papovavirus or HIV.[108] In PDL, there is multifocal, severe, occasionally symmetrical necrosis of long white matter tracts (e.g. the internal capsules) with calcification and reactive astrogliosis, although typical papovavirus intranuclear inclusions are not necessarily present. The clinical correlate of this appears to be a rapidly progressive dementia with spasticity and hyperreflexia. The single case we have encountered also showed extensive MGN and CMV encephalitis throughout the central neuraxis, as well as HIV type giant cells (see below).[109] Other similar forms of long tract degeneration have been described, also without proof as to the etiology.[110]

Since this classification was presented, a fairly definite association has been made between direct HIV infection of brain and a subcortical leukoencephalopathy of variable severity, the clinical correlate of which has been termed the AIDS dementia complex (ADC).[19,20] It is still not certain that direct HIV infection of CNS causes all examples of the commonly observed regions of poorly demarcated demyelination and gliosis in AIDS brains. CMV has also been implicated as a cause of similar structural abnormalities within subcortical white matter.[38]

One of the best characterized abnormalities of white matter in patients with AIDS is a vacuolar myelopathy that pathologically is very similar to subacute combined degeneration of the spinal cord, i.e., with prominent vacuolization and degeneration (caused by both axon and myelin loss) in the lateral corticospinal tracts and dorsal columns.[111,112] This has a well defined clinical correlate and has been seen in up to 25% of AIDS patients in one series, though the frequency in our material has been substan-

tially lower. The suggestion that the vacuolar myelopathy is caused by a neurotropic
form of HIV that infects the spinal cord has
been disputed.[113] Many patients with this
type of myelopathy have dementia and
MGN encephalitis. A histologically similar
vacuolar encephalopathy has been described
in some AIDS patients.[114]

We have described a lesion of the pons
(focal pontine leukoencephalopathy, [FPL])
that was initially found in two patients with
AIDS and has subsequently been seen in
patients immunosuppressed for other reasons (Fig. 13).[115] The pathology shows multifocal areas of vacuolization, axon injury
with swelling (i.e., neuroaxonal spheroids),
and focally prominent calcification within
the basis pontis, in particular the pontocere-
bellar fibers. This lesion has been described
in other clinical settings (e.g., cancer pa-

tients treated with chemotherapy and CNS
radiotherapy)[116,117] and is often not confined
to the pons (i.e., microscopically similar foci
are noted in white matter tracts throughout
the brain e.g., the internal capsules). The
clinical common denominator in most cases
has been some form of immunosuppression.
Since our initial report, we have found
FPL in a patient with lymphoma and a
woman with the Shwachman-Diamond
syndrome.[118]

The reasons why this form of leukoencephalopathy should be most prominent
within the basis pontis and occur almost
exclusively in immunosuppressed patients
remain a mystery. The abnormality has not
been correlated with systemic metabolic or
biochemical abnormalities. Central pontine
myelinolysis (CPM) — morphologically dis-
similar to FPL — has been noted in a hand-

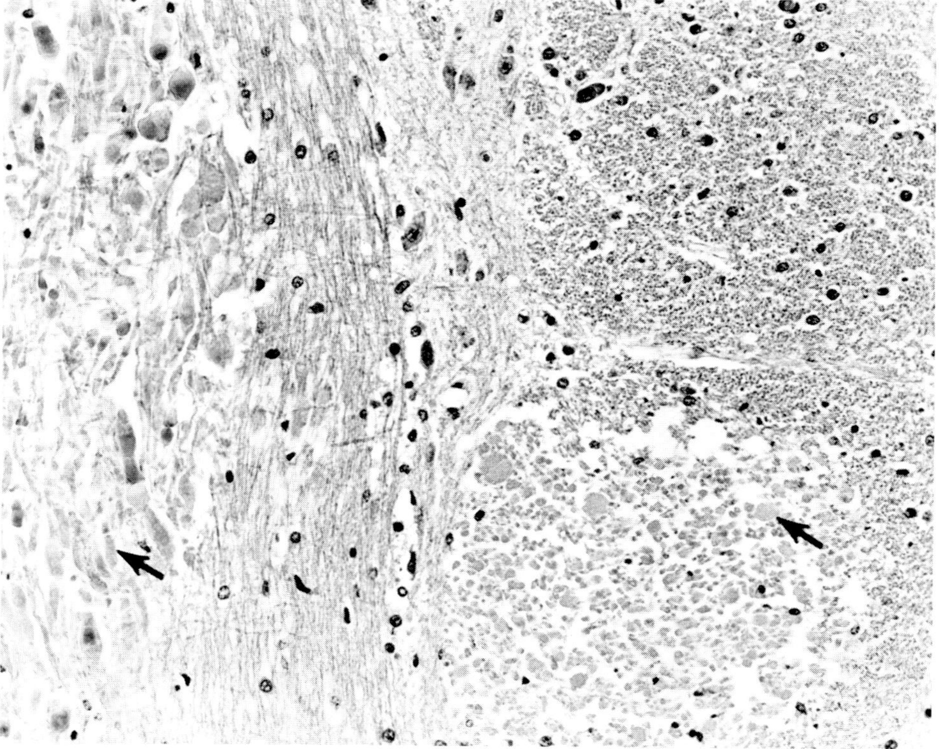

Figure 13. Focal pontine leukoencephalopathy. Both transversely oriented crossing fibers and descending long
tracts seen in cross section show enlarged dystrophic axons (arrows) and spongy change. Calcification is not seen in
this section (H&E, original magnification ×150).

ful of patients with AIDS, usually without a history of the primary risk factor for CPM (i.e., a rapid correction of profound hyponatremia).[2] The clinical correlate of FPL remains obscure.

ABNORMALITIES OF NERVE AND MUSCLE

Clinical features indicating disease of peripheral and/or cranial nerves and skeletal muscle are commonly found in AIDS patients, and include syndromes of chronic inflammatory polyneuropathy, Bell's palsy, distal symmetrical neuropathy, HZV radiculitis, persistent myalgias, myopathy, and polymyositis.[7,44] Despite this, early attention to the neurologic/neuropathologic complications of AIDS focused on CNS pathology, virtually to the exclusion of a consideration of abnormalities of the PNS. This oversight is in the process of being rectified (Table 3).

Some of the above syndromes can clearly result from CNS parenchymal or meningeal lymphoma (e.g. affecting the brainstem and thus cranial nerve nuclei or existing fibers), or opportunistic infections (e.g cryptococcosis) that cause meningitis with resultant infiltration of cranial nerves as they exit the brainstem or spinal nerve roots as they leave the spinal cord. A careful search for such an explanation must be made when the neuropathologist assesses the brain and spinal

cord at necropsy. Herpes viruses, such as CMV and HZV, can cause a radiculitis or radiculopathy. The ability of CMV to produce an ascending polyneuropathy (GBP) by infiltration of nerve roots, subarachnoid space, and spinal cord (with extensive necrosis and inflammation) has already been described and illustrated.[39,40] CMV has been implicated as the causal agent of more extensive polyneuropathy in AIDS patients, though the association is based on circumstantial evidence.

An inflammatory demyelinating neuropathy (IDP) without CMV infection has recently been described in patients harboring HIV but without clinical features of AIDS in all cases.[119,120] Of nine patients, three presented with GBP, whereas six had chronic neuropathy. Affected patients had moderately elevated CSF protein and small numbers of white blood cells within the CSF. Nerve biopsies[119] showed intense inflammatory cell infiltrates and macrophage-mediated demyelination, suggesting an immunopathogenetic mechanism for development of the IDP. Preliminary data indicate that the patients' neuropathies improve with steroid treatment or plasmapheresis.

Other studies of sural nerve biopsies in AIDS patients with overt symptoms referable to the PNS showed segmental demyelination, axon loss, and endoneurial or epineurial mononuclear cell infiltrates.[121] In one nerve biopsy, viral particles suggestive of HIV were found within the axoplasm and were assumed to have been transported there from the neuronal perikaryon[122]—a hypothesis that seems contradictory to the fact that HIV rarely, if ever, invades neurons, despite its overall affinity for the CNS. Acute or subacute neuropathy and polyradiculopathy associated with seroconversion for HIV or elevated CSF titers of anti-HIV have been described, but the pathology has not.[123,124] Solid evidence for the presence of HIV within peripheral nerve has not yet been presented. Autonomic neuropathy has also been seen in AIDS patients,[125,126] though without neuropathologic confirmation of the functional abnormality.

TABLE III

Clinicopathologic Syndromes Affecting the Peripheral Nervous System in Patients with HIV Infection

	References
1. *Peripheral nerve/roots:*	
a. CMV-induced polyradiculoneuropathy	39,40
b. Inflammatory demyelinating neuropathy (? autoimmune)	119,120
c. Autonomic neuropathy	125,126
2. *Muscle:*	
a. Noninflammatory myopathy	128,129
b. Myositis (incl. polymyositis)	130,131

In an attempt to ascertain the frequency with which peripheral nerve abnormalities might be expected in the AIDS population in general, we have sampled the sural nerves in 20 unselected AIDS or ARC patients who came to autopsy, none of whom had had major complaints referable to the PNS.[127] Simple morphometric studies and fiber teasing carried out on glutaraldehyde-fixed plastic-embedded or glycerinated material showed that eight patients had some degree of peripheral nerve pathology, usually consisting of a diminution in density of myelinated fibers, with a disproportionately greater loss of large myelinated fibers. A single patient without other major risk factors for peripheral neuropathy showed a profound loss of myelinated fibers, with approximately a 40% loss in total myelinated fibers and a 65% loss of large myelinated fibers. Osmicated teased fiber preparations demonstrated evidence of axon and myelin breakdown but no definite segmental demyelination. Despite this, the patient was apparently asymptomatic with respect to peripheral nerve complaints or findings, though his complicated terminal course may have precluded detailed clinical assessment of such lesions. The specimens had not been specifically examined for the presence of HIV, and the question of whether neuropathy results from direct HIV infection of peripheral nerve axons or Schwann cells remains unanswered.

Sporadic reports of a myopathy, without specific histologic features, in AIDS patients have appeared.[128,129] More commonly, myositis, sometimes with features of polymyositis, has been reported, although the number of such cases is very small.[130,131] In one study,[130] polymyositis was the presenting clinical feature of HIV infection, though typical ARC and AIDS ensued in the patients. HIV viral antigen was found in OKT4 positive lymphoid cells around muscle fibers and within endomysial septa. Polymyositis was also found in 50% of primates with acquired immunodeficiency caused by a Type D retrovirus (SAIDS D), and again virus was shown to be present within inflammatory lymphoid cells in the muscle and adjacent connective tissues.[132]

MISCELLANEOUS NEUROPATHOLOGIC CHANGES

Nodular subependymal glial proliferations (granular ependymitis) with loss or attenuation of overlying ependyma are frequently encountered and may represent a reparative response to prior infection of the CSF. These lesions are of uncertain etiology, however. Similarly, occasional individuals have slight thickening of the subarachnoid or perivascular spaces by a nonspecific infiltrate of lymphocytes and histiocytes, without identifiable organisms. This may be related to direct HIV infection of the nervous system or CSF. Occasionally, Alzheimer Type II astrocytes are noted. Rarely, small intraparenchymal calcifications are found, as is patchy Bergmann gliosis (focal sclerosis) of the cerebellum.[2]

PEDIATRIC AIDS

Risk factors for AIDS in children include: Parents at high risk (with infection of the child in utero or early postnatal life), hemophilia, and blood transfusion therapy. The rate of transmission is high since infants are essentially immunoincompetent. Marion et al.[133] have described a pattern of congenital anomalies thought secondary to congenital HIV infection. This syndrome, known as HTLV-III embryopathy, is characterized by growth failure, microcephaly, and craniofacial abnormalities. Other features of pediatric AIDS include a diminished T-helper cell population, serum hypergammaglobulinemia with circulating immune complexes, low birth weight, failure to thrive, lymphadenopathy, hepatosplenomegaly, and recurrent (opportunistic) viral and bacterial infections.[134]

Clinically, some of these children have a

progressive encephalopathy with lethargy, seizures, dementia, spastic quadriparesis, and pyramidal tract signs. Neuroradiologic studies show a markedly increased incidence of calcification of basal ganglia and cerebral atrophy.[107] Pathologic evaluation shows a calcific vasculopathy (siderocalcinosis) involving both large- and medium-sized vessels primarily in the basal ganglia, but occasionally involving the centrum semiovale. These mineralized vascular deposits stain positively for iron and calcium. Pyramidal tract degeneration may be seen, as may occasional MGNs, HIV-type giant cells,[2] and toxoplasmosis.[135]

HIV WITHIN THE CENTRAL NERVOUS SYSTEM

Since the publication of the landmark paper by Shaw et al.,[136] which showed clear-cut evidence of HIV infection of the nervous system in AIDS patients, numerous laboratories have (using various methods) confirmed the presence of the pathogenic retrovirus or its genome in neural tissues, with resultant production of HIV antigen and/or HIV-specific antibodies within the CSF of infected patients.[2,26,99,137-146] The molecular biology of HIV and related retroviruses, their mechanisms of replication and effects on cell metabolism have been reviewed at length[147-151] and a discussion of these topics is far beyond the scope of this review. Several important questions have emerged from these studies:

1. In what cell type(s) in the neuraxis does HIV survive and replicate?
2. What effects does HIV have on neural tissue?
3. How does HIV get from the bloodstream through the BBB into the brain?

These questions, most of which have at least partial answers, will be the focus of this section.

The tissue marker of HIV infection in brain appears to be a multinucleated cell, sometimes a giant cell of possible microglial origin, often with very little cytoplasm or foamy or granular cytoplasm, and usually situated just outside the adventitia of small cerebral blood vessels (Fig. 14).[152-155] The brain surrounding the multinucleated cells is often hypercellular due to an increase of microglial or microglia-like cells and to a lesser extent of astrocytes. HIV genome and/or antigen have been localized to the multinucleate cells using in situ hybridization and immunocytochemistry, and typical viral particles have rarely been seen ultrastructurally in the multinucleated cell cytoplasm.[156-158]

Viral genome or antigen has most commonly been found within white matter and deep central grey matter rather than cortex.[139] Most studies confirm that HIV is localized to microglia, macrophages, and giant cells — the latter may derive, as noted, from the former two — and is rarely (if ever) found within other glial cells or neurons.[159,160] One group, however, has reported the frequent finding of HIV within astrocytes and oligodendrocytes of brain biopsies from AIDS patients.[157] The presence of HIV within cerebral capillary endothelium (i.e., cells that constitute the BBB)[99] suggests one mechanism whereby HIV might penetrate this barrier to enter the brain. HIV, however, may enter brain within infected lymphoid and/or mononuclear cells circulating in the blood.[161]

The AIDS virus seems to infect cells after initial interaction with the T4 or CD4 receptor, and this receptor is shared by the cell surfaces of lymphoid and neural cells, particularly neurons and astrocytes.[162-164] An elegant scenario is thus proposed whereby the AIDS virus exhibits the propensity to affect both the nervous system and lymphocytes. This hypothesis is challenged, however, by the observation that neurons and glia are seldom invaded by HIV (at least so far as we can detect with the power of resolution of existing techniques).

Infection of the nervous system by AIDS

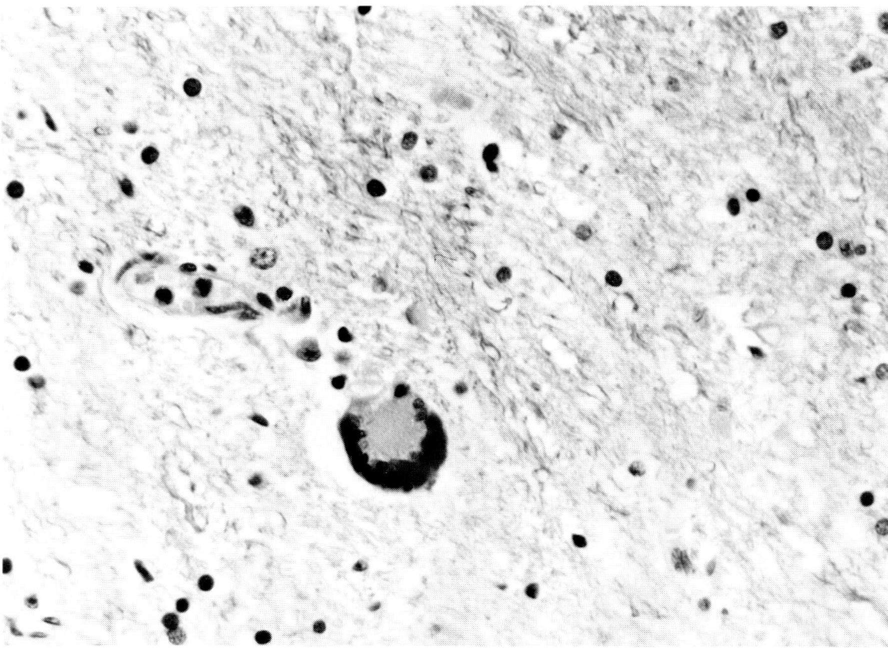

Figure 14. HIV type multinucleate cell. Multinucleate giant cell with eccentrically clustered nuclei is located adjacent to a microvessel, as are two smaller macrophages (H&E, original magnification ×300).

viruses with distinct cell tropisms has been demonstrated,[165] i.e. two genetically distinct but related viruses were isolated from one patient with AIDS and progressive diffuse leukoencephalopathy,[109] from two different sources in the CNS: brain and CSF. HIV infection of brain-derived cells in vitro has been successfully achieved in other laboratories.[166] Findings such as this suggest that treatment of the systemic manifestations of AIDS, when such therapy becomes available, may not always be effective in the treatment of its neurologic complications (i.e., those caused directly by HIV infection).

HIV infection of the CNS produces a syndrome now referred to as the AIDS dementia complex (ADC).[19-21] Clinicopathologic investigation of patients with this disorder suggests that the dementing illness correlates with a subcortical leukoencephalopathy,[20] though it is not understood how the presence of HIV in a relatively small number of macrophages or microglia within the brain, associated with minimal inflammation, can induce the relatively severe degree of myelin loss, spongy change, and astrogliosis that is frequently seen within the white matter. Even in the most detailed clinicopathologic series, the correlation between the presence of HIV within brain and the evidence of a clinical dementia is sometimes a poor one.[20,99] A recent study has suggested that HIV may cause dementia in part by suppression of neuronal responses to neurotrophic factors.[167]

As mentioned above, many cases of MGN encephalitis are now also attributed to HIV infection of brain.[168] A remarkable finding within large series, including our own, is that the relative proportion of AIDS brains with evidence of direct HIV infection (using the multinucleate cell as a footprint of this) has increased dramatically within the past 2–3 years.[3] This might also suggest the evolution of a more neurotropic form of HIV, though other explanations for the rise are plausible. A small population of patients with HIV infection, often with no visceral manifestation of AIDS, are now presenting exclusively with clinical features of the ADC.[14] It must even be considered in the differential diagnosis of more elderly patients with dementia.[169]

Other unexpected sequelae of direct HIV infection of the CNS (and possibly PNS) are, unfortunately, almost certain to emerge within the coming months and years. Neuropathologists will have to be vigilant in anticipation of finding, describing, and categorizing such diseases, since this can serve to guide basic researchers in deciphering the mechanisms by which HIV injures the nervous system.

ACKNOWLEDGMENTS

The following individuals provided invaluable assistance in various aspects of the study and preparation of the manuscript: Scott Brooks, Roy Bailey, Beverly Chandler, Laurel Reed, Carol Appleton, Alice Nakanishi, Charlotte Preston, Paula Berger, Walter Grant, and Gary Ono. Work in Dr. Vinters' laboratory supported in part by grant #000369 from the American Foundation for AIDS Research, and a U.C.L.A. Biomedical Research Support Grant.

LIST OF ABBREVIATIONS

ADC	AIDS dementia complex
AIDS	Acquired immune deficiency syndrome
ARC	AIDS related complex
BBB	Blood-brain barrier
CMV	Cytomegalovirus
CNS	Central nervous system
CPM	Central pontine myelinolysis
CSF	Cerebrospinal fluid
CT	Computerized tomography
EBV	Epstein-Barr virus
FPL	Focal pontine leukoencephalopathy
GBP	Guillain-Barré polyneuropathy
HIV	Human immunodeficiency virus
HSV	Herpes simplex virus
HZV	Herpes zoster virus
IDP	Inflammatory demyelinating neuropathy
MAI	Mycobacterium avium-intracellulare
MGN	Microglial nodule
MRI	Magnetic resonance image
PML	Progressive multifocal leukoencephalopathy
PNS	Peripheral nervous system
TB	Mycobacterium tuberculosis

REFERENCES

1. Anders K, Steinsapir KD, Iverson DJ, et al: Neuropathologic findings in the acquired immunodeficiency syndrome (AIDS). Clin Neuropathol 1986; 5:1–20
2. Anders KH, Guerra WF, Tomiyasu U, et al: The neuropathology of AIDS. UCLA experience and review. Am J Pathol 1986; 124:537–558
3. Petito CK, Cho E-S, Lemann W, et al: Neuropathology of acquired immunodeficiency syndrome (AIDS): An autopsy review. J Neuropathol Exp Neurol 1986; 45:635–646
4. Fischer P-A, Enzensberger W: Neurological complications in AIDS. J Neurol 1987; 234:269–279
5. Britton CB, Miller JR: Neurologic complications in acquired immunodeficiency syndrome (AIDS). Neurol Clin 1984; 2:315–339
6. Snider WD, Simpson DM, Nielsen S, et al: Neurological complications of acquired immune deficiency syndrome: Analysis of 50 patients. Ann Neurol 1983; 14:403–418
7. Levy RM, Bredesen DE, Rosenblum ML: Neurological manifestations of the acquired immunodeficiency syndrome (AIDS): Experience at UCSF and review of the literature. J Neurosurg 1985; 62:475–495
8. Fenelon G, Bolgert F, Dehen H: Les manifestations neurologiques du syndrome d'immuno-dépression acquise (SIDA). Rev Neurol (Paris) 1986; 142:97–106
9. Rosemberg S, Lopes MBS, Tsanaclis AM: Neuropathology of acquired immunodeficiency syndrome (AIDS). Analysis of 22 Brazilian cases. J Neurol Sci 1986; 76:187–198
10. Helweg-Larsen S, Jakobsen J, Boesen F, Arlien-Søborg P.: Neurological complications and concomitants of AIDS. Acta Neurol Scand 1986; 74:467–474
11. Kato T, Hirano A, Llena JF, Dembitzer HM: Neuropathology of acquired immune deficiency syndrome (AIDS) in 53 autopsy cases with particular emphasis on microglial nodules and multi-

nucleated giant cells. Acta Neuropathol (Berlin) 1987; 73:287–294

12. Rhodes RH: Histopathology of the central nervous system in acquired immunodeficiency syndrome. Hum Pathol 1987; 18:636–643

13. Koppel BS, Wormser GP, Tuchman AJ, et al: Central nervous system involvement in patients with acquired immune deficiency syndrome (AIDS). Acta Neurol Scand 1985; 71:337–353

14. Navia BA, Price RW: The acquired immunodeficiency syndrome dementia complex as the presenting or sole manifestation of human immunodeficiency virus infection. Arch Neurol 1987; 44:65–69

15. Davtyan DG, Vinters HV: Wernicke's encephalopathy in AIDS patient treated with zidovudine. (letter). Lancet 1987; 1:919–920

16. Elkin CM, Leon E, Grenell SL, Leeds NE: Intracranial lesions in the acquired immunodeficiency syndrome. Radiologic (computed tomographic) features. JAMA 1985; 253:393–396

17. Levy RM, Rosenbloom S, Perrett LV: Neuroradiologic findings in AIDS: A review of 200 cases. AJNR 1986; 7:833–839

18. DeLaPaz R, Floris R, Brant-Zawadzki M, et al: MRI of CNS complications of acquired immune deficiency syndrome (AIDS). (abstract) AJNR 1986; 7:541

19. Navia BA, Jordan BD, Price RW: The AIDS dementia complex: I. Clinical features. Ann Neurol 1986; 19:517–524

20. Navia BA, Cho E-S, Petito CK, Price RW: The AIDS dementia complex: II Neuropathology. Ann Neurol 1986; 19:525–535

21. Price RW, Navia BA, Cho E-S: AIDS encephalopathy. Neurol Clin 1986; 4:285–301

22. Nath A, Jankovic J, Pettigrew LC: Movement disorders and AIDS. Neurology 1987; 37:37–41

23. Berger JR, Bender A, Resnick L, Perlmutter D: Spinal myoclonus associated with HTLV III/LAV infection. Arch Neurol 1986; 43:1203–1204

24. Faulstich ME: Psychiatric aspects of AIDS. Am J Psychiatry 1987; 144:551–556

25. Gudesblatt M, Gerber O, Vaillancourt PD, Bronster D: Liquide céphalo-rachidien quasi-normal chez des patients atteints du syndrome d'immunodéficience acquise et d'une méningite a cryptocoque. Rev Neurol (Paris) 1987; 143:290–293

26. Resnick L, DiMarzo-Veronese F, Schüpbach J, et al: Intra-blood-brain-barrier synthesis of HTLV-III-specific IgG in patients with neurologic symptoms associated with AIDS or AIDS-related complex. N Engl J Med 1985; 313:1498–1504

27. Ackermann R, Nekic M, Jürgens R: Locally synthesized antibodies in cerebrospinal fluid of patients with AIDS. J Neurol 1986; 233:140–141

28. Goudsmit J, Wolters EC, Bakker M, Smit L, et al: Intrathecal synthesis of antibodies to HTLV-III in patients without AIDS or AIDS related complex. Br Med J 1986; 292:1231–1234

29. Pepose JS, Hilborne LH, Cancilla PA, Foos RY: Concurrent herpes simplex and cytomegalovirus retinitis and encephalitis in the acquired immune deficiency syndrome (AIDS). Ophthalmology 1984; 91:1669–1677

30. Post MJD, Hensley GT, Moskowitz LB, Fischl M: Cytomegalic inclusion virus encephalitis in patients with AIDS: CT, clinical and pathologic correlation. AJNR 1986; 7:275–280

31. Morgello S, Cho E-S, Nielsen S, et al: Cytomegalovirus encephalitis in patients with acquired immunodeficiency syndrome: An autopsy study of 30 cases and a review of the literature. Hum Pathol 1987; 18:289–297

32. Edwards RH, Messing R, McKendall RR: Cytomegalovirus meningoencephalitis in a homosexual man with Kaposi's sarcoma: Isolation of CMV from CSF cells. Neurology 1985; 35:560–562

33. Vital C, Vital A, Vignoly B, et al: Cytomegalovirus encephalitis in a patient with acquired immunodeficiency syndrome. Arch Pathol Lab Med 1985; 109:105–106

34. Muñoz DG, Perl DP, Pendlebury WW, Highland, RA: Comparison of cytomegalovirus infection of brain and lung in a patient with subacute encephalopathy of acquired immunodeficiency syndrome. Arch Pathol Lab Med 1987; 111:234–237

35. Nielsen SL, Petito CK, Urmacher CD, Posner JB: Subacute encephalitis in acquired immune deficiency syndrome: A postmortem study. Am J Clin Pathol 1984; 82:678–682

36. Vinters HV, Kwok MK, Ho HW, et al: Cytomegalovirus in the nervous system of patients with the acquired immune deficiency syndrome. Brain 1988; in press

37. Wiley CA, Schrier RD, Denaro FJ, et al: Localization of cytomegalovirus proteins and genome during fulminant central nervous system infection in an AIDS patient. J Neuropathol Exp Neurol 1986; 45:127–139

38. Moskowitz LB, Gregorios JB, Hensley GT, Berger JR: Cytomegalovirus-induced demyelination associated with acquired immune deficiency syndrome. Arch Pathol Lab Med 1984; 108:873–877

39. Eidelberg D, Sotrel A, Vogel H, et al: Progressive polyradiculopathy in acquired immune deficiency syndrome. Neurology 1986; 36:912–916

40. Behar R, Wiley C, McCutchan JA: Cytomegalovirus polyradiculoneuropathy in acquired immune deficiency syndrome. Neurology 1987; 37:557–561

41. Goodman MD, Porter DD: Cytomegalovirus vasculitis with fatal colonic hemorrhage. Arch Pathol Lab Med 1973; 96:281–284

42. Koeppen AH, Lansing LS, Peng S-K, Smith RS: Central nervous system vasculitis in cytomegalovirus infection. J Neurol Sci 1981; 51:395–410

43. Leonard JC, Tobin J O'H, Heyworth B, et al: Polyneuritis associated with cytomegalovirus infections. Quart J Med 1971; 40:435–442

44. Janssen RS, Saykin AJ, Kaplan JE, et al: Neurologic complications of lymphadenopathy syndrome associated with human immunodeficiency virus infection (abstract). Neurology 1987; 37:344

45. Dix RD, Waitzman DM, Follansbee S, et al: Herpes simplex virus type 2 encephalitis in two homosexual men with persistent lymphadenopathy. Ann Neurol 1985; 17:203–206

46. Britton CB, Mesa-Tejada R, Fenoglio CM, et al:

A new complication of AIDS: thoracic myelitis caused by herpes simplex virus. Neurology 1985; 35:1071–1074

47. Ryder JW, Croen K, Kleinschmidt-DeMasters BK, et al: Progressive encephalitis three months after resolution of cutaneous zoster in a patient with AIDS. Ann Neurol 1986; 19:182–188

48. Hochberg FH, Miller G, Schooley RT, et al: Central-nervous-system lymphoma related to Epstein-Barr virus. N Engl J Med 1983; 309:745–748

49. Rosenberg NL, Hochberg FH, Miller G, et al: Primary central nervous system lymphoma related to Epstein-Barr virus in a patient with acquired immune deficiency syndrome. Ann Neurol 1986; 20:98–102

50. Brooks BR, Walker DL: Progressive multifocal leukoencephalopathy. Neurol Clin 1984; 2:299–313

51. Tomiyasu U, Baker RN, Wollman J: Progressive multifocal leukoencephalopathy and the "slow viruses". Bull LA Neurol Soc 1968; 33:59–69

52. ZuRhein GM: Association of papova-virions with a human demyelinating disease (progressive multifocal leukoencephalopathy). Progr Med Virol 1969; 11:185–247

53. Aksamit AJ Jr, Gendelman HE, Pezeshkpour GH, Orenstein JM: PML in AIDS: Comparison to non-AIDS cases by in situ hybridization and immunohistochemistry. (abstract) Neurology 1987; 37:345

54. Greenlee JE, Stroop WG: Progressive multifocal leukoencephalopathy in patients with the acquired immunodeficiency syndrome: Study of the infection by in situ hybridization methods. (abstract) Ann Neurol 1986; 20:141–142

55. Schlitt M, Morawetz RB, Bonnin J, et al: Progressive multifocal leukoencephalopathy: Three patients diagnosed by brain biopsy, with prolonged survival in two. Neurosurgery 1986; 18:407–414

56. Anders KH, Chandrasoma P, Connelly S, Vinters HV: Surgical neuropathology in patients with AIDS. (In preparation, 1988)

57. Shapshak P, Tourtellotte WW, Wolman M, et al: Search for virus nucleic acid sequences in postmortem human brain tissue using in situ hybridization technology with cloned probes: Some solutions and results on progressive multifocal leukoencephalopathy and subacute sclerosing panencephalitis tissue. J Neurosci Res 1986; 16:281–301

58. Jakobsen J, Diemer NH, Gaub J, et al: Progressive multifocal leukoencephalopathy in a patient without other clinical manifestations of AIDS. Acta Neurol Scand 1987; 75:209–213

59. Berger JR, Kaszovitz B, Post MJD, Dickinson G: Progressive multifocal leukoencephalopathy associated with human immunodeficiency virus infection. A review of the literature with a report of sixteen cases. Ann Intern Med 1987; 107:78–87

60. Kovacs JA, Kovacs AA, Polis M, et al: Cryptococcosis in the acquired immunodeficiency syndrome. Ann Intern Med 1985; 103:533–538

61. Zuger A, Louie E, Holzman RS, et al: Cryptococcal disease in patients with the acquired immunodeficiency syndrome. Diagnostic features and outcome of treatment. Ann Intern Med 1986; 104:234–240

62. Johnson PC, Sarosi GA: AIDS and progressive disseminated histoplasmosis. (letter) JAMA 1987; 258:202

63. Johnson PC, Sarosi GA, Septimus EJ, Satterwhite TK: Progressive disseminated histoplasmosis in patients with the acquired immune deficiency syndrome: A report of 12 cases and a literature review. Sem Respiratory Infect 1986; 1:1–8

64. Bronnimann DA, Adam RD, Galgiani JN, et al: Coccidioidomycosis in the acquired immunodeficiency syndrome. Ann Intern Med 1987; 106:372–379

65. Navia BA, Petito CK, Gold JWM, et al: Cerebral toxoplasmosis complicating the acquired immune deficiency syndrome: Clinical and neuropathological findings in 27 patients. Ann Neurol 1986; 19:224–238

66. Luft BJ, Brooks RG, Conley FK, et al: Toxoplasmic encephalitis in patients with acquired immune deficiency syndrome. JAMA 1984; 252:913–917

67. Farkash AE, Maccabee PJ, Sher JH, et al: CNS toxoplasmosis in acquired immune deficiency syndrome: A clinical-pathological-radiological review of 12 cases. J Neurol Neurosurg Psychiatry 1986; 49:744–748

68. Conley FK, Jenkins KA, Remington JS: Toxoplasma gondii infection of the central nervous system: Use of the peroxidase-antiperoxidase method to demonstrate Toxoplasma in formalin fixed, paraffin embedded tissue sections. Hum Pathol 1981; 12:690–698

69. Tang TT, Harb JM, Dunne WM Jr, et al: Cerebral toxoplasmosis in an immunocompromised host. A precise and rapid diagnosis by electron microscopy. Am J Clin Pathol 1986; 85:104–110

70. Fischl MA, Pitchenik AE, Spira TJ: Tuberculous brain abscess and Toxoplasma encephalitis in a patient with the acquired immunodeficiency syndrome. JAMA 1985; 253:3428–3430

71. Bahls F, Sumi SM: Cryptococcal meningitis and cerebral toxoplasmosis in a patient with acquired immune deficiency syndrome. J Neurol Neurosurg Psychiatry 1986; 49:328–330

72. Gonzalez MM, Gould E, Dickinson G, et al: Acquired immunodeficiency syndrome associated with Acanthamoeba infection and other opportunistic organisms. Arch Pathol Lab Med 1986; 110:749–751

73. Wiley CA, Safrin RE, Davis CE: Acanthamoeba meningoencephalitis in a patient with AIDS. J Infect Dis 1987; 155:130–133

74. Kuo T, Hsueh S, Wu J-L, Wang A-M: Cutaneous protothecosis. A clinicopathologic study. Arch Pathol Lab Med 1987; 111:737–740

75. Sharer LR, Kaminski Z, Cho E-S, Ambros R: Case 1, 28th Annual Diagnostic Slide Session, American Association of Neuropathologists, Seattle, Washington, June, 1987

76. Witt DJ, Craven DE, McCabe WR: Bacterial infections in adult patients with the acquired immune deficiency syndrome (AIDS) and AIDS-related complex. Am J Med 1987; 82:900–906

77. Eng RHK, Bishburg E, Smith SM, et al: Bactere-

mia and fungemia in patients with acquired immune deficiency syndrome. Am J Clin Pathol 1986; 86:105–107

78. Klatt EC, Jensen DF, Meyer PR: Pathology of *Mycobacterium avium-intracellulare* infection in acquired immunodeficiency syndrome. Hum Pathol 1987; 18:709–714

79. Hawkins CC, Gold JWM, Whimbey E, et al: *Mycobacterium avium* complex infections in patients with the acquired immunodeficiency syndrome. Ann Intern Med 1986; 105:184–188

80. Bishburg E, Sunderam G, Reichman LB, Kapila R: Central nervous system tuberculosis with the acquired immunodeficiency syndrome and its related complex. Ann Intern Med 1986; 105:210–213

81. Jacobs JL, Murray HW: Why is *Listeria monocytogenes* not a pathogen in the acquired immunodeficiency syndrome? Arch Intern Med 1986; 146:1299–1300

82. Mullin GE, Sheppell AL: *Listeria monocytogenes* and the acquired immunodeficiency syndrome. (letter) Arch Intern Med 1987; 147:176

83. Koziol K, Rielly KS, Bonin RA, Salcedo JR: *Listeria monocytogenes* meningitis in AIDS. Can Med Assoc J 1986; 135:43–44

84. Jankovic J: Whipple's disease of the central nervous system in AIDS. (letter) N Engl J Med 1986; 315:1029–1030

85. Zaidman GW: Neurosyphilis and retrobulbar neuritis in a patient with AIDS. Ann Ophthalmol 1986; 18:260–261

86. Levine AM, Gill PS, Meyer PR, et al: Retrovirus and malignant lymphoma in homosexual men. JAMA 1985; 254:1921–1925

87. Ciobanu N, Wiernik PH: Malignant lymphomas, AIDS, and the pathogenic role of Epstein-Barr virus. Mt Sinai J Med 1986; 53:627–638

88. Mernick MH, Malamud SC, Haubenstock A, et al: Non-Hodgkin's lymphoma in AIDS: Report of 11 cases and literature review. Mt Sinai J Med 1986; 53:664–667

89. Gill PS, Levine AM, Meyer PR, et al: Primary central nervous system lymphoma in homosexual men. Clinical, immunologic, and pathologic features. Am J Med 1985; 78:742–748

90. So YT, Beckstead JH, Davis RL: Primary central nervous system lymphoma in acquired immune deficiency syndrome: A clinical and pathological study. Ann Neurol 1986; 20:566–572

91. Song SK, Schwartz IS, Breakstone BA: Lymphoproliferative disorder of the central nervous system in AIDS. Mt Sinai J Med 1986; 53:686–689

92. Verity MA, Wolfson WL: Cerebral lymphomatoid granulomatosis. A report of two cases, with disseminated necrotizing leukoencephalopathy in one. Acta Neuropathol (Berlin) 1976; 36:117–124

93. Verity MA: Cerebral lymphomatoid granulomatosis. In: (Vinken PJ, Bruyn GW, eds.) *Handbook of Clinical Neurology (vol. 39): Neurological Manifestations of Systemic Diseases, part II.* North-Holland Publishing Co., Amsterdam 1980; 517–536

94. Cammarosano C, Lewis W: Cardiac lesions in acquired immune deficiency syndrome (AIDS). J Am Coll Cardiol 1985; 5:703–706

95. Velji AM: Leukocytoclastic vasculitis associated with positive HTLV-III serological findings. JAMA 1986; 256:2196–2197

96. Yankner BA, Skolnik PR, Shoukimas GM, et al: Cerebral granulomatous angiitis associated with isolation of human T-lymphotropic virus type III from the central nervous system. Ann Neurol 1986; 20:362–364

97. Schwartz ND, So YT, Hollander H, et al: Eosinophilic vasculitis leading to amaurosis fugax in a patient with acquired immunodeficiency syndrome. Arch Intern Med 1986; 146:2059–2060

98. Vinters HV, Guerra WF, Eppolito L, Keith PE III: Necrotizing vasculitis of the nervous system in a patient with AIDS-related complex. Neuropathol Appl Neurobiol 1988; in press

99. Wiley CA, Schrier RD, Nelson JA, et al: Cellular localization of human immunodeficiency virus infection within the brains of acquired immune deficiency syndrome patients. Proc Natl Acad Sci USA 1986; 83:7089–7093

100. Doyle PW, Gibson G, Dolman CL: Herpes zoster ophthalmicus with contralateral hemiplegia: Identification of cause. Ann Neurol 1983; 14:84–85

101. Phinney PR, Fligiel S, Bryson YJ, Porter DD: Necrotizing vasculitis in a case of disseminated neonatal herpes simplex infection. Arch Pathol Lab Med 1982; 106:64–67

102. Cho E-S, Sharer LR, Peress NS, Little B: Intimal proliferation of leptomeningeal arteries and brain infarcts in subjects with AIDS. (abstract) J Neuropathol Exp Neurol 1987; 46:385

103. Stafford CR, Bogdanoff BM, Green L, Spector HB: Mononeuropathy multiplex as a complication of amphetamine angiitis. Neurology 1975; 25:570–572

104. Citron BP, Halpern M, McCarron M, et al: Necrotizing angiitis associated with drug abuse. N Engl J Med 1970; 283:1003–1011

105. Takashima S, Becker LE: Basal ganglia calcification in Down's syndrome. J Neurol Neurosurg Psychiatry 1985; 48:61–64

106. Slager UT, Wagner JA: The incidence, composition, and pathological significance of intracerebral vascular deposits in the basal ganglia. J Neuropathol Exp Neurol 1956; 15:417–431

107. Belman AL, Lantos G, Horoupian D, et al: AIDS: Calcification of the basal ganglia in infants and children. Neurology 1986; 36:1192–1199

108. Kleihues P, Lang W, Burger PC, et al: Progressive diffuse leukoencephalopathy in patients with acquired immune deficiency syndrome (AIDS). Acta Neuropathol (Berlin) 1985; 68:333–339

109. Clark GL, Vinters HV: Dementia and ataxia in a patient with AIDS. West J Med 1987; 146:68–72

110. Horoupian DS, Pick P, Spigland I, et al: Acquired immune deficiency syndrome and multiple tract degeneration in a homosexual man. Ann Neurol 1984; 15:502–505

111. Petito CK, Navia BA, Cho E-S, et al: Vacuolar myelopathy pathologically resembling subacute combined degeneration in patients with the ac-

quired immunodeficiency syndrome. N Engl J Med 1985; 312:874–879

112. Goldstick L, Mandybur TI, Bode R: Spinal cord degeneration in AIDS. Neurology 1985; 35:103–106

113. Sharer LR, Epstein LG, Cho E-S, Petito CK: HTLV-III and vacuolar myelopathy. (letter) N Engl J Med 1986; 315:62–63

114. De La Monte SM, Moore T, Hedley-Whyte ET: Vacuolar encephalopathy of AIDS. (letter) N Engl J Med 1986; 315: 1549–1550

115. Vinters HV, Anders KH, Barach P: Focal pontine leukoencephalopathy in immunosuppressed patients. Arch Pathol Lab Med 1987; 111:192–196

116. Breuer AC, Blank NK, Schoene WC: Multifocal pontine lesions in cancer patients treated with chemotherapy and CNS radiotherapy. Cancer 1978; 41:2112–2120

117. Rubinstein LJ, Herman MM, Long TF, Wilbur JR: Disseminated necrotizing leukoencephalopathy: A complication of treated central nervous system leukemia and lymphoma. Cancer 1975; 35:291–305

118. Mah V, Nelson L, Vinters HV: Focal pontine leukoencephalopathy in a patient with the Shwachman-Diamond syndrome. Can J Neurol Sci 1987; 14:608–610

119. Cornblath DR, McArthur JC, Kennedy PGE, et al: Inflammatory demyelinating peripheral neuropathies associated with human T-cell lymphotropic virus type III infection. Ann Neurol 1987; 21:32–40

120. Mishra BB, Sommers W, Koski CL, Greenstein JI: Acute inflammatory demyelinating polyneuropathy in the acquired immune deficiency syndrome. (abstract) Ann Neurol 1985; 18:131–132

121. Lipkin WI, Parry G, Kiprov D, Abrams D: Inflammatory neuropathy in homosexual men with lymphadenopathy. Neurology 1985; 35:1479–1483

122. Bailey RO, Singh JK, Bishop MB: AIDS neuropathy: The role of axoplasmic transport. (abstract) Neurology 1987; 37(Suppl 1):356

123. Przedborski S, Liesnard C, Hildebrand J: Letter to the editor. N Engl J Med 1986; 315:63

124. Piette AM, Tusseau F, Vignon D, et al: Acute neuropathy coincident with seroconversion for anti-LAV/HTLV-III. (letter) Lancet 1986; 1:852

125. Lin-Greenberg A, Taneja-Uppal N: Dysautonomia and infection with the human immunodeficiency virus. (letter) Ann Intern Med 1987; 106:167

126. Craddock C, Bull R, Pasvol G, et al: Cardiorespiratory arrest and autonomic neuropathy in AIDS. Lancet 1987; 2:16–18

127. Mah V, Vartavarian L, Akers MA, Vinters HV: Abnormalities of peripheral nerve in patients with HIV infection. Ann Neurol 1988; (in press)

128. Stern R, Gold J, DiCarlo EF: Myopathy complicating the acquired immune deficiency syndrome. Muscle Nerve 1987; 10:318–322

129. Simpson DM, Bender AN: HTLV-III-associated myopathy. (abstract) Neurology 1987; 37 (Suppl 1):319

130. Dalakas MC, Pezeshkpour GH, Gravell M, Sever JL: Polymyositis associated with AIDS retrovirus. JAMA 1986; 256:2381–2383

131. Bailey RO, Turok DI, Jaufmann BP, Singh JK: Myositis and acquired immunodeficiency syndrome. Hum Pathol 1987; 18:749–751

132. Dalakas MC, London WT, Gravell M, Sever JL: Polymyositis in an immunodeficiency disease in monkeys induced by a type D retrovirus. Neurology 1986; 36:569–572

133. Marion RW, Wiznia AA, Hutcheon RG, Rubinstein A: Human T-cell lymphotropic virus type III (HTLV-III) embryopathy. A new dysmorphic syndrome associated with intrauterine HTLV-III infection. Am J Dis Child (1986); 140:638–640

134. Rubinstein A: Acquired immunodeficiency syndrome in infants. Am J Dis Child 1983; 137:825–827

135. Biggemann B, Voit Th, Neuen E, et al: Neurological manifestations in three German children with AIDS. Neuropediatrics 1987; 18:99–106

136. Shaw GM, Harper ME, Hahn BH, et al: HTLV-III infection in brains of children and adults with AIDS encephalopathy. Science 1985; 227:177–182

137. Vazeux R, Brousse N, Jarry A, et al: AIDS subacute encephalitis. Identification of HIV-infected cells. Am J Pathol 1987; 126:403–410

138. Koenig S, Gendelman HE, Orenstein JM, et al: Detection of AIDS virus in macrophages in brain tissue from AIDS patients with encephalopathy. Science 1986; 233:1089–1093

139. Stoler MH, Eskin TA, Benn S, et al: Human T-cell lymphotropic virus type III infection of the central nervous system. A preliminary in situ analysis. JAMA 1986; 256:2360–2364

140. Gabuzda DH, Ho DD, de la Monte SM, et al: Immunohistochemical identification of HTLV-III antigen in brains of patients with AIDS. Ann Neurol 1986; 20:289–95

141. Goudsmit J, Paul DA, Lange JMA, et al: Expression of human immunodeficiency virus antigen (HIV-Ag) in serum and cerebrospinal fluid during acute and chronic infection. Lancet 1986; 2:177–180

142. Epstein LG, Goudsmit J, Paul DA, et al: Expression of human immunodeficiency virus in cerebrospinal fluid of children with progressive encephalopathy. Ann Neurol 1987; 21:397–401

143. Pumarola-Sune T, Navia BA, Cordon-Cardo C, et al: HIV antigen in the brains of patients with the AIDS dementia complex. Ann Neurol 1987; 21:490–496

144. Ward JM, O'Leary TJ, Baskin GB: Immunohistochemical localization of human and simian immunodeficiency viral antigens in fixed tissue sections. Am J Pathol 1987; 127:199–205

145. Gartner S, Markovits P, Markovitz DM, et al: Virus isolation from and identification of HTLV-III/LAV-producing cells in brain tissue from a patient with AIDS. JAMA 1986; 256:2365–2371

146. Hollander H, Levy JA: Neurologic abnormalities and recovery of human immunodeficiency virus from cerebrospinal fluid. Ann Intern Med 1987; 106:692–695

147. Gallo RC: The AIDS virus. Sci Am 1987; 256(1):47–56
148. Chen ISY: Regulation of AIDS virus expression. Cell 1986; 47:1–2
149. Barre-Sinoussi F, Chermann J-C: The etiologic agent of AIDS. Mt Sinai J Med 1986; 53:598–608
150. Wong-Staal F, Gallo RC: Human T-lymphotropic retroviruses. Nature 1985; 317:395–403
151. Ho DD, Pomerantz RJ, Kaplan JC: Pathogenesis of infection with human immunodeficiency virus. N Engl J Med 1987; 317: 278–286
152. Budka H: Multinucleated giant cells in brain: A hallmark of the acquired immune deficiency syndrome (AIDS). Acta Neuropathol (Berlin) 1986; 69:253–258
153. Dickson DW: Multinucleated giant cells in acquired immunodeficiency syndrome encephalopathy. Origin from endogenous microglia? Arch Pathol Lab Med 1986; 110:967–968
154. Sharer LR, Epstein LG, Cho E-S, et al: Pathologic features of AIDS encephalopathy in children: Evidence for LAV/HTLV-III infection of brain. Hum Pathol 1986; 17:271–284
155. Vinters HV: The AIDS dementia complex. (letter) Ann Neurol 1987; 21:612
156. Meyenhofer MF, Epstein LG, Cho E-S, Sharer LR: Ultrastructural morphology and intracellular production of human immunodeficiency virus (HIV) in brain. J Neuropathol Exp Neurol 1987; 46:474–484
157. Gyorkey F, Melnick JL, Gyorkey P: Human immunodeficiency virus in brain biopsies of patients with AIDS and progressive encephalopathy. J Infect Dis 1987; 155:870–876
158. Kato T, Dembitzer HM, Hirano A, Llena JF: HTLV-III-like particles within a cell process surrounded by a myelin sheath in an AIDS brain. Acta Neuropathol (Berlin) 1987; 73:306–308
159. Gartner S, Markovits P, Markovitz DM, et al: The role of mononuclear phagocytes in HTLV-III/LAV infection. Science 1986; 233:215–219
160. Streicher HZ, Joynt RJ: HTLV-III/LAV and the monocyte/macrophage. JAMA 1986; 256:2390–2391
161. Wiley CA, Oldstone MBA, Nelson JA: Pathogenesis of AIDS encephalitis. (abstract) J Neuropathol Exp Neurol 1987; 46:348
162. Funke I, Hahn A, Rieber EP, et al: The cellular receptor (CD4) of the human immunodeficiency virus is expressed on neurons and glial cells in human brain. J Exp Med 1987; 165:1230–1235
163. Maddon PJ, Dalgleish AG, McDougal JS, et al: The T4 gene encodes the AIDS virus receptor and is expressed in the immune system and the brain. Cell 1986; 47:333–348
164. Hill JM, Farrar WL, Pert CB: Autoradiographic localization of T4 antigen, the HIV receptor, in human brain. Int J Neurosci 1987; 32:687–693
165. Koyanagi Y, Miles S, Mitsuyasu RT, et al: Dual infection of the central nervous system by AIDS viruses with distinct cellular tropisms. Science 1987; 236:819–822
166. Chiodi F, Fuerstenberg S, Gildlund M, et al: Infection of brain-derived cells with the human immunodeficiency virus. J Virol 1987; 61: 1244–1247
167. Lee MR, Ho DD, Gurney ME: Functional interaction and partial homology between human immunodeficiency virus and neuroleukin. Science 1987; 237:1047–1051
168. De la Monte SM, Ho DD, Schooley RT, et al: Subacute encephalomyelitis of AIDS and its relation to HTLV-III infection. Neurology 1987; 37:562–569
169. Mirra SS, Anand R, Spira TJ: HTLV-III/LAV infection of the central nervous system in a 57-year-old man with progressive dementia of unknown cause. N Engl J Med 1986; 314:1191–1192

8

Neuropathology of HIV Infection:
Adults versus Children

Leroy R. Sharer
Eun-Sook Cho

A LARGE PROPORTION OF ADULTS and children who die of human immunodeficiency virus (HIV) related illnesses have neuropathologic abnormalities at postmortem examination.[1,2] Several large autopsy series have numerated the findings in adult patients.[1,3-5] The findings in a smaller number of pediatric cases have been similarly detailed,[6-8] reflecting in part the smaller number of cases of children with HIV infection that have been seen thus far in the United States. The material presented has mirrored the clinical experience of the various centers from which the cases have been reported, with regard to the preponderance of adult or pediatric cases, and to a lesser extent, the interests of the reporting neuropathologists. A comparison of the range of findings in adults versus children has not been attempted previously.

The major neuropathologic findings in subjects dying with HIV infection can be broadly grouped into one of the following categories: opportunistic or reactivated latent infections, neoplasms, vacuolar myelopathy, and primary infection of the central nervous system (CNS) by HIV itself. The latter mentioned disorder has proven to be one of the most important and least well understood aspects of HIV infection; it is in this area in particular that neuropathology has made an invaluable contribution. Our own observations indicate that there are subtle differences in findings related to primary HIV infection of the CNS in adults versus children, in addition to more obvious differences in the other categories. Such differences may have a bearing on the pathogenesis of primary HIV infection of the CNS.

This chapter will examine some of the differences that we and others have encountered concerning the pathologic findings in the CNS of adults and children with HIV infection, based in part on the literature as well as on the experience of Eun-Sook Cho in examining brains of adults both at New Jersey Medical School and Memorial Sloan Kettering Cancer Center (cases from the latter were reported by Petito et al.).[1] Leroy R. Sharer has concentrated on findings in the CNS of children, and the chapter will draw extensively from an autopsy series of 26 brains from children with HIV infection of which the first 11 cases have been previously reported.[6]

131

OPPORTUNISTIC AND REACTIVATED LATENT INFECTIONS

In adult patients, opportunistic and reactivated latent infections have constituted the largest single category of neuropathological abnormalities in the various reported series. There has been some difference in the reported incidence of certain common opportunistic pathogens, particularly *Toxoplasma gondii* and *Cryptococcus neoformans*, related either to the geographical location of the reporting center or to the type of patient with HIV infection seen at the center. For example, in the series reported from New York and Memorial Hospitals,[1] cryptococcal meningitis was relatively uncommon, while the UCLA series had relatively few cases of cerebral toxoplasmosis.[4] Nevertheless, four infections have been commonly reported in most of the series: cytomegalovirus (CMV), *T. gondii*, *C. neoformans*, and progressive multifocal leukoencephalopathy (PML) due to a papova virus. Several other organisms have also been seen, although less frequently, including: *Candida* sp., *Herpes simplex hominis* Type 1, *Herpes zoster* (varicella-zoster virus, VZV), *Mycobacterium tuberculosis hominis (M. tuberculosis* complex), *Histoplasma capsulatum*, *Coccidioides immitis*, and *Escherichia coli*. There is also a long list of other organisms that have been reported, generally in single cases, including: *Herpes simplex* virus Type 2,[5] *Treponema pallidum*,[9] *Nocardia asteroides*,[10] *Salmonella* sp.,[10] *Listeria monocytogenes*,[5] and the alga *Prototheca wickerhamii*.[11]

The number of reported opportunistic or reactivated latent CNS infections in children with HIV infection has been much smaller than that in adults, probably due to the shorter time of exposure of children, particularly infants and young children, to the various opportunistic agents. In our own material, which includes neuropathology from autopsies of 26 children with HIV infection, the only pathogens that we have identified have been CMV (two cases) and *Candida* sp. (one case). This last patient, a four-year-old girl, also had a large necrotic lesion that was felt to represent a healed *Toxoplama gondii* abscess, although no organisms were seen and an immunoperoxidase reaction for *Toxoplasma* antigen was negative. One other patient, also a four-year-old girl, had a focus of acute, necrotizing, hemorrhagic encephalitis in the basal ganglia; no inclusion bodies were recognized in this lesion, and an immunoperoxidase reaction for *Herpes simplex* Type 1 antigen gave equivocal results.

We have not identified any cases of definite cerebral toxoplasmosis in our series of children with HIV infection, although one such case has recently been reported.[12] One premature infant not included in our series had evidence of congenital CNS toxoplasmosis at birth, with many large, necrotizing lesions containing encysted bradyzoites at death three months later; the mother, an intravenous drug abuser, also died with CNS toxoplasmosis. We have seen no cases of cryptococcal meningitis, and our clinical colleagues have not as yet documented a single instance in over 100 children with HIV infection whom they have followed.* Likewise, no cases of PML have been seen. Seroconversion to JC virus, which causes this white matter disease, has been found to occur in late childhood or adolescence, in epidemiologic studies.[13] PML, even in other clinical settings, is unusual in children, with the youngest case reported in a five-year-old child who had congenital combined immunodeficiency.[13]

NEOPLASMS

The most common CNS neoplasm seen in adult patients with HIV infection is primary lymphoma, usually of the B cell type. An etiologic role for Epstein-Barr virus

---

*L.G. Epstein, personal communication

(EBV) has been suggested in primary CNS lymphoma,[14] raising the possibility that it might represent another form of opportunistic or reactivated latent infection.[15] Petito et al.[1] reported an incidence for this tumor of 6% in their large series of adult subjects with AIDS, the majority of whom were homosexual men. It has been suggested that this lesion is less frequent in subjects who were intravenous drug abusers.[16]

Few cases of primary CNS lymphoma have been mentioned previously in children with HIV infection.[17] We have seen three such neoplasms, two of which were proven on biopsy (both patients, a five-year-old boy and an eleven-year-old boy, eventually died of progressive brain lymphomas, but autopsies could not be obtained), and one was discovered at autopsy in a two-year-old girl.[18] The cell types were large cell lymphoma (two cases) and immunoblastic sarcoma (one case), similar to the results in the adult series of So et al.[19] The incidence of primary lymphoma is 1 : 25 (4%) in our autopsy series, or 3 : 100 (3%) of all pediatric cases of HIV infection, living and dead, seen at this institution, suggesting that this neoplasm is a less frequent complication of HIV infection in children than it is in adults.

Although Kaposi's sarcoma is a common neoplasm in adults, particularly in homosexual men with HIV infection, few cases of central nervous system involvement by this disease have been reported.[9] We have seen no cases of Kaposi's sarcoma in children at this institution, either outside or inside the CNS, and no cases of CNS involvement by this tumor have been reported in children with HIV infection.

VACUOLAR MYELOPATHY

Petito et al.[20] reported the first series of patients with a lesion characterized by spinal cord signs and symptoms and vacuolar degeneration of myelin in the lateral and dorsal columns of the spinal cord (Fig. 1).

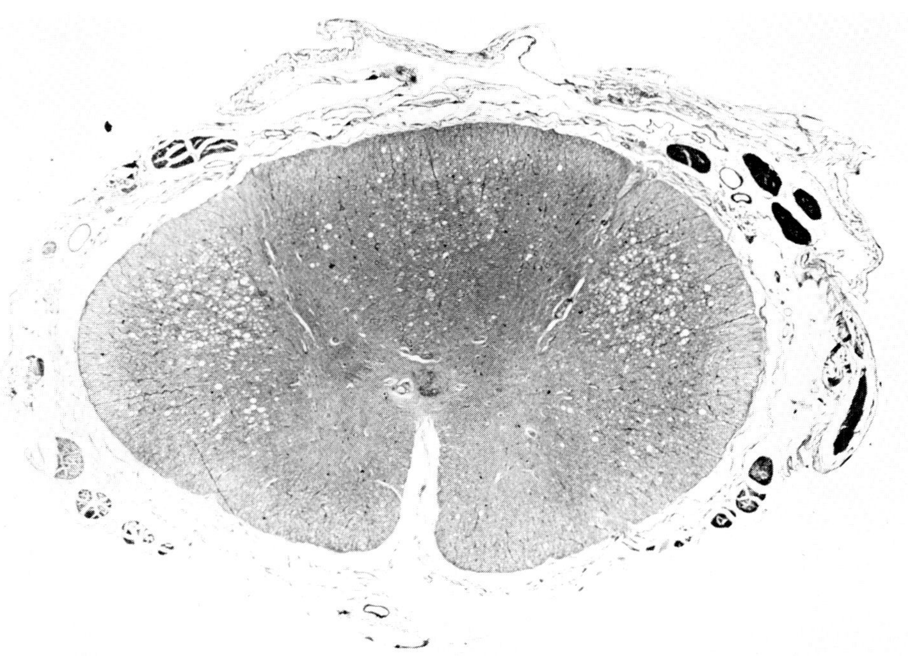

Figure 1. Vacuolar myelopathy in a 44-year-old homosexual man. Note vacuolation in the posterior and lateral columns without respect for fiber tracts. (Luxol fast blue-PAS stain, original magnification ×12.)

These authors noted a resemblance to the classical neuropathological changes of subacute combined degeneration, due to vitamin B_{12} deficiency, although none of the patients who were studied had low serum B_{12} levels. The incidence of this disorder was greater than 20% in subjects coming to autopsy, and more recent data from a larger series of subjects from the same institution have confirmed this figure.[1] The etiology has been controversial, with some authors favoring direct infection of the spinal cord with HIV,[21,22] while others have suggested other factors, such as metabolic derangements.[1,5,20,23]

We have examined 20 spinal cords in our own series of autopsy material in children with HIV infection and have been able to find only two cases of vacuolar myelopathy, one in a two-year-old boy who developed an acute spinal cord syndrome, and the other in a nine-year-old girl with progressive dementia and spasticity. However, about one third of our cases have shown in the gray and white matter of the spinal cord histopathological features (see below), which we and others have associated with primary HIV infection, without concurrent vacuolar myelopathy,[23] leading us to conclude that it is unlikely that primary HIV infection of the spinal cord is the cause of the myelopathy. It has recently been proposed[24] that this lesion is due to the presence of another retrovirus, human T-leukemia virus Type I (HTLV-I), producing a lesion in patients with HIV infection similar to that seen in patients with HTLV-I infection alone (tropical spastic paraparesis and variants).[25,26] It is likely that the etiology of vacuolar myelopathy in subjects with HIV infection will be resolved in the near future.

PRIMARY HIV INFECTION OF THE CNS

The pathological findings of HIV encephalitis have been reported in several previous papers.[1,6,27,28] In summary, the brain was frequently atrophic and the centrum semiovale showed diffuse myelin pallor. The microscopical hallmark has been the presence of multinucleated giant cells (MGC),[28-30] which have been reported to contain HIV particles on ultrastructural examination, with evidence of budding or replication in and from these cells.[31-33] The MGC have been seen in the perivascular space and in the parenchyma of both gray and white matter, often in association with round cell infiltrates, including macrophages, lymphocytes, and occasional plasma cells. In addition, there are many findings that are nonspecific, yet prevalent, in the brains of patients with HIV infection . Even though most of these findings are observed in the brains of both adults and children with HIV infection, the extent and topography of some of these findings differ in the two groups.

A. Multinucleated Giant Cells

Multinucleated giant cells are the most characteristic microscopical finding of HIV infection of the brain. However, not all brains that have evidence of virus (by hybridization techniques, immunocytochemistry, or electron microscopy) have been reported to contain MGC.[28,34-36] Failure to demonstrate MGC in such cases may represent insufficient tissue sampling or perhaps an earlier stage of HIV infection, before the formation of MGC. Although the MGC themselves were occasionally found singly, without other cells, they usually were located amid loose collections of other chronic inflammatory cells, including many macrophages and variable numbers of lymphocytes and plasma cells (Fig. 2). Lymphocytes tended to be abundant in these cellular infiltrates in children, while they were less conspicuous in adults, except for occasional cases with a shorter and more fulminant clinical course of dementia.[28] In adults, MGC were frequent in the centrum semiovale, basal ganglia, external capsule, thalamus, and pons, with involvement of the ce-

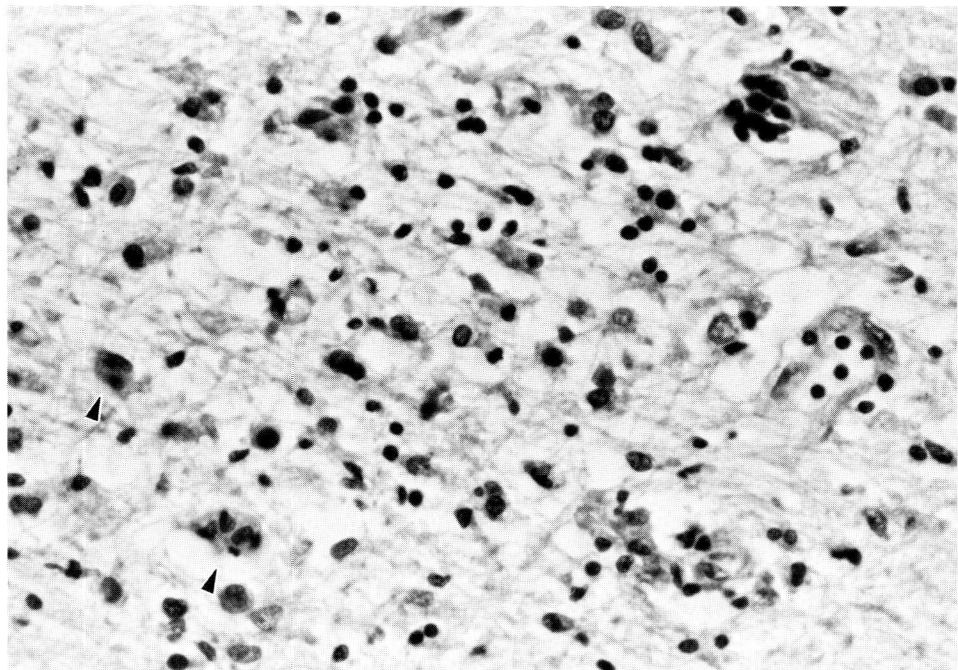

Figure 2. Inflammatory infiltrate in the centrum semiovale of a 34-year-old man who was an intravenous drug abuser. This loose cellular collection includes macrophages, lymphocytes, plasma cells, and multinucleated cells (arrowheads). (H&E, original magnification ×500.)

rebral cortex only in more severe cases.[28] In children, the cerebral cortex frequently contained these cells, although they were also prominent in the same regions as in the adult cases.[6] The appearance of the MGC suggested that they had resulted from both cell fusion[6,37] and amitotic division of nuclei.[38] Those MGC that appeared to have partially fused cell membranes (Fig. 3) were frequently noted in the brains of adults, while those that appeared to arise by amitotic division were more readily observed in children. The latter often attained huge sizes, with a granular, densely eosinophilic center surrounded by a ring of nuclei or a cluster of nuclei in a horseshoe shape. It was in such MGC that HIV particles were most readily observed by electron microscopy.[31] In some instances, the nuclei of these large MGC had tails that could be traced to other nuclei (nuclear bridging) (Fig. 4).[38]

B. Mineralization

Mineralization is prevalent and extensive in the brains of children with HIV infection, constituting the most frequently encountered microscopical finding.[6] The most commonly involved areas have been the basal ganglia, particularly the putamen and globus pallidus, and the frontal white matter, regions that exhibit increased density with computerized tomographic scans.[6,7] Small mineralizations were present as extracellular, basophilic concretions located about or adjacent to small blood vessels. Larger vessel mineralization, involving the walls of medium-sized arteries (Fig. 5), has also been noted, similar to the calcific arteriopathy observed in the systemic organs of some children with HIV infection.[39] In some instances, the larger CNS vessels also had inflammation of their walls, but usually

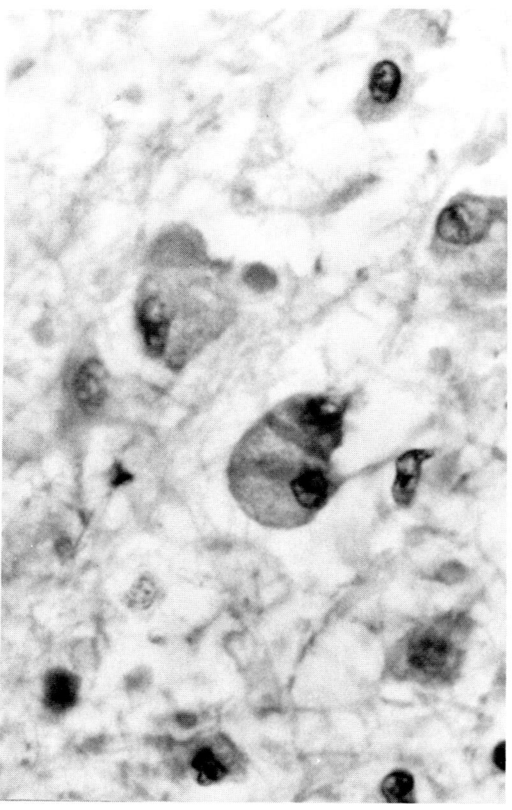

Figure 3. Multinucleated giant cell with an appearance suggesting cell fusion, in internal capsule of a 34-year-old intravenous drug abuser. (H&E, original magnification ×800.)

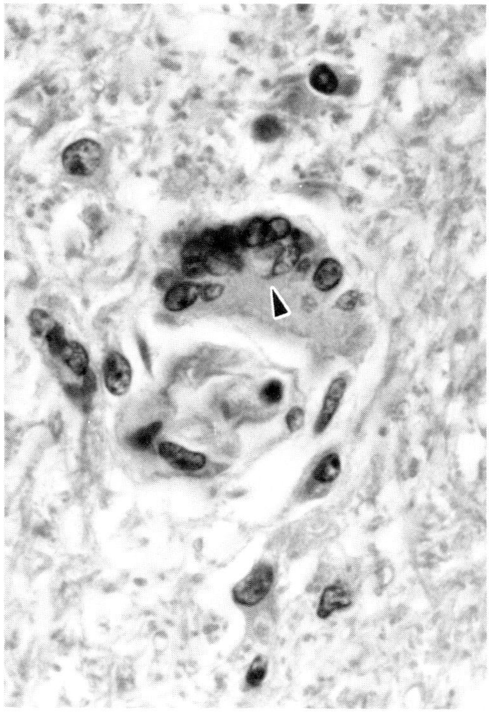

Figure 4. Multinucleated giant cell with a nuclear tail (arrowhead), in cerebellar white matter of a 9-year-old girl with HIV infection. Note also the horseshoe arrangement of the numerous nuclei as well as the dense cytoplasm. (H&E, original magnification ×800.)

there was no apparent inflammation associated with either the large or small vessel mineralizations. In a few cases, we have also encountered small, juxtavascular mineralizations in the cerebral cortex, occasionally associated with inflammatory cell infiltrates and MGC. With special staining techniques, the mineralizations can be demonstrated to contain both calcium and iron.

Mineralization was noted in the brains of adult subjects as well, but was usually minimal or moderate in amount, occurring as vascular calcification or as calcium droplets in the basal ganglia and hippocampus. These changes were similar in appearance and in extent to the mineralization encountered in the brains of elderly individuals without HIV infection.[40]

C. Perivascular Brown Pigment

Perivascular brown pigment was the most prevalent finding in the brains of adults who died with AIDS. This pigment was seen in both atrophic and nonatrophic brains and in brains both with and without inflammatory changes. The pigment was usually located in the cerebral cortex, within perivascular macrophages, but occasionally it was free in the perivascular space. Some of this pigment was clearly iron on Prussian blue staining, suggesting previous extravasation of red blood cells. However, in some instances the pigment was Prussian blue negative, but was periodic acid-Schiff (PAS) positive and appeared to be lipofuscin, suggesting an origin from degenerating cells, of which the most likely source was neurons. The presence of PAS positive pigment ap-

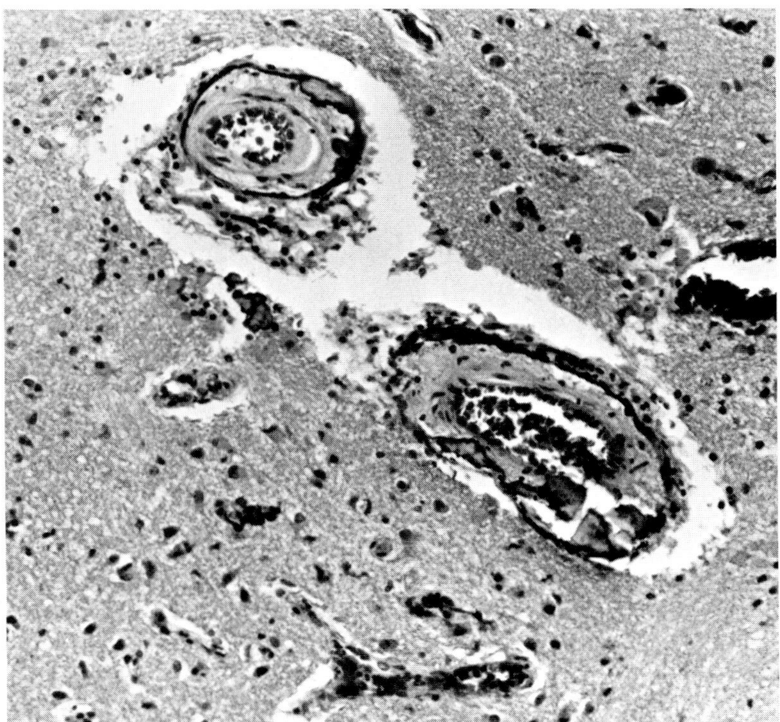

Figure 5. Mineralization of medium sized arteries in the basal ganglia of a 2-year-old boy with HIV infection. (H&E, original magnification ×200.)

peared to correlate with the frequent presence of atrophic, darkly staining neurons with shrunken, pyknotic nuclei in the cerebral cortex of adult patients with HIV infection.*

Perivascular brown pigment was infrequently encountered in the brains of children with HIV infection, and when it occurred, it usually consisted of iron rather than lipofuscin. This difference may simply be a reflection of a relative lack of lipofuscin in the neurons of young children.

D. White Matter Changes

White matter pallor (Fig. 6) appeared to be the most common finding in the brains of adult subjects with HIV infection and

AIDS-dementia complex (ADC).[28] The pathogenesis of this pallor is not yet clear. The degree of pallor was usually beyond what would be expected from the extent of the cellular infiltrates. In many brains of adult subjects with ADC, white matter pallor was the sole finding, with no associated cellular infiltrates or MGC.[28] In children, the centrum semiovale usually had a loose appearance;[6] however, interpretation of this change has been difficult, since myelination is an ongoing process that continues for several years of postnatal life. The childhood cases usually exhibited white matter astrocytosis on immunoperoxidase stain for glial fibrillary acidic protein (GFAP).[6] This gliosis was clearly pathologic in children who were over two years of age, whereas in children less than two years of age there was a similar "myelination gliosis" in the white matter in controls, limiting the usefulness of this finding.

____

*E.-S. Cho, unpublished observations

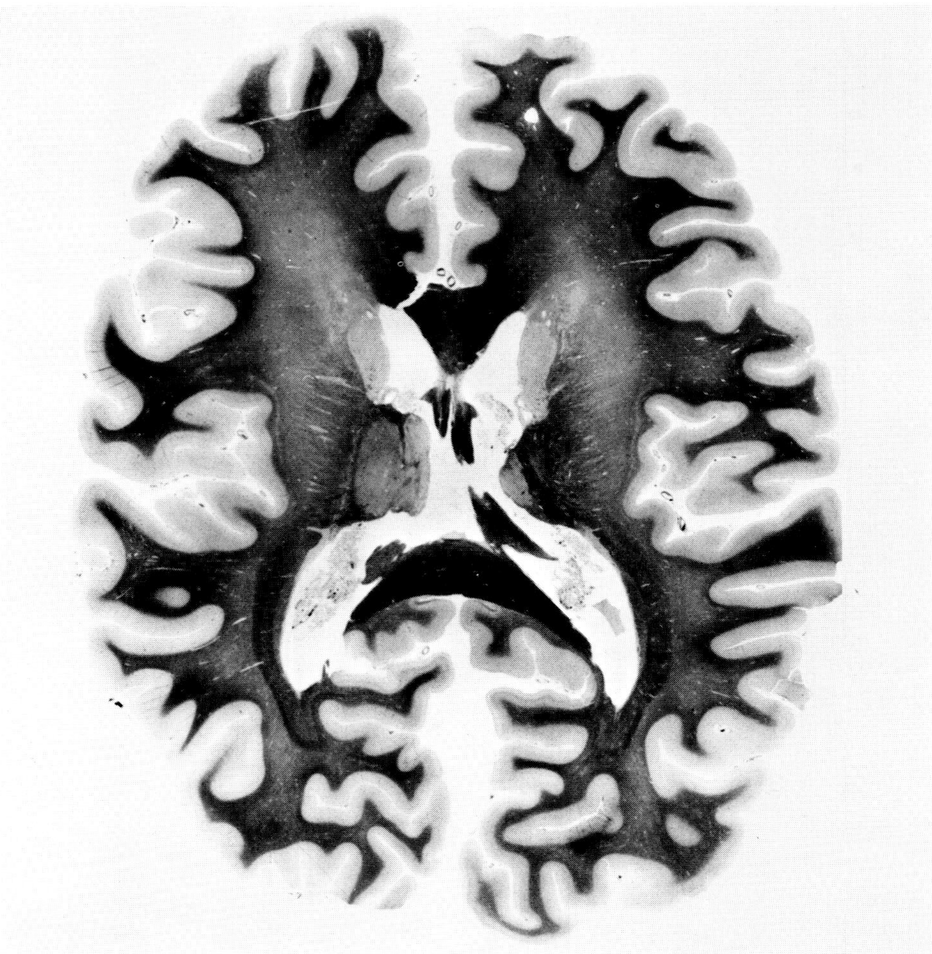

Figure 6. Moderately atrophic brain with diffuse myelin pallor in the centrum semiovale of a 44-year-old homosexual man. (Weigert myelin stain)

DISCUSSION

Children dying with HIV infection, particularly infants, have far fewer opportunistic infections of the CNS than do adults with this disease. The most obvious explanation for this difference, although possibly not the only one, is the shorter time of exposure of children to the various pathogens that are usually seen in HIV-infected adults. In addition, there is a lower incidence in children of primary infection with certain otherwise benign microorganisms, such as *Toxoplasma gondii* and cytomegalovirus, that in adults result in reactivated infection at a later time due to the immunodeficient state associated with HIV infection. Although the mechanisms of infection are not well understood, it would appear that exposure to such pathogens as *T. gondii* and *Cryptococcus neoformans* is unusual in children in industrialized, Western countries, even among children from a lower socioeconomic background. A different pattern of exposure might be expected in developing countries, such as those in central Africa, where HIV infection is endemic and where there is a large number of perinatally acquired cases.

The situation is clearest with regard to JC virus exposure. Epidemiologic studies have identified the age of seroconversion to this papovavirus as being predominantly in late childhood after the age of five years and in adolescence.[41] Thus it is not surprising that as yet no cases of PML have been reported in children with HIV infection. On the other hand, CMV infection is prevalent in children and young children in general, and it is this agent that we have identified twice in the CNS in our series of autopsies of children with HIV infection.

Until now, the overwhelming majority of children over the age of five years who have had clinically manifest HIV infection have acquired the infection by receiving a transfusion of blood products from an HIV infected donor.[42] However, an increasingly older population of children with perinatally acquired HIV is being seen, with the oldest reported case being seven years at clinical presentation.[42] The oldest patient with perinatally acquired disease to come to autopsy in our series was age nine years (we had previously reported findings in an 11-year-old boy who was a hemophiliac, who interestingly had CMV lesions in the brain).[43] It is likely that we will see more opportunistic infections, and possibly neoplasms, involving the CNS in these children, as time goes on. It is also possible that the incidence of vacuolar myelopathy might be higher in these older children, since the nine-year-old patient had this spinal cord disorder. As the spectrum of HIV infection in children widens and as older children with perinatally acquired disease survive, it is likely that some of them will have the same complications as adults with HIV infection, unless preventive measures or antiretroviral therapies prove adequate to control the disease.

SUMMARY

The lower incidence of complicating opportunistic and reactivated latent infections in the CNS of children with HIV infection has resulted in a "cleaner" system, allowing better appreciation of the lesions associated with primary HIV brain infection. The most striking differences that we have seen in the CNS of children, when compared to adults with regard to primary HIV infection, have been the following: More florid inflammation and more frequent MGC in the children; more frequent localization of MGC in the cerebral cortex in children; more basophilic mineralization in the children; more perivascular brown pigment in the adults; and more obvious white matter change in the adults. It has been noted that the median survival time for children under one year of age with AIDS is significantly less than that for older children (6.5 months vs. 19.7 months).[42] Thus the tempo of HIV infection would seem to be more rapid in children, particularly young children. Our own neuropathological observations would support the hypothesis of a more fulminant CNS disease in children, in keeping with the well-known phenomenon of increased virulence of viral infections in the immature central nervous system.[44]

ACKNOWLEDGMENTS

The authors wish to thank Dr. Leon G. Epstein for reviewing the manuscript. This project has been supported by Public Health Service Grants NS 25121 and AI 23242.

REFERENCES

1. Petito CK, Cho E-S, Lemann W, et al: Neuropathology of acquired immunodeficiency syndrome (AIDS): An autopsy review. J Neuropathol Exp Neurol 1986; 45:635–646
2. Epstein LG, Sharer LR, Oleske JM, et al: Neurologic manifestations of HIV infection in children. Pediatrics 1986; 78:678–687
3. Moskowitz LB, Hensley GT, Chan JC et al: The neuropathology of acquired immune deficiency syndrome. Arch Pathol Lab Med 1984; 108:867–872
4. Anders KH, Guerra WF, Tomiyasu U, et al: The neuropathology of AIDS: UCLA experience and review. Am J Pathol 1986; 124:537–558
5. Rhodes RH: Histopathology of the central nervous system in the acquired immunodeficiency syndrome. Hum Pathol 1987; 18:636–643

6. Sharer LR, Epstein LG, Cho E-S, et al: Pathologic features of AIDS encephalopathy in children: Evidence for LAV/HTLV-III infection of brain. Hum Pathol 1986; 17:271–284

7. Belman AL, Lantos G, Horoupian D, et al: Calcification of the basal ganglia in infants and children with AIDS. Neurology 1986; 36:1129–1199

8. Anderson VM, Kaufmann SL, Sher JH, et al: The pathology of pediatric AIDS: A review of 33 cases. Presented at Third International Conference on AIDS, Washington, D.C. June 3, 1987

9. Levy RM, Bredesen DE, Rosenblum ML: Neurological manifestations of the acquired immunodeficiency syndrome (AIDS): Experience at UCSF and review of the literature. J Neurosurg 1985; 62:475–495

10. Sharer LR, Kapila R: Neuropathologic observations in acquired immunodeficiency syndrome (AIDS). Acta Neuropathol (Berlin) 1985; 66:188–198

11. Kaminski ZC, Kapila R, Sharer LR, et al: *Prototheca wickerhamii* meningitis in a patient with acquired immunodeficiency syndrome. Submitted for publication

12. Biggemann B, Voit T, Neuen E, et al: Neurologic manifestations in three German children with AIDS. Neuropediatrics 1987; 18:99–106

13. Walker DL: Progressive multifocal leukoencephalopathy. In: Koetsier JC, ed, Handbook of Clinical Neurology, Vol 3 (47): Demyelinating Diseases, Amsterdam, Elsevier, 1985; 503–524

14. Hochberg FH, Miller G, Schooley RT, et al: Central-nervous-system lymphoma related to Epstein-Barr virus. N Engl J Med 1983; 309:745–748

15. Rosenberg NL, Hochberg FH, Miller G, Kleinschmidt-DeMasters BK: Primary central nervous system lymphoma related to Epstein-Barr virus in a patient with acquired immune deficiency syndrome. Ann Neurol 1986; 20:98–102

16. Ambros RA, Lee E-Y, Sharer LR, et al: The acquired immunodeficiency syndrome in intravenous drug abusers and patients with a sexual risk: Clinical and postmortem comparisons. Hum Pathol 1987; 18:1109–1114

17. Andiman WA, Eastman R, Martin K, et al: Opportunistic lymphoproliferations associated with Epstein-Barr viral DNA in infants and children with AIDS. Lancet 1985; 2:1390–1392

18. Epstein LG, Di Carlo FJ, Joshi VV, et al: Primary lymphoma of the central nervous system in children with AIDS. Pediatrics (in press, 1988)

19. So YT, Beckstead JH, Davis RL: Primary central nervous system lymphoma in acquired immune deficiency syndrome: A clinical and pathological study. Ann Neurol 1986; 20:566–572

20. Petito CK, Navia BA, Cho E-S, et al: Vacuolar myelopathy pathologically resembling subacute combined degeneration in patients with the acquired immunodeficiency syndrome. N Engl J Med 1985; 312:874–879

21. Ho DD, Rota TR, Schooley, et al: Isolation of HTLV-III from CSF and neural tissues of patients with AIDS related neurologic syndromes. N Engl J Med 1985; 313:1493–1497

22. de la Monte SM, Ho DD, Schooley RT, et al: Subacute encephalomyelitis of AIDS and its relation to HTLV-III infection. Neurology 1987; 37:562–569

23. Sharer LR, Epstein LG, Cho E-S, Petito CK: HTLV-III and vacuolar myelopathy (Letter). N Engl J Med 1986; 315:62–63

24. Petito CK: Review of central nervous system pathology in human immunodeficiency virus infection. Ann Neurol 1988; 23(Suppl):54–57

25. Johnson RT, McArthur JC; Myelopathies and retroviral infections (Editorial). Ann Neurol 1987; 21:113–116

26. Roman GC: Retrovirus-associated myelopathies. Arch Neurol 1987; 44:659–663

27. Snider WD, Simpson DM, Nielsen SL, et al: Neurological complications of acquired immune deficiency syndrome: Analysis of 50 patients. Ann Neurol 1983; 14:403–418

28. Navia BA, Cho E-S, Petito CK, Price RW: The AIDS dementia complex.: II Neuropathology. Ann Neurol 1986; 19:525–535

29. Sharer LR, Cho E-S, Epstein LG: Multinucleated giant cells and HTLV-III in AIDS encephalopathy. Hum Pathol 1985; 16:760

30. Budka H: Multinucleated giant cells in brain: A hallmark of the acquired immune deficiency syndrome (AIDS). Acta Neuropathol (Berlin) 1986; 69:253–258

31. Epstein LG, Sharer LR, Cho E-S, et al: HTLV/III/LAV-like retrovirus particles in the brains of patients with AIDS encephalopathy. AIDS Res 1985; 1:447–454

32. Koenig S, Gendelman HE, Orenstein JM, et al: Detection of AIDS virus in macrophages in brain tissue from AIDS patients with encephalopathy. Science 1986; 233:1089–1093

33. Meyenhofer MF, Epstein LG, Cho E-S, Sharer LR: Ultrastructural morphology and intracellular production of human immunodeficiency virus (HIV) in brain. J Neuropathol Exp Neurol 1987; 46:474–484

34. Gabuzda DH, Ho DD, de la Monte SM, et al: Immunohistochemical identification of HTLV-III antigen in brains of patients with AIDS. Ann Neurol 1986; 20:289–295

35. Vazeux R, Brousse N, Jarry A, et al: AIDS subacute encephalitis: Identification of HIV-infected cells. Am J Pathol 1987; 126:403–410

36. Gyorkey F, Melnick JL, Gyorkey P: Human immunodeficiency virus in brain biopsies of patients with AIDS and progressive encephalopathy. J Infect Dis 1987; 155:870–876

37. Kato T, Hirano A, Llena JF, Dembitzer HM: neuropathology of acquired immune deficiency syndrome (AIDS) in 53 autopsy cases with particular emphasis on microglial nodules and multinucleated giant cells. Acta Neuropathol 1987; 73:287–294

38. Mizusawa H, Hirano H, Llena JF, Kato T: Nuclear bridges in multinucleated giant cells associated with primary lymphoma of the brain in acquired immunodeficiency syndrome (AIDS). Acta Neuropathol (Berlin) 1987; 75:23–26

39. Joshi VV, Pawel B, Connor E, et al: Arteriopathy

in children with acquired immune deficiency syndrome. Ped Pathol 1987; 7:261–275

40. Oppenheimer DR: Diseases of the basal ganglia, cerebellum and motor neurons. In: Adams JH, Corsellis JAN, Duchen LW (eds.): Greenfield's Neuropathology, 4th ed., New York, John Wiley and Sons, 1984; 709–712

41. Padgett BL, Walker DL: Prevalence of antibodies in human sera against JC virus, an isolate from a case of progressive multifocal leukoencephalopathy. J Infect Dis 1973; 127:467–470

42. Rogers MF, Thomas PA, Starcher ET, et al: Acquired immunodeficiency syndrome in children: Report of the Centers for Disease Control national surveillance, 1982 to 1985. Pediatrics 1987; 79:1008–10014

43. Epstein LG, Sharer LR, Joshi VV, et al: Progressive encephalopathy in children with acquired immune deficiency syndrome. Ann Neurol 1985; 17:488–496

44. Johnson RT: Viral Infections of the Nervous System. New York, Raven Press 1982

9

Polyradiculopathy and Sensory Ganglionitis due to Cytomegalovirus in Acquired Immune Deficiency Syndrome (AIDS)*

Gleb N. Budzilovich
Ann Avitabile
George Niedt
Slobodan N. Aleksic
Marc K. Rosenblum

A CAUSE AND EFFECT RELATIONSHIP between cytomegalovirus (CMV) infection and a syndrome of subacute symmetric progressive polyradiculoneuropathy was initially suggested by Klemola et al.[1] who in 1967 reported two adult male patients presenting with characteristic clinical features of Guillain-Barré syndrome (GBS) and serologic evidence of a recently acquired CMV infection. A number of subsequent clinical case reports and epidemiologic surveys provided additional and rather compelling, albeit indirect, evidence of a link between CMV infection and various neurologic syndromes suggesting involvement of the peripheral nervous system (PNS). These syndromes include brachial plexus neuropathy,[2] polyneuritis,[3] GBS,[4,5] distal symmetric neuropathy, and chronic inflammatory polyneuropathy,[6] the latter two disorders occurring in the setting of acquired immune deficiency syndrome (AIDS).

The pertinent pathologic studies of the PNS carried out on patients suffering from AIDS are few. In one of these, no etiologic agent could be identified,[7] while in the additional three studies, in which CMV was demonstrated in the PNS, the scope of the pathologic examination was limited in two,[8,9] the exception being only one adequately studied case of Eidelberg et al.[10] In the following, results of complete post mortem examinations of the general organs and central and peripheral nervous systems of three patients with AIDS are reported. A

*Presented in part at X International Congress of Neuropathology, September 7–12, 1986, Stockholm, Sweden.

detailed description of pathologic changes in various subdivisions of the PNS, including the hitherto unreported findings in the peripheral sensory ganglia, will be presented and diverse pathogenetic mechanisms operative in the production of CMV-induced injury to the PNS discussed.

CASE REPORTS

CASE 1: This 38-year-old man, a homosexual with AIDS for 10 months manifested by cutaneous Kaposi's sarcoma and an episode of *Pneumocystis carinii* pneumonia, was admitted to the hospital for evaluation of diarrhea, new skin lesions, and weakness. One and a half months ante mortem he developed a neurologic disorder characterized by shooting pains in his legs and progressive loss of the ability to walk. Neurologic examination revealed that he was barely able to overcome gravity with his lower extremities, which lacked deep tendon reflexes, while sensation and upper extremity strength and reflexes remained essentially intact. Lumbar puncture, x-ray examination of the lumbosacral spine, and myelography failed to establish a diagnosis. Electromyography demonstrated diffuse hyperirritability in both lower extremities without florid abnormal spontaneous activity. On attempted volitional activation, the patient could scarcely muster a single unit interference pattern, but prompt responses of good amplitude were elicited on more proximal stimulation. Conduction velocities were basically intact, though a moderate attenuation in sensory potential amplitudes was present in the lower extremities. He became increasingly confused, disoriented, and weak to the point where he could barely move either leg and developed pulmonary infiltrates accompanied by tachypnea, hypothermia, and hypotension shortly before death.

At general autopsy, the pertinent findings included: multiple necrotizing lesions due to CMV in bronchi, stomach, colon, gallbladder, adrenal glands, and testes. No necrosis was associated with the presence of CMV in the pulmonary parenchyma, thyroid, or kidneys. There was widespread infestation of the spleen and lymph nodes with *Mycobacterium avium-intracellulare* (MAI) and severe lymphoid depletion. Multiple foci of Kaposi's sarcoma were found involving the skin and both lungs.

Gross examination of the central (brain and spinal cord) and peripheral nervous systems (cranial and spinal nerve roots and nerves; Gasserian and dorsal root ganglia; brachial and lumbosacral plexuses; lumbar sympathetic, stellate and celiac ganglia) revealed only conspicuous thickening and fine granularity of the ventricular ependymal lining (Fig. 1).

Microscopically, there was focal loss of ependymal cells often associated with frank necrosis of subependymal tissues. Both large intranuclear (Cowdry's type A) and smaller intracytoplasmic amphophilic or eosinophilic inclusion bodies were readily identified in many of the surviving ependymal cells (Fig. 2), and in some of the greatly hypertrophied astrocytes in edematous subependymal tissues around the foci of necrosis. Small veins in the vicinity of the latter showed infiltrates of mononuclear inflammatory cells. Scattered "microglial" nodules, some containing large unidentified cells with intranuclear and/or cytoplasmic viral inclusion bodies, were encountered in the grisea and white matter of the cerebrum and lower brain stem. Some motoneurons of lumbar segments of spinal cord displayed central chromatolysis.

The changes in the cranial nerves (III & V) and spinal nerve roots ranged from active degeneration (swelling, vacuolation, fragmentation or loss) of

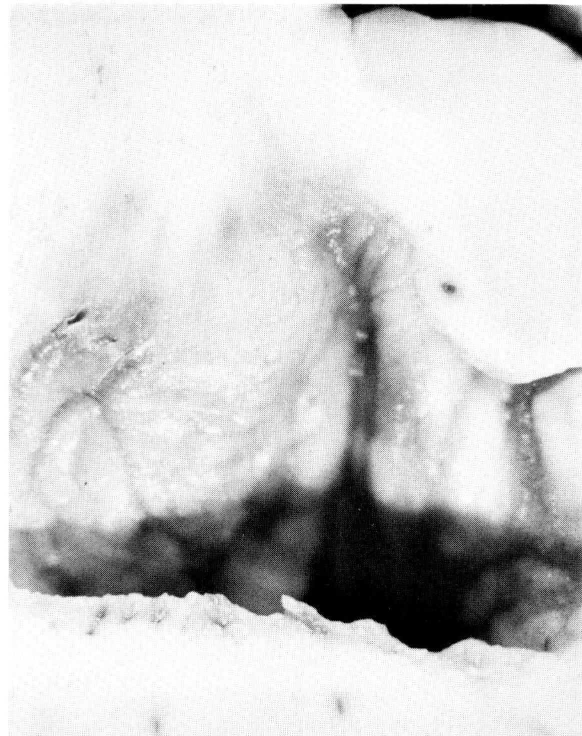

Figure 1. (Case 1) The ependymal lining of temporal horn of left lateral ventricle is thickened, dull, and granular.

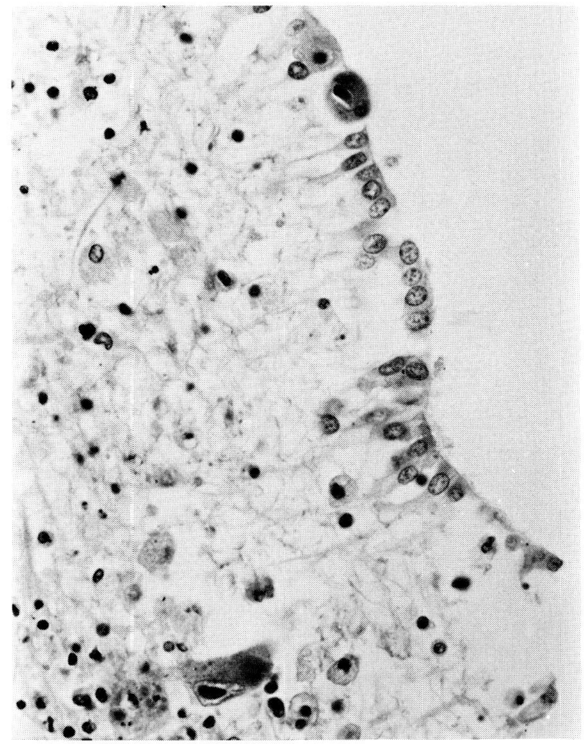

Figure 2. (Case 1) Intranuclear and cytoplasmic CMV inclusion bodies in two ependymal cells (top) and enlarged astrocyte (bottom) in edematous, slightly inflamed subependymal tissue. (H&E, original magnification ×100.)

myelin sheaths with axonal preservation, to frank recent necrosis involving all tissue constituents. Such changes were accompanied by a relatively mild and predominantly chronic inflammatory response. Intranuclear and cytoplasmic inclusions as described above were noted frequently in Schwann cells and only occasionally in endoneurial and perineurial fibroblasts (Fig. 3). The walls of some small blood vessels, probably veins, adjacent to foci of frank necrosis, and, occasionally, at some distance from them, were edematous and infiltrated by inflammatory cells or replaced by fibrin. No viral inclusions were identified in such blood vessels. The extent and degree of the involvement of the anterior and posterior spinal nerve roots differed strikingly, the former bearing the brunt of the injury, which was most pronounced in the lumbosacral anterior roots (Figs. 4 & 5). Central chromatolysis and necrosis

of rare ganglion cells were noted in the lumbar spinal ganglia. No specific changes were recognized in the sympathetic ganglia or their processes, save for a few small lymphocytic infiltrates in some of the gray rami. A small number of nerve fibers in samples of the lumbosacral plexus showed active Wallerian degeneration.

Case 2: This 41-year-old man, a homosexual with AIDS for 11 months manifested by repeated bouts of *Pneumocystis carinii* pneumonia, developed lower back pain with radiation into the right leg and paresthesias in April 1983. By June, this required narcotic analgesics. Neurologic examination at that time revealed decrease in all sensory modalities in the right lower extremity in an L5-S1 root distribution and absent ankle jerk. He then noted the onset of new low thoracic back pains with shock-like radiations to the chest and abdomen as well as increasing numb-

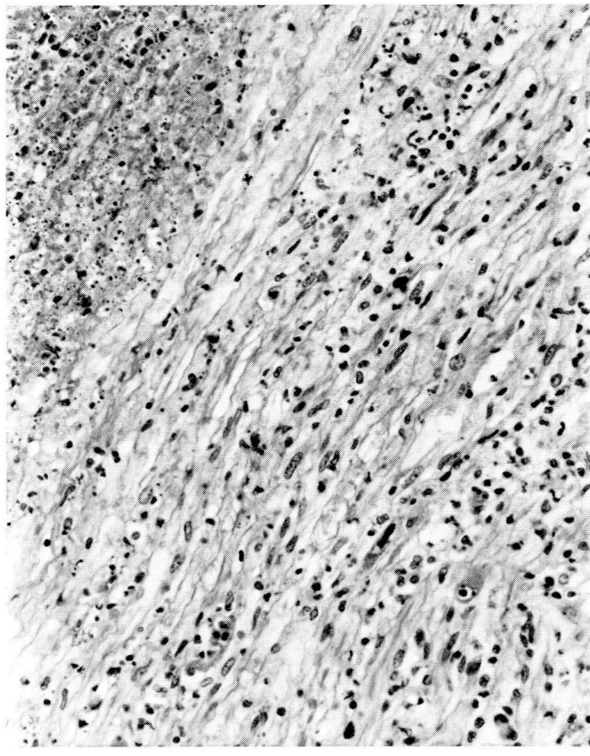

Figure 3. (Case 1) Anterior spinal nerve root, lumbar level. Viral inclusion bodies in two Schwann cells, diffuse rarefaction, and mononuclear infiltrate in root. Area of total necrosis in left upper corner. (H&E, original magnification ×60.)

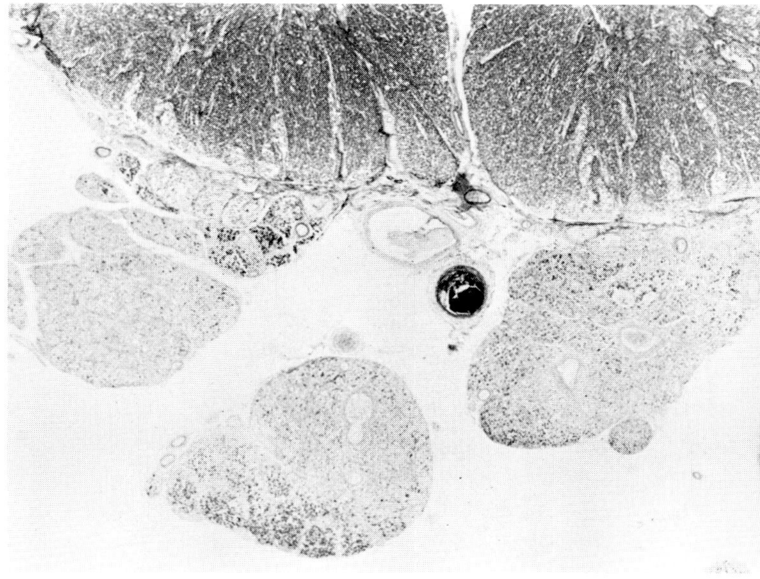

Figure 4. (Case 1) Anterior spinal roots, lumbar level. There is almost total loss of myelin sheaths. (LFB-PAS stain for myelin, original magnification ×5.)

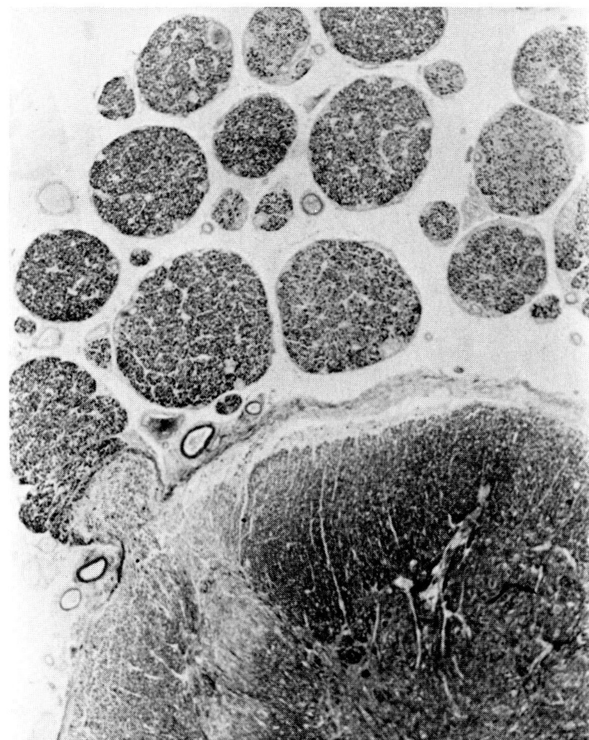

Figure 5. (Case 1) Posterior spinal root, same level as Fig. 4. Slight loss of myelin sheaths in two fascicles (right upper corner). (LFB-PAS stain for myelin, original magnification ×5.)

ness of both legs. When examined in July, lower extremity strength was relatively preserved, but there was circumferential loss of pin-prick sensation in both lower extremities as well as decreased vibratory sense and proprioception. Ankle jerks could not be elicited and knee jerks were 1+. Electromyography and nerve conduction studies suggested a sensorimotor polyneuropathy with prominent demyelinating features. Diffuse hyperirritability of the lumbar paraspinal muscles was thought to represent a superimposed radiculopathy. CMV was documented in bronchial washings and suspected in a liver biopsy in September. The patient developed progressive respiratory failure and died in October 1983.

At general autopsy, pertinent findings included: widely disseminated CMV infection involving lungs (severe necrotizing bronchopneumonia, combined weight of lungs 2,450 grams), liver, pancreas, spleen, adrenal, thyroid and parathyroid glands, esophagus, stomach, colon and rectum; pneumonitis with abscess formation and necrotizing laryngo-tracheobronchitis due to *Aspergillus fumigatus*; esophagitis due to *Candida albicans*; severe lymphoid depletion of spleen and lymph nodes, and MAI infection of the lymphoid tissues.

Grossly, the brain and spinal cord were normal. The lumbosacral spinal nerve roots appeared dark tan. The dorsal root ganglia and spinal nerves from the thoracic and lumbosacral regions were unremarkable.

Microscopically, "microglial" nodules were numerous in the cerebrum, cerebellum, and lower brain stem, and rare in the spinal cord, which showed moderate loss of fibers in the fasciculi graciles (Fig. 6) and central chromatolysis of occasional motoneurons in the lumbosacral segments. The sensory ganglia of the low thoracic and particularly the lumbosacral regions showed a 30–75% loss of their neurons associated with formation of residual nod-

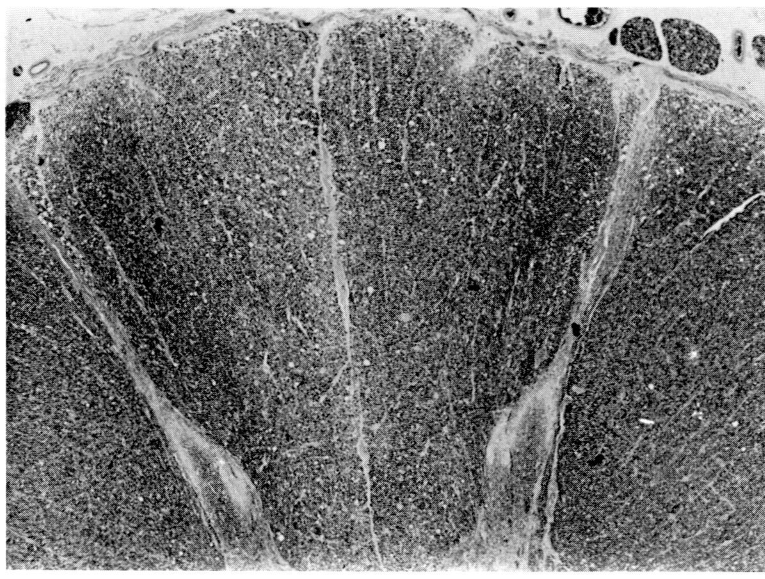

Figure 6. (Case 2) Spinal cord, posterior columns, upper thoracic level. Moderate pallor and vacuolation of fasciculi graciles. (LFB-PAS stain for myelin, original magnification ×5.)

ules of Nageotte (Fig. 7). Viral inclusion bodies were detected in the capsule cells of some of the surviving neurons and in "stromal" cells (Schwann cells and fibroblasts). Active neuronophagia of an occasional ganglion cell was also seen. There was a mild mixed inflammatory response. Secondary (Wallerian) degeneration of the posterior nerve roots was commensurate with the degree of neuronal loss at different levels involved, ranging from slight to moderate at low thoracic levels to near total in the cauda equina (Figs. 8 & 9). Neither viral inclusion bodies nor inflammation were present in the posterior roots, which only showed a conspicuous infiltration by lipid-laden macrophages. In contrast, there was only focal, slight to moderate demyelination of the anterior roots (Fig. 10). Typical viral inclusion bodies were seen in rare Schwann cells and endoneurial and perineurial fibro-

blasts of the anterior roots and proximal portions of the spinal nerves.

Case 3: This 30-year-old man, a homosexual with AIDS for 5 months manifested by cutaneous and gastrointestinal Kaposi's sarcoma, atypical mycobacteriosis (MAI) and an episode of *Pneumocystis carinii* pneumonia, was admitted to the hospital for evaluation of progressive weakness, fever, and dyspnea. Neurologic examination revealed muscle atrophy, areflexia of the lower extremities, and a loss of sensation in the 4th and 5th digits of the right hand. Five days after admission he could no longer walk. Nerve conduction studies were within normal limits, however, abnormal spontaneous activity was present on electromyography. Repetitive stimulation tests were normal and the impression was lumbar root disease or axonal neuropathy. Within 2 weeks, the patient became

Figure 7. (Case 2) Dorsal root ganglion, lumbar level. Severe loss of neurons and numerous residual nodules of Nageotte. (Nissl, original magnification ×25.)

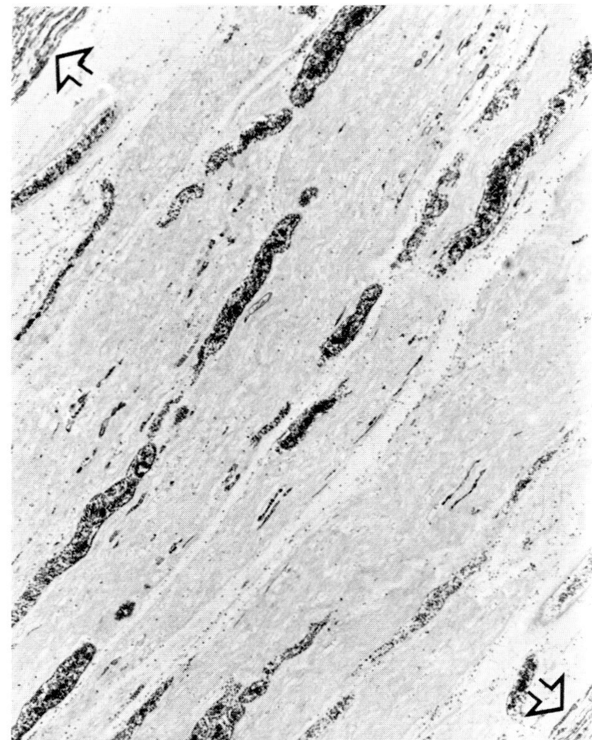

Figure 8. (Case 2) Cauda equina. Compare near total loss of myelin staining in a fascicle of posterior root (center) with well preserved myelin sheaths of anterior root fascicles (hollow arrows) in left upper and right lower corners. (LFB-PAS stain for myelin, original magnification ×30.)

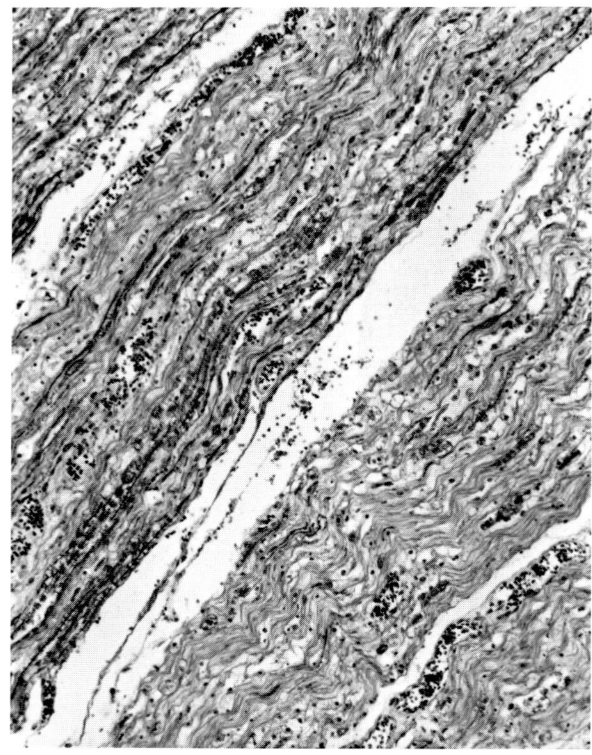

Figure 9. (Case 2) Cauda equina, posterior root. Note severe loss of nerve fibers and active Wallerian degeneration (fragmentation of axons and their myelin sheaths) of a few surviving nerve fibers. (Combined silver impregnation for axons and LFB-PAS stain for myelin, original magnification ×30.)

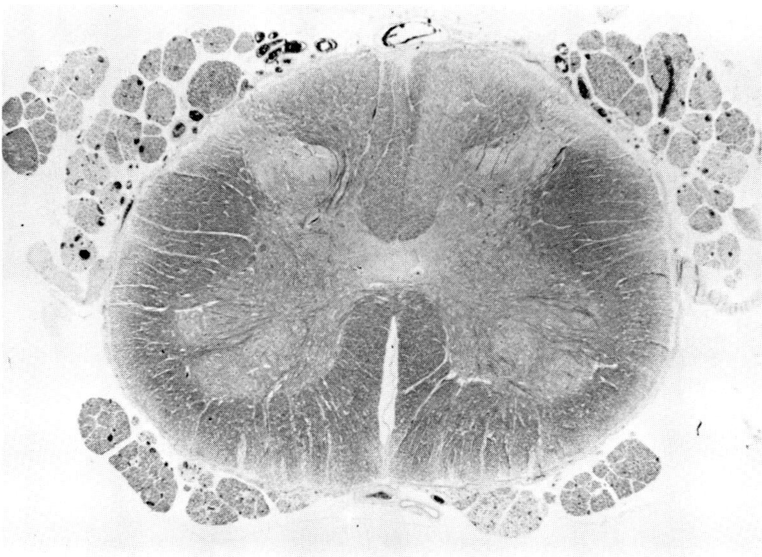

Figure 10. (Case 2) Spinal cord, lumbar level. Loss of myelin staining in majority of fascicles of posterior roots is contrasted by similar changes in only a few small fascicles of anterior roots. (LFB-PAS stain for myelin, original magnification ×2.5.)

paraplegic with a bilateral loss of proprioception in the lower extremities extending to the level of L1. He became progressively dyspneic and died 1 month after admission.

At general autopsy, significant findings included: disseminated CMV infection involving lungs (diffuse bilateral necrotizing and hemorrhagic pneumonia), thyroid gland, liver, spleen, lymph nodes, and colon (including mucosa, smooth muscle coats, and rare ganglion cells of the plexus of Auerbach); focal bilateral bronchopneumonia due to *Aspergillus fumigatus*; granulomatous lymphadenitis and splenitis secondary to MAI infection; Kaposi's sarcoma involving skin of head and extremities, esophagus, rectum, and hilar lymph nodes.

Gross examination of the central (brain and spinal cord) and peripheral nervous systems (cranial and spinal nerve roots: cervical, thoracic and lumbosacral dorsal root ganglia with spinal nerves; brachial and lumbosacral plex-

uses; sural nerves; and paravertebral sympathetic ganglia) revealed no changes.

Microscopic examination of the central nervous system revealed characteristic CMV inclusion bodies in cells of the pia-arachnoid of the brain and spinal cord, and ependyma of the former. The ependymal lining was focally destroyed and there were viral inclusion bodies in hypertrophied astrocytes of the subjacent periventricular tissues. No "microglial" nodules were recognized in the brain or spinal cord. A majority of the motoneurons of the lumbosacral segments of the latter showed central chromatolysis (Fig. 11). The fasciculi graciles showed a moderate, active Wallerian degeneration throughout their length (Fig. 12).

In the spinal nerve roots and proximal portions of spinal nerves, viral inclusion bodies were seen in Schwann cells, perineurial and endoneurial fibroblasts (Fig. 13), and endothelial cells lining some thin-walled blood vessels,

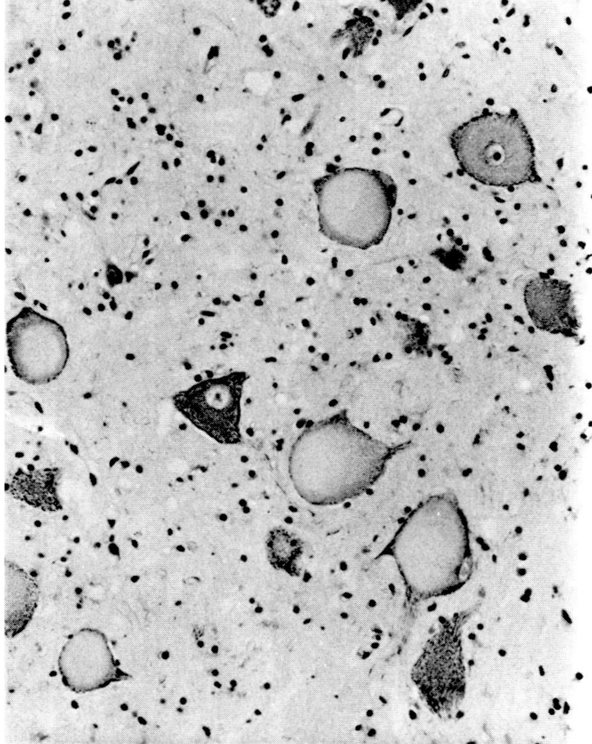

Figure 11. (Case 3) Anterior horn, low lumbar spinal cord. Marked central chromatolysis of majority of motoneurons. (Nissl, original magnification ×50.)

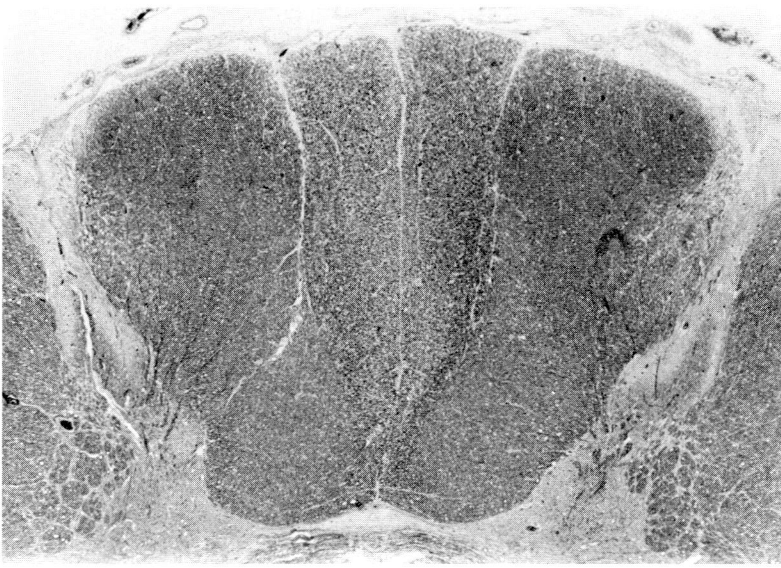

Figure 12. (Case 3) Posterior columns, upper cervical spinal cord. Moderate loss of fibers in fasciculi graciles. (LFB-PAS stain for myelin, original magnification ×5.)

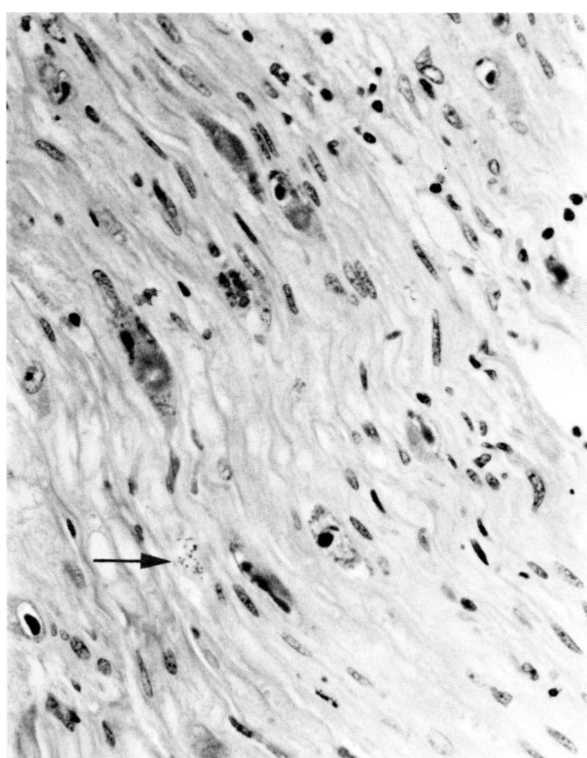

Figure 13. (Case 3) Proximal spinal nerve, low lumbar level. Note intranuclear and cytoplasmic viral inclusion bodies in several enlarged Schwann cells. A mitotic figure (attempt at regeneration) is indicated by arrow. No overt degenerative changes are seen at this early stage of infection. (H&E, original magnification ×100.)

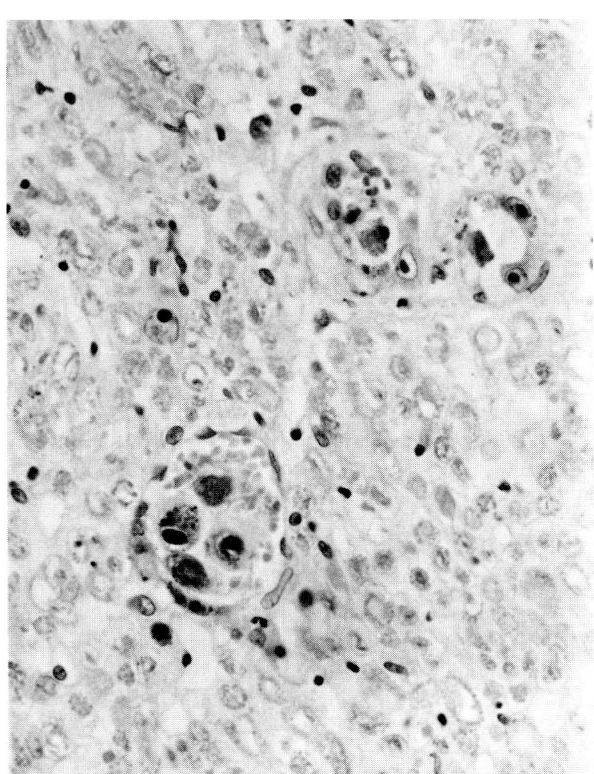

Figure 14. (Case 3) Anterior nerve root, cauda equina. Endothelial cells of three small veins contain viral inclusion bodies; similar inclusion bodies are seen in several unidentified large cells within vascular lumina. Interstitial edema and swelling of myelin sheaths are evident. (H&E, original magnification ×100.)

presumably small veins (Fig. 14). The degree and extent of the infection ranged from only slight and focal at the cervicothoracic levels to severe in the lumbosacral roots. Some affected blood vessels showed acute mural necrosis with partial or complete thrombosis, resulting in multiple variably extensive recent hemorrhages and/or infarcts. Both posterior and anterior roots were affected to an approximately equal degree. Additional changes in the nerve roots and the proximal segments of the spinal nerves included either pure demyelination or Wallerian degeneration (Fig. 15), neither accompanied by a significant inflammatory reaction. In the dorsal root ganglia viral inclusions were seen in the satellite cells, Schwann cells, and interstitial fibroblasts (Fig. 16). No inclusions were detected within the somata of the ganglion cells. Focal fresh hemorrhages associated with vascular

changes as above were seen in the lumbar spinal ganglia. Focal loss of neurons, occasional residual nodules of Nageotte, and rare instances of central chromatolysis were observed in the low thoracic and lumbosacral sensory ganglia (Fig. 17).

Samples of the brachial and lumbar plexuses showed only widely scattered viral inclusion bodies in Schwann cells and endoneurial fibroblasts at times accompanied by a minimal chronic inflammatory infiltrate. In addition, active Wallerian degeneration of small groups of nerve fibers was noted.

DISCUSSION

In agreement with previous reports,[8,9,10] we found the most frequent and widespread form of PNS damage secondary to CMV to

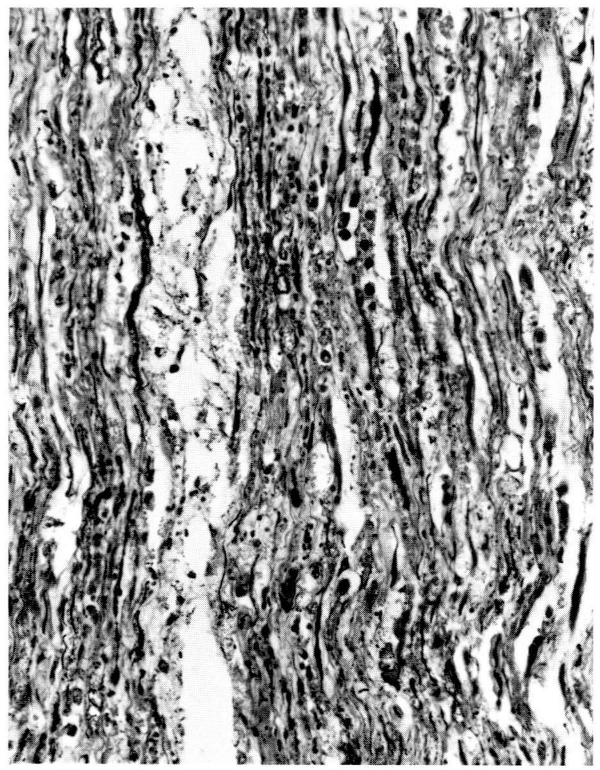

Figure 15. (Case 3) Cauda equina. Moderate loss of nerve fibers and active Wallerian degeneration (beading and fragmentation of axons and myelin sheaths) are seen. (Combined silver impregnation for axons and LFB-PAS stain for myelin, original magnification ×50.)

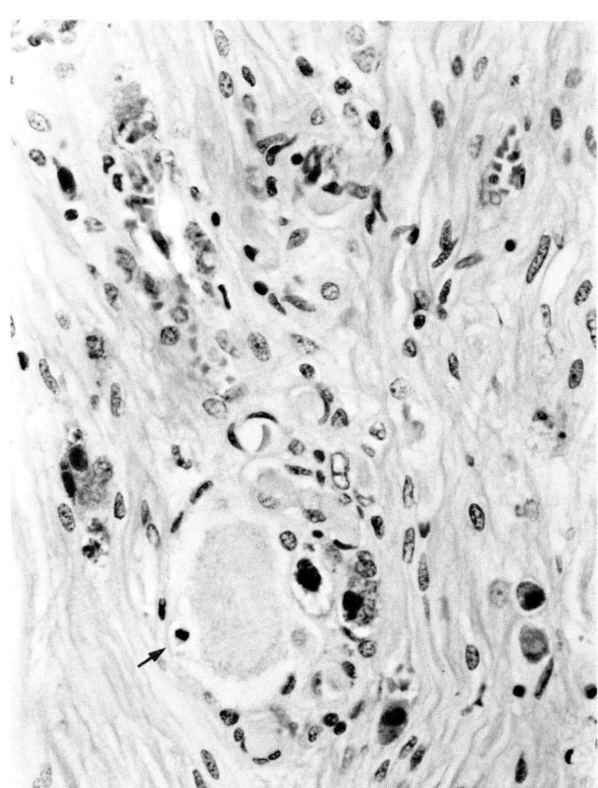

Figure 16. (Case 3) Dorsal root ganglion, lumbar level. Note viral inclusion bodies in a satellite cell and several unidentified "stromal" cells. A mitotic figure (arrow) within the capsule is indicative of attempted regenerative activity on part of satellite cells in early stages of viral attack upon sensory neurons. (H&E, original magnification ×100.)

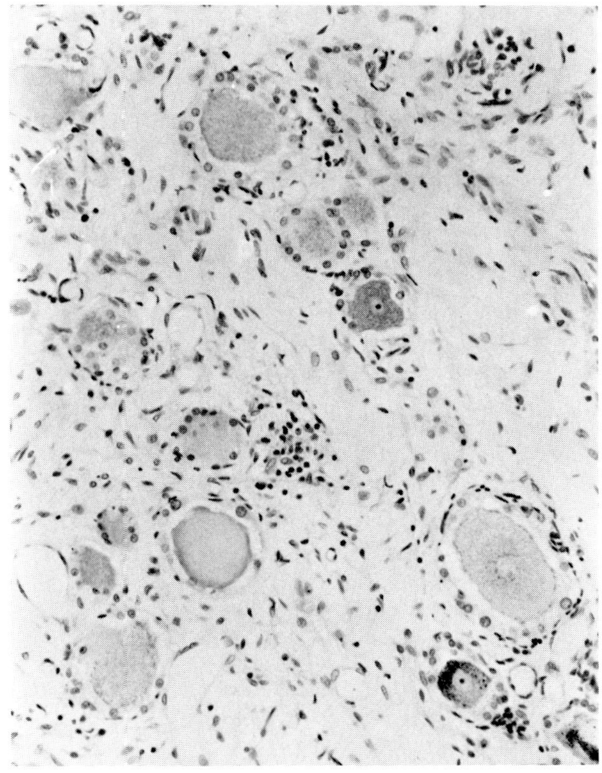

Figure 17. (Case 3) Dorsal root ganglion, lumbar level. Note focal loss of neurons, active neuronophagia, central chromatolysis, and slight mononuclear inflammatory reaction. (Nissl, original magnification ×50.)

155

be a primarily demyelinating polyradiculoneuropathy attributable to direct viral infection and destruction of the elements responsible for the production and maintenance of peripheral myelin-Schwann cells. The conspicuous vulnerability of the spinal nerve roots in general, and those at the lumbosacral level in particular, implicates the cerebrospinal fluid (CSF) pathway in the dissemination of virus to these divisions of the PNS, probably from primary foci of blood-borne infection at higher levels of the neuraxis. That the ependyma may play an important role as a primary site of infection has been suggested,[9,10] and it is perhaps significant in this regard that a destructive CMV ependymitis was present in two of our three cases (patients 1 and 3). In contrast to the striking involvement of the spinal nerve roots and proximal spinal nerves, we found only scattered foci of infection in major peripheral nerves, implicating a hematogenous, "embolic" mode of dissemination of the virus and providing additional, albeit indirect, evidence that the former pattern of injury is best explained by the presence of virus in the CSF that bathes proximal divisions of the PNS.

Two of our cases (patients 2 and 3) evidenced, in addition, a sensory ganglionitis that, to the best of our knowledge, had not been previously documented. Intranuclear and intracytoplasmic inclusion bodies typical of CMV were present in Schwann cells, endoneurial fibroblasts and, most importantly, capsule or satellite cells. Our failure to detect viral inclusions in the somata of ganglion cells, despite clear evidence of their prior and ongoing degeneration, suggests that these sensory neurons sustain indirect, but irreparable damage secondary to a viral attack on the supporting satellite cells that exert a trophic effect on them. In both cases, the degree and extent of Wallerian degeneration in the posterior columns and roots correlated well with the anatomic localization and severity of the primary injury to the dorsal root ganglia. In case 3, however, as discussed below, focal ischemic lesions further contributed to the damage. Retrograde degeneration following ischemic injury to the spinal roots may explain the neuronal changes in case 1, in which CMV was not demonstrable within the ganglia.

Multiple foci of recent hemorrhage and/or necrosis of all tissue elements were observed in the cranial and spinal nerve roots, proximal spinal nerves, and sensory ganglia of patients 1 and 3. Blood vessels, probably venous, adjacent to such lesions demonstrated vasculitis ranging from mural edema and chronic inflammatory infiltration to fibrinoid necrosis and acute thrombosis. Endothelial cells lining some of these vessels, notably in case 3, contained viral inclusions illustrating yet another mechanism by which this pantropic agent[11] can inflict injury on the PNS. Such ischemic lesions are similar to those recently described by Eidelberg et al.[10] in polyradiculoneuropathy complicating AIDS.

The patients described here manifested various clinical forms of neurologic dysfunction including a motor, Guillain-Barré-like syndrome (case 1), a predominantly sensory, pseudotabetic syndrome (case 2), and a sensorimotor polyradiculoneuropathy (case 3) that were shown to result from predominant infection of particular subdivisions of the PNS by CMV. Given the high prevalence of this virus in AIDS sufferers, it is likely that physicians will continue to encounter such patients in the years to come. Therefore, an appreciation of the spectrum of the pathological changes that can be produced by CMV in various subdivisions of the PNS is essential for an understanding of resulting diverse clinical syndromes, and a timely arrival at a precise diagnosis in each individual case.

ACKNOWLEDGMENTS

The authors are greatly indebted to Ms. Laura Anderson and Ms. Goulette Zamor for expert technical assistance, and Ms. Cathy Britt and Ms. Rosalyn Klein for preparation of the manuscript. Mr. Robert A. Feinberg produced the microphotographs. Our thanks are also due to colleagues who generously shared with us their clinical observations and general autopsy findings.

REFERENCES

1. Klemola E, Weckman N, Haltia K, Kaariainen L: The Guillain-Barré syndrome associated with acquired cytomegalovirus infection. Acta Med Scand 1967; 181:603–607
2. Duchovny M, Caplan L, Siber G: Cytomegalovirus infection of the adult nervous system. Ann Neurol 1979; 5:458–461
3. Leonard JC, Tobin JO: Polyneuritis associated with cytomegalovirus: A report from various centers. Quat Med 1971; 40:135
4. Schmitz H, Enders G: Cytomegalovirus as a frequent cause of Guillain-Barré syndrome. J Med Virol 1977; 1:21–27
5. Dowling PC, Cook SD: Role of infection in Guillain-Barré syndrome: Laboratory confirmation of herpesviruses in 41 cases. Ann Neurol 1981; 9:44–55
6. Levy RM, Bredesen DE, Rosenblum ML: Neurological manifestations of the acquired immunodeficiency syndrome (AIDS): Experience at UCSF and review of literature. J Neurosurg 1985; 62:475–495
7. Lipkin WI, Parry G, Kiprov E, Abrams D: Inflammatory neuropathy in homosexual men with lymphadenopathy. Neurology 1985; 35: 1475–1483
8. Moscowitz LB, Gregorios JB, Hensley GT, Berger JR: Cytomegalovirus-induced demyelination associated with acquired immunodeficiency syndrome. Arch Pathol Lab Med 1984; 108:873–877
9. Morgello S, Cho ES, Nielsen S, et al: Cytomegalovirus encephalitis in patients with acquired immunodeficiency syndrome: An autopsy study of 30 cases and a review of literature. Hum Pathol 1987; 18:289–297
10. Eidelberg D, Sotrel A, Vogel H, et al: Progressive polyradiculopathy in acquired immune deficiency syndrome. Neurology 1986; 36:912–916
11. Ho M: Cytomegalovirus: Biology and infection, New York, Plenum Press, 1982

10

Motor Disorders in Patients with Human Immunodeficiency Virus Infection

Avindra Nath

Joseph Jankovic

MOTOR DISORDERS are relatively common neurological complications of acquired immune deficiency syndrome (AIDS). Hemichorea, ballismus, myoclonus, dystonia, tremor, and parkinsonism have been documented in patients with AIDS[1-10] (Tables 1 and 2). In most cases a specific cause, such as toxoplasma abscess in the basal ganglia, can be identified, but in many, no specific cause for the movement disorder, except the AIDS virus, can be found.

HEMICHOREA-BALLISMUS

The combination of hemichorea and hemiballismus was seen in three patients with AIDS due to toxoplasma brain abscesses in the basal ganglia and confirmed at autopsy in one patient (Fig. 1).[8] In two patients the

hyperkinetic movement disorder was the first manifestation of AIDS (Fig. 2A,B and C). Navia et al.[3] reported chorea in two of 27 patients with cerebral toxoplasmosis and AIDS. Therefore, all five patients reported so far with AIDS and chorea-ballismus have had lesions of toxoplasmosis. To our knowledge, movement disorders caused by *Toxoplasma gondii* have not been described in the non-AIDS population. This suggests that the human immunodeficiency virus (HIV) may make the basal ganglia more susceptible to attack by *Toxoplasma gondii*.

MYOCLONUS

We described two AIDS patients with segmental myoclonus. The first case had facial (branchial) myoclonus along with supranuclear ophthalmoplegia, parkinsonism and CNS Whipple's disease, but a negative jejunal biopsy.[8] Cases with cerebral Whipple's disease and AIDS, as well as cerebral Whipple's disease, and negative jejunal biopsy were previously described, but this was the first case of AIDS with cerebral Whipple's

Address all correspondence to: Joseph Jankovic, MD, Professor of Neurology, Baylor College of Medicine, Department of Neurology, One Baylor Plaza, Houston, Texas 77030

Avindra Nath, MD, Neurology Fellow, University of Texas Health Science Center, Houston, Texas.

TABLE I
Clinical Features of Patients with HIV Infection and Motor Disorders

Pt. No./ Sex/Age	Neurologic Manifestations	Latency Between Onset of AIDS and Neurologic Manifestations* (Months)	Neuroimaging Studies	Comments
1/M/57	Branchial myoclonus, parkinsonian tremor in right hand, bradykinesia, retropulsion, supranuclear ophthalmoparesis, bulbar palsy, peripheral neuropathy	−17	CT—normal, MRI—two small areas of increased density in right frontal lobe angiogram-normal	CSF protein 65 mg/dl, brain biopsy showed Whipple's disease
2/M/35	Mild right hemiparesis, dystonic posturing of both hands, postural tremor	+4	CT—normal, MRI—small lesion in left thalamus and posterior internal capsule, angiogram-normal	Serum titers: EBV 1:640 CMV 1:64 Herpes 1:80 increased CSF IgG
3/M/37	Segmental myoclonus in both legs, more on the left, parkinsonian tremor in right hand, generalized cogwheel rigidity	−22	CT—normal	CSF 7 lymphocytes increased CSF IgG
4/F/26	Left-sided headaches, choreic-ballistic movements of right arm and leg	+3	CT—contrast enhancing lesion in left frontal lobe and basal ganglia	CSF toxoplasmosis titer 1:60
5/F/32	Paroxysmal dystonia, exudates in retina characteristic of toxoplasmosis	+14	MRI—lesion in both hemispheres (Fig. 3A,B)	
6/M/56	Ballistic movements of right arm and leg	0	CT—normal	CSF toxoplasmosis titer 1:512 Serum EBV 1:160 CMV 1:512 Toxoplasmic brain abscess in left subthalamus (Fig. 1)
7/M/47	Choreic-ballistic movements of right arm and leg	0	CT—multiple abscesses involving mainly left cerebral hemisphere, including left basal ganglia (Fig. 2A,B,C)	CSF 11 cells (95% mononuclear) Protein 79 mg/dl Serum toxoplasmosis titer 1:256
8/M/32	Retropulsion, bradykinesia, dysarthria, intention tremor	+12	CT and MRI—mild atrophy	

*(−) neurologic symptoms started before diagnosis of AIDS; (+) after diagnosis of AIDS

160

TABLE II
Movement Disorders in Patients with
HIV Infection

Movement Disorders	Number of Patients Reported	Reference
Tremor	27	1,2,6,8,10
Myoclonus	11	2,6–8
Dystonia	9	4,5,8,10
Hemichorea-ballismus	5	3,8
Parkinsonism	4	8–11

disease and negative jejunal biopsy.[12,15] While most of the neurologic findings in this patient may have been attributed to cerebral Whipple's disease, it is possible that the associated AIDS may have contributed to the motor symptoms, and CNS Whipple's disease may be an opportunistic infection in AIDS.[16] The second patient had segmental myoclonus affecting one leg, probably triggered by laminectomy. The myoclonic movements progressed to involve the arms, suggesting an underlying spinal cord pathology. In addition, the patient had levodopa-responsive parkinsonism. Other opportunistic infections developed 22 months after the onset of the neurological manifestations.

Myoclonus restricted to one particular region is usually due to pathology at that level of the spinal cord.[17-22] The spinal cord may be involved by opportunistic viral infections in AIDS.[23-25] A vacuolar myelopathy has been described at autopsy in patients with AIDS. The vacuoles are surrounded by a thin myelin sheath and seem to arise from the myelin sheath.[26-28] The pathologic changes are more severe in the lateral and posterior columns of the thoracic cord. Further, HIV has been isolated from the spinal

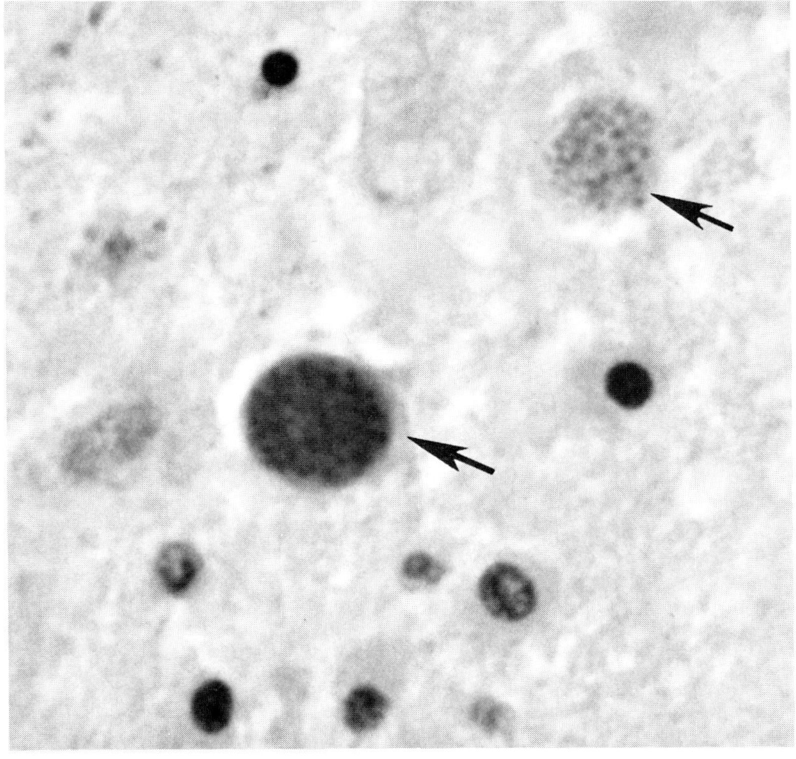

Figure 1. Patient 6 (Table 1). Autopsy material from left subthalamus showing *Toxoplasma gondii* cyst and trophozoites (arrows). (H&E, original magnification ×425.)

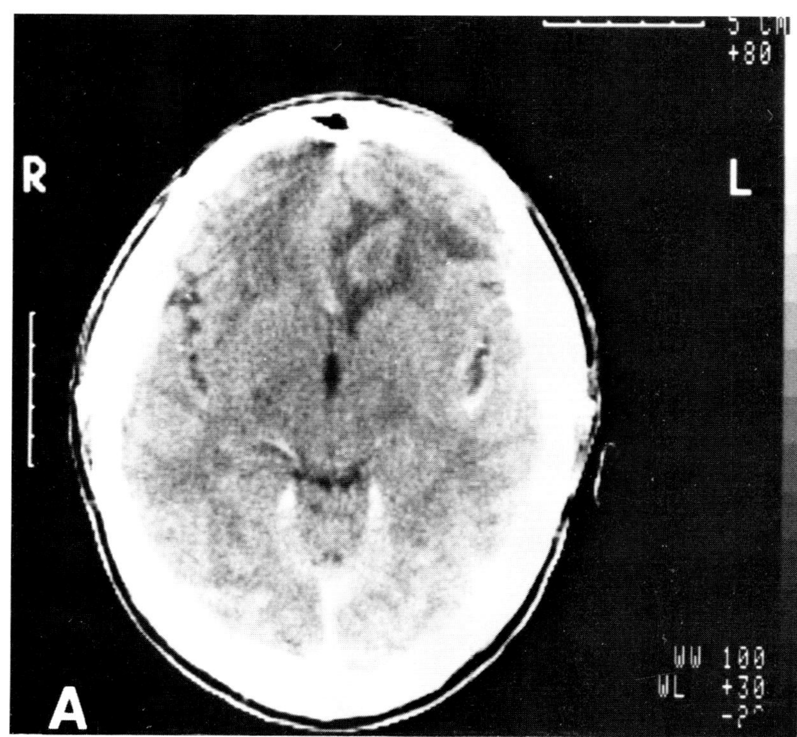

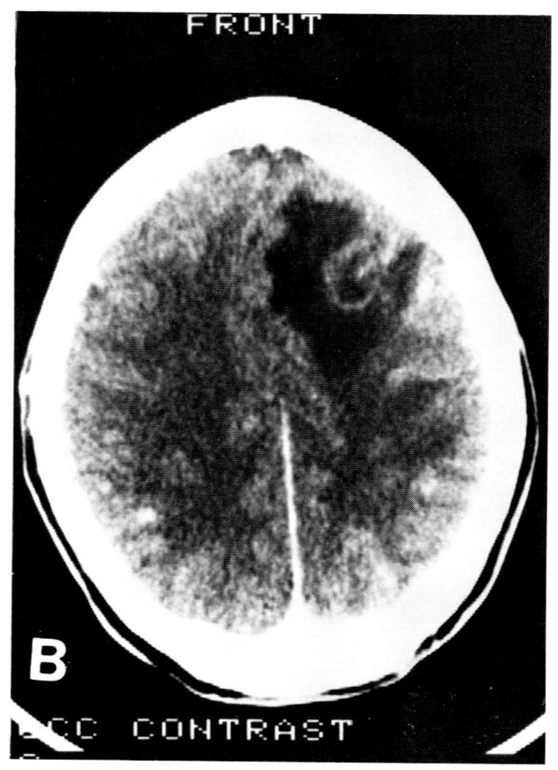
FRONT
CC CONTRAST

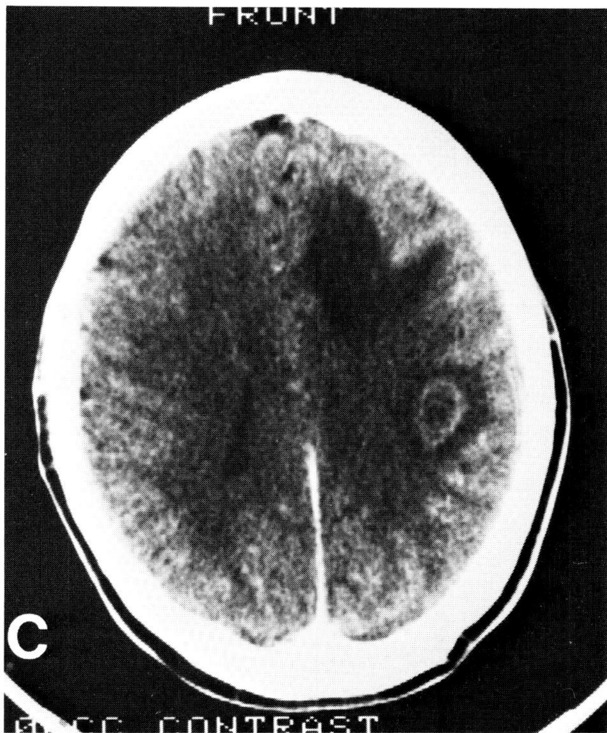

Figure 2A,B,C. Patient 7 (Table 1). Axial CT with contrast demonstrating multiple toxoplasma abscesses in left hemisphere.

cord in an AIDS patient with myelopathy,[29] suggesting that spinal myoclonus could be due to direct involvement with the HIV virus. Navia et al.[2] also reported myoclonus in 9 of 45 patients in advanced stages of the AIDS dementia complex, but they failed to characterize it further, although at autopsy 7 of the 9 patients had a vacuolar myelopathy. Myoclonus along with action tremor has been described in an adult patient with AIDS.[6] This patient had calcification of the arteries in the basal ganglia at autopsy. Another patient with myoclonus had clusters of HIV infected cells in the white matter, basal ganglia, brainstem, and thoracic posterior columns.[7]

mide or chlorpromazine given as an antiemetic during therapy with cotrimoxole or pentamidine isethionate for *Pneumocystis* pneumonia. All reactions occurred within the first 48 hours after the first dose and ranged from mild to severe dystonia.[5] Dystonia was also reported in three adults and one child with AIDS who had no prior exposure to neuroleptics[4,8,10] The first adult had dystonia of both hands (Fig. 3A and B), the second had paroxysmal dystonia (Fig. 2A,B and C), and the third had torticollis.[8,10] The child with dystonia and AIDS had calcification of the basal ganglia.[4] All these patients had other manifestations of AIDS.

DYSTONIA

Dystonia was described in 6 of 7 AIDS patients treated with low dose metoclopra-

TREMOR

Navia et al.[2] reported a rapid postural tremor in 7 of 44 patients as an early mani-

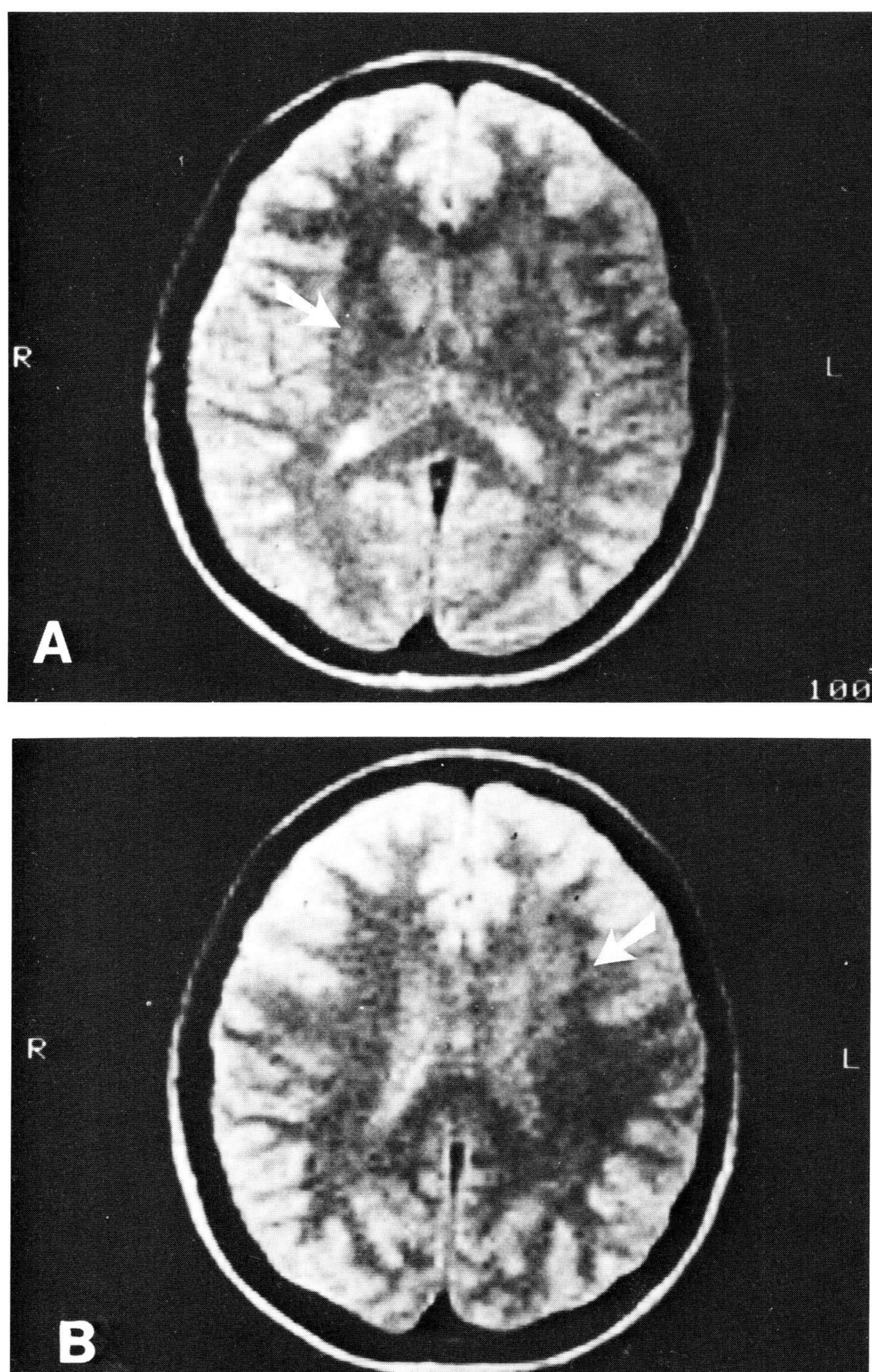

Figure 3A,B. Patient 5 (Table 1). Spin echo magnetic resonance (T2 weighted) images showing multiple foci (arrows) of high signal intensity in both hemispheres.

festation of the AIDS dementia complex, while 20 of 45 patients had tremor during the late stages of the illness. Berger et al.[1] reported tremor in 3 of 62 patients with AIDS and neurological symptoms. However, the tremor was not well characterized. Tremor has been described in four other patients who had various neurological manifestations of AIDS. One had a parkinsonian tremor, another an action tremor with myoclonus, but details on the tremor seen in the other two patients were not reported.[6] We reported a unilateral parkinsonian tremor in two patients; one of whom as described above had ipsilateral bradykinesia, retropulsion, and was associated with CNS Whipple's disease.[8] The other patient had generalized cogwheel rigidity and segmental myoclonus of both legs; CT scan of the brain was normal. Another patient had a postural tremor in both hands associated with dystonic posturing.[8]

We have since seen another patient, 32 years old, with HIV infection who had marked retropulsion and bradykinesia. He developed a rapid intention tremor in both hands seven days after starting trazodone. The tremor disappeared when trazodone was stopped, while the retropulsion and bradykinesia persisted. Hollander et al.[11] have described a patient with a parkinsonian syndrome and dementia with HIV isolated from the CSF. He had a generalized lymphadenopathy but no opportunistic infection. Metzer[10] described a 28-year-old patient who had a bilateral 3–5 Hz resting tremor and rigidity accompanied by segmental dystonia manifested as torticollis 3 years after the onset of AIDS. He had no known exposure to neuroleptics. Epstein et al.[9] described extrapyramidal rigidity in some children with HIV infection.

PATHOGENESIS OF MOTOR DISORDERS IN AIDS PATIENTS

Opportunistic infections are a common cause of neurological syndromes in AIDS, but motor disorders can occur even without opportunistic infection.[8] HIV can be isolated from the CSF, brain, and spinal cord of AIDS patients.[9,23,28,29,31,32] Direct involvement by HIV of the basal ganglia, brainstem, or spinal cord may result in a movement disorder. Ninety percent of autopsied adult patients with AIDS have histological evidence of subacute encephalitis, and 77% of these patients have involvement of the basal ganglia, mainly the putamen.[28,30] A calcific vasculopathy has been described in the basal ganglia, predominantly involving the putamen and the outer segment of the globus pallidus, on postmortem examination in four children.[4] Cells immunoreactive to HIV viral antigen have been found in the basal ganglia of patients with AIDS at autopsy.[7,28,30,33] Also, relative hypermetabolism in the basal ganglia and thalamus, as analyzed by [^{18}F] fluorodeoxyglucose positron emission tomography, is characteristic of early AIDS dementia complex with motor disorders. HIV infection may enhance any drug-induced movement disorders.[5] Ninety-six percent of patients with neurologic complications of AIDS or AIDS-related complex (ARC) have evidence of central synthesis of HIV specific IgG.[34] Moreover, Visna virus, which has sequence homology of and morphologic characteristics similar to HIV, can cause involuntary movements with paraplegia in sheep.[35–39]

In conclusion, there is strong clinical, pathological, and metabolic evidence to suggest that HIV plays an important role in the manifestation of motor disorders in AIDS patients. Besides, motor disorders may be the initial manifestation of AIDS.

REFERENCES

1. Berger JR, Moskowitz L, Fischl M, Kelley LE: The neurologic complications of AIDS: Frequently the initial manifestation. Neurology 1984; 34: 134–135
2. Navia BA, Jordan BD, Price RW: The AIDS dementia complex: I. Clinical features. Ann Neurol 1986; 19:517–524
3. Navia BA, Petito CK, Gold JWM, et al: Cerebral

toxoplasmosis complicating AIDS. Clinical and neuropathological findings in 27 patients. Ann Neurol 1986; 19:224–238

4. Belman AL, Lantos G, Horoupian D, et al: AIDS: Calcification of the basal ganglia in infants and children. Neurology 1986; 36:1192–1199

5. Hollander H, Golden J, Mendelson T, Cortland D: Extrapyramidal symptoms in AIDS patients given low-dose metoclopramide or chlorpromazine. Lancet 1985; 2:1186

6. Anders K, Steinsapir KD, Iverson DJ, et al: Neuropathologic findings in the acquired immunodeficiency syndrome (AIDS). Clin Neuropathol 1986; 5:1–20

7. Vazeux R, Brousse N, Jarry A, et al: AIDS subacute encephalitis: Identification of HIV infected cells. Am J Pathol 1987; 126:403–410

8. Nath A, Jankovic J, Pettigrew LC: Movement disorders and AIDS. Neurology 1987; 37:37–41

9. Epstein LG, Goudsmit J, Paul DA, et al: Expression of human immunodeficiency virus in cerebrospinal fluid of children with progressive encephalopathy. Ann Neurol 1987; 21:397–401

10. Metzer WS: Movement disorders with AIDS encephalopathy: Case report. Neurology 1987; 37:1438

11. Hollander H, Levy JA: Neurologic abnormalities and recovery of human immunodeficiency virus from cerebrospinal fluid. Ann Intern Med 1987; 106:692–695

12. Feurle GE, Volk B, Waldherr R: Cerebral Whipple's disease with negative jejunal biopsy. N Engl J Med 1979; 300:907–908

13. Autran BR, Govin I, Leibowitch M, et al: AIDS in a Haitian woman with cardiac Kaposi's sarcoma and Whipple's disease. Lancet 1983; 1:767–768

14. Schwartz MA, Selhorst JB, Ochs AL, et al: Oculomasticatory myorhythmia: A unique movement disorder occurring in Whipple's disease. Ann Neurol 1986; 20:677–683

15. Adams M, Rhyner PA, Day J, et al: Whipple's disease confined to the central nervous system. Ann Neurol 1987; 21:104–108

16. Jankovic J: Whipple's disease of the central nervous system in AIDS. N Engl J Med 1986; 315:1029–1030

17. Swanson PD, Luttrell CN, Magladery JM: Myoclonus: A report of 67 cases and review of literature. Medicine 1962; 41:339–356

18. Castaigne P, Cambur J, Laplane D, et al: Myoclonus rythmées segmentaires d'orgine medullaire: à propos de deux observations. Rev Otoneuroophthalmol 1969; 41:241–250

19. Frenken CWGM, Korten JJ, Gasreels FJM, et al: Spinal myoclonus. Clin Neurol Neurosurg 1974; 1:44–53

20. Hoehn NM, Cherington M: Spinal myoclonus. Neurology 1977; 27:942–946

21. Shivapour E, Teasdall RD: Spinal myoclonus with vacuolar degeneration of anterior horn cells. Arch Neurol 1980; 37:451–453

22. Jankovic J, Pardo R: Segmental myoclonus: Clinical and pharmacologic study. Arch Neurol 1986; 43:1025–1031

23. Levy JA, Hollander H, Shimabukuro J, et al: Isolation of AIDS associated retroviruses from cerebro-spinal fluid and brain of patients with neurological symptoms. Lancet 1985; 2:586–588

24. Tucker T, Dix RD, Katzen L, et al: Cytomegalovirus and herpes simplex virus ascending myelitis in a patient with acquired immune deficiency syndrome. Ann Neurol 1985; 18:74–79

25. Britton CB, Mesa-Tejada R, Fenoglio CM, et al: A new complication of AIDS: Thoracic myelitis caused by herpes simplex. Neurology 1985; 35:1071–1074

26. Petito CK, Navia BA, Cho ES, et al: Vacuolar myelopathy pathologically resembling subacute combined degeneration in patients with acquired immunodeficiency syndrome. N Engl J Med 1985; 312:874–879

27. Goldstick L, Mandybeer TI, Bode R: Spinal cord degeneration in AIDS. Neurology 1985; 35:103–106

28. de la Monte SM, Ho DD, Schooley RT, et al: Subacute encephalomyelitis of AIDS and its relation to HTLV-III infection. Neurology 1987; 37:562–569

29. Ho DD, Rota TR, Schooley RT, et al: Isolation of HTLV III from cerebrospinal fluid and neural tissues of patients with neurologic syndromes related to acquired immunodeficiency syndrome. N Engl J Med 1985; 313:1493–1497

30. Navia BA, Cho ES, Petito CK, Price RW: The AIDS dementia complex II. Neuropathology Ann Neurol 1986; 19:525–535

31. Shaw GM, Harper ME, Hahn BH: HTLV-III infection in brains of children and adults with AIDS encephalopathy. Science 1985; 227:177–181

32. Gabuzda DH, Ho DD, de la Monte SM, et al: Immunohistochemical identification of HTLV-III antigen in brains of patients with AIDS. Ann Neurol 1986; 20:289–295

33. Ward JM, O'Leary TJ, Baskin GB, et al: Immunohistochemical localization of human and simian immunodeficiency viral antigens in fixed tissue sections. Am J Pathol 1987; 127:199–205

34. Resnick L, di Mazo-Veronese F, Schiipbach J, et al: Intra blood-brain barrier synthesis of HTLV-III specific IgG in patients with neurologic symptoms associated with AIDS or AIDS related complex. N Engl J Med 1985; 313:1498–1504

35. Sigurdsson B, Palsson PA, Grimbson H: Visna, a demyelinating transmissible disease of sheep. J Neuropathol 1957; 16:389–403

36. Gonda MA, Staal FW, Gallo RC, et al: Sequence homology and morphologic similarity of HTLV-III and Visna virus, a pathogenic lentivirus. Science 1985; 227:173–177

37. Stephens RM, Casey JW, Rice NR: Equine infectious anemia virus *gag* and *pol* genes: Relatedness to Visna and AIDS virus. Science 1986; 228:589–594

38. Sonigo P, Alizon M, Stakus K: Nucleotide sequences of the Visna lentivirus: Relationship to the AIDS virus. Cell 1985; 42:369–382

39. Georgsson G, Houwers DJ, Stefansson K, et al: Immunohistochemical staining of cells in the brain of a patient with acquired immune deficiency syndrome (AIDS) with a monoclonal antibody to Visna virus. Acta Neuropathologica 1987; 73:406–408

11

Immunohistochemistry of Human Immunodeficiency Virus in the Central Nervous System and an Hypothesis Concerning the Pathogenesis of AIDS Meningoencephalomyelitis

Roy H. Rhodes
Jerrold M. Ward*

LOCALIZATION OF human immunodeficiency virus (HIV) by immunostaining or in situ hybridization in the central nervous system (CNS) of acquired immunodeficiency syndrome (AIDS) patients has been correlated with white-matter pallor and gliosis, and with chronic inflammatory foci that may contain monocyte-macrophages, multinucleated cells, and lymphocytes.[1-7] HIV meningoencephalomyelitis has been demonstrated in frozen sections in most of these studies, and in fixed tissue by immunostaining with a rabbit antiserum to whole disrupted HIV and with a monoclonal antibody to core protein p24.[6] Immunostaining for HIV is found in subarachnoid and par-

enchymal monocyte-macrophages, in capillary and venular endothelial cells, in astrocytes and other glial cells, and possibly in neurons. About 25% of our AIDS patients with CNS pathology have opportunistic infections. A third problem, that of hypersensitivity disease in the CNS in AIDS may be present but the frequency of mixed neuropathologic findings in most autopsy cases has obscured this process.[8]

Autopsy studies of the CNS in AIDS often reveal isolated or clustered macrophages or multinucleated cells in the subarachnoid space or parenchyma. The parenchymal macrophages are commonly in perivascular regions, but they may also infiltrate otherwise normal appearing white matter or cortex. In our series of 200 cases, 28% had relatively small to medium-size multinucleated cells, so that HIV meningoencephalomyelitis, in a minority of instances, is a

*Supported in part by PHS Contract NO1-CO-12910 to Program Resources, Inc., and PHS Grant No. RR-00164 from the Division of Research Resources, NIH.

form of granulomatous disease. Multinucleated giant cells were present in about 30% of the cases that contained the smaller variety of multinucleated cells. Forty-five percent of our total cases had gliomesenchymal-cell (microglial) nodules, some of which were immunoreactive for HIV antigens, both in the brain and in the spinal cord.[6,9] The macrophages in the brain, including their multinucleated variants, have been double-labeled for antigens of blood-derived monocyte-macrophages and for HIV nucleic acid.[10,11]

The degree of immunoreactivity against HIV is not very high in the CNS, yet significant dementia can be present. How might this come about? Key neural centers may be involved, such as subcortical nuclei and white matter;[12,13] CNS damage is caused by opportunistic infections in many cases; there might be hypersensitivity damage;[8,14–16] HIV encephalitis may initially be more widespread with antigen largely cleared from parenchymal cells before death, as in herpes simplex virus type 1 encephalitis;[17] a combination of lesions may alter the blood-brain barrier to cause CNS dysfunction; and infiltrating macrophages could be secreting toxic factors (e.g., prostaglandins, proteolytic enzymes and hydrogen ions) that damage myelin and perhaps neurons and glial cells.[15,18] Other possibilities will arise, no doubt, as more is learned about HIV.

Recent studies, including our own, have emphasized the predominance of HIV antigens within infiltrating macrophages in the CNS. However, prominent endothelial-cell, astrocytic, and perineuronal glial-cell HIV immunoreactivity can be seen in the cortex or white matter where little or no necrosis is present (vide infra). Most studies have used autopsy tissues from patients whose AIDS encephalitis had likely been present for months to years, and the finding of HIV antigens and nucleic acid mostly in infiltrating cells from the blood may only indicate that CNS parenchymal damage had occurred remotely, and the immunolabeled cells present in the CNS at the time of the patient's death would then only be an indication of past damage.

A new area of concern and investigation, and one that particularly could involve autoallergic phenomena, is the immune response to viral proteins that have sequence homologies to natural CNS products, such as the partial sequence homology of HIV envelope glycoprotein gp120 and neuroleukin.[16] The regional homologies of HIV p17 with thymosin α_1[19,20] and HIV *env* antigen with interleukin-2[21,22] provide another means of allergic response. There may also be an immune response against cells with a viral protein on their surface (Fig. 1), even when these cells contain no productive infection.[23,24] HIV gp120 is one of the products shed in abundance by infected cells,[25] and neither immunostaining nor an immune reaction would be likely to distinguish between gp120 as an isolated gene product, gp120 covering an infectious viral particle on a cellular surface, or a cross-reacting host sequence.

CD4 PROTEIN ANTIGEN

Lymphocytes (T4 cells) and monocyte-macrophages that have the CD4 cell-surface antigen are susceptible to HIV infection because the CD4 protein is the receptor molecule, or so far as is known the major receptor molecule, for HIV.[26–29] Once infected with HIV, CD4$^+$ cells downregulate this surface protein,[30] perhaps making CD4 protein only an early marker for cells susceptible to an HIV infection. Frozen-section immunolocalization of CD4 protein in a normal human brain shows that it is found in many areas, with some subcortical concentrations in regions known to harbor HIV in AIDS patients.[31] For this reason, a further detailed study of normal tissue may prove even more revealing than our limited results in lymph nodes and brain, since the tissue we have studied for the presence of CD4 protein has previously been positively immunostained for HIV antigens. Our preliminary results of

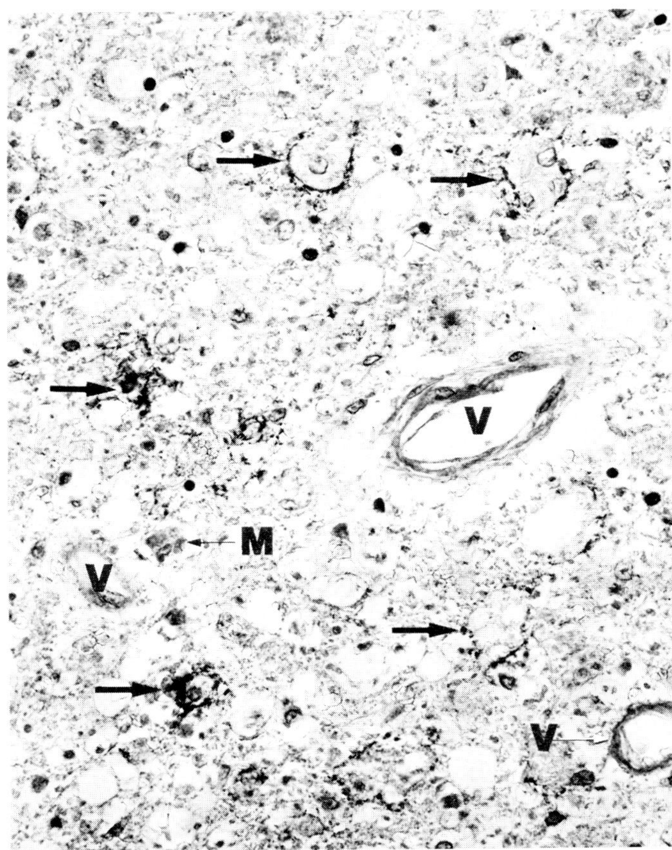

Figure 1. A formalin-fixed, paraffin-embedded area in one of the pyramids in the medulla of an AIDS patient with vacuolar myelopathy is shown here immunostained with the avidin-biotin-peroxidase method using a primary monoclonal antibody to HIV p24. Several glial cells have cell-surface immunoreactivity for p24 (arrows). There is one negative foamy macrophage (M). Three venules (V) with endothelial-cell hypertrophy are present and have no immunoreactivity. (Original magnification ×400. Monoclonal antibody M26, diluted 1:1000; courtesy of Dr. F. DiMarzo Veronese. A #47 Wratten blue filter was used for photomicrography to prevent transmission of any of the blue hematoxylin counterstain.)

CD4 protein immunostaining show this antigen on the luminal and abluminal surfaces of venous endothelial cells and in the Golgi areas of these cells in some, but not all, of the formalin-fixed lymphoid and brain sections studied with the Leu 3 monoclonal antibody (Fig. 2).

The endothelial cell-surface CD4 protein, expressed normally or by induction, could be an important route for parenchymal HIV infection. CD4 protein immunolocalization might also be related to the relatively high antigenic load of HIV in lymph nodes and cerebrum compared to other organs studied.[6] An induction (or increase) of CD4-protein expression by endothelial cells, particularly in subsets of endothelial cells, might also explain why deep white matter, basal ganglia,[3,6] and spinal cord white matter are favored sites of tissue degeneration in AIDS patients.[17,32,33] The CD4 protein itself, at least on T4 cells, has been shown to be affected by interactions with antigen-presenting cells[34] and to enhance T4 cell activity.[35,36] Interestingly, and perhaps related to the pathogenesis of AIDS encephalomye-

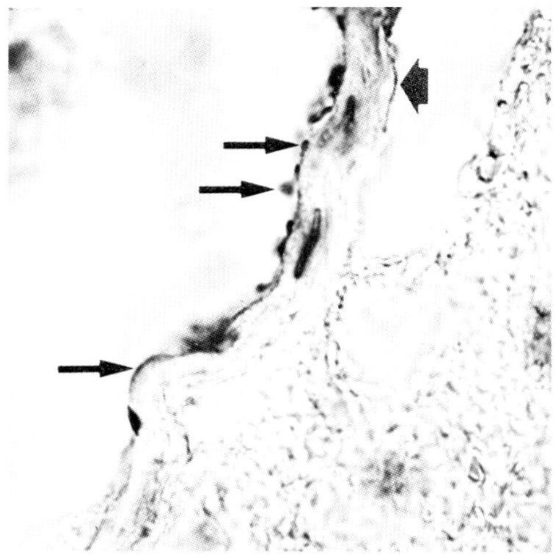

Figure 2. Formalin-fixed, paraffin-embedded venular endothelium is shown here in the white matter (external capsule) between the putamen and claustrum in a non-demented young woman with AIDS. Many glio-mesenchymal-cell nodules and multinucleated cells in both her brain and spinal cord and some capillary endothelial cells in the insular cortex were immunoreactive in other sections with an HIV polyclonal antiserum and a monoclonal antibody to p24. The venular endothelium is immunostained in this section with a monoclonal antibody to the cell-surface CD4 protein. Punctate and linear luminal cell-surface immunoreactivity (arrows) and some abluminal staining can be seen (arrowhead). (Original magnification ×1,000. Leu 3a+b, 1:50. Blue filter.)

litis, cerebral endothelial cells and astrocytes can present antigens.[37] Also, there is some evidence for differences between subsets of endothelial cells in relation to immune function.[38] A temporal relationship of spinal cord symptoms with decreased mental status in AIDS patients who have HIV antigens in the spinal cord and cerebrum is an indication that HIV encephalomyelitis can occur by infection of specific and distant regions of the CNS at about the same time.[9] A possible relationship between immune functions of CNS endothelial cells and HIV infection of the CNS needs close scrutiny.

HIV ANTIGENS IN CNS

The line of progression to HIV encephalitis has not yet been directly demonstrated. Pathogenesis may involve an endothelial cell infection initially, and endothelial cell damage might result in an opening of the blood-brain barrier followed by lymphocyte and macrophage attraction to the CNS. There is no evidence of widespread endothelial cell degeneration, but in some cases of AIDS encephalitis, there is perivascular hemorrhage that could be a result of HIV damage or of a hypersensitivity response.[8] Over one third of our cases have chronic perivasculitis and 6% have chronic vasculitis. Whatever the origin of the vascular lesions, the blood-brain barrier is often compromised in AIDS, as indicated by perivasculitis and vasculitis, by perivascular hemorrhages and by the numerous small or large areas of CNS pallor and necrosis.

The most striking HIV immunoreactivity has been in some networks of astrocyte-like cells ringing capillaries or small venules.[3] This type of perivascular HIV+ web of astrocytes can be found in areas that have no structural lesions (Fig. 3). Occasionally, this web is not clearly defined, and some immunoreactive macrophages are seen among the apparently discontinuous (degenerating?) cellular processes (Fig. 4). HIV infection of vascular endothelial cells, or spread of HIV from the blood between endothelial cells,[2] may eventually involve perivascular astrocytes and evoke little inflammatory response except for that of macrophages that presumably phagocytose the infected astrocytic debris and infectious HIV. The macrophages may be the source of the perivascular multinucleated cells so commonly seen in the CNS in AIDS. Infected macrophages, which can live for several days in culture,[10] might then become attracted to other HIV lesions in the CNS such as gliomesenchymal-cell nodules, and sites of opportunistic infections or primary lymphomas (Fig. 5). They may migrate toward endogenous

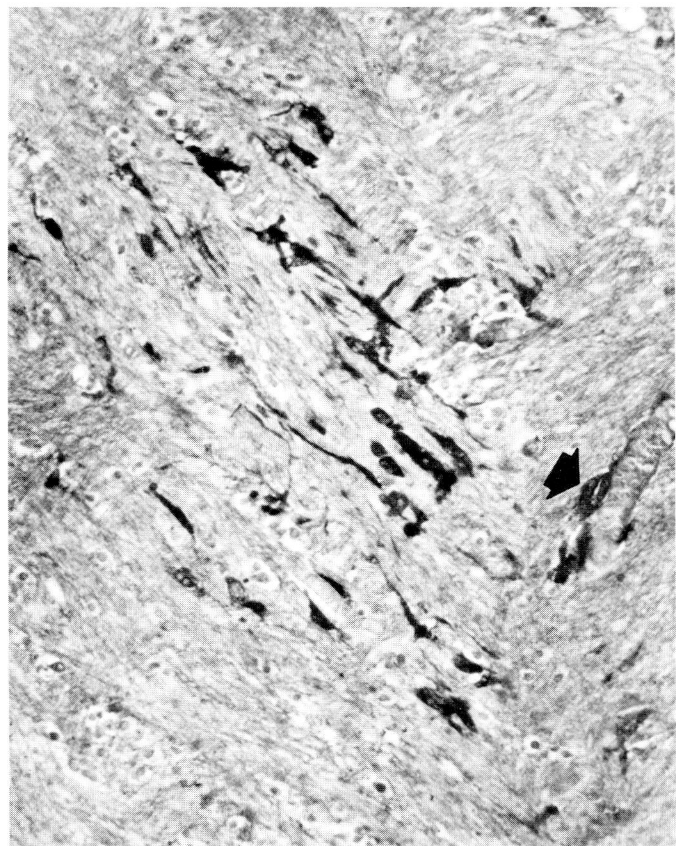

Figure 3. The internal capsule of the brain shown in Fig. 2 is immunostained with antiserum to HIV. An enlarged capillary has some positive cells closely associated with it (arrowhead). The network of immunoreactive cells with long processes has two key morphologic features. That is, these cells appear to be a network of astrocytes, and no structural lesion is evident. (Original magnification ×180. FRE-3 (#762) antiserum to whole disrupted HIV, 1 : 150. Blue filter.)

neuropeptides that provide a chemotactic stimulus to macrophages,[39,40] or toward self-antigens or cross-reacting antigens recognized by macrophages once they have crossed the blood-brain barrier.[41-43] The macrophages may also be infected with HIV before they enter the CNS in their response to any of a variety of lesions.[7,10]

The brain weight in AIDS patients may be lower than expected for a relatively young patient,[13,44] with gross thinning of the neocortical strip commonly being found. No neuronal loss has been demonstrated in the neocortex in AIDS, but astrocytes and peri-neuronal glial cells in the neocortex can have HIV antigens in them (Figs. 6 and 7). Degeneration of these neocortical cells might leave neurons in place, but their functioning at a reduced level of activity. Chemotherapy for HIV with 3′-azido-3′-deoxythymidine (AZT) has been shown to improve brain metabolism as seen in a few patients with positron emission tomography.[45] Perhaps an effect on HIV transcrip-

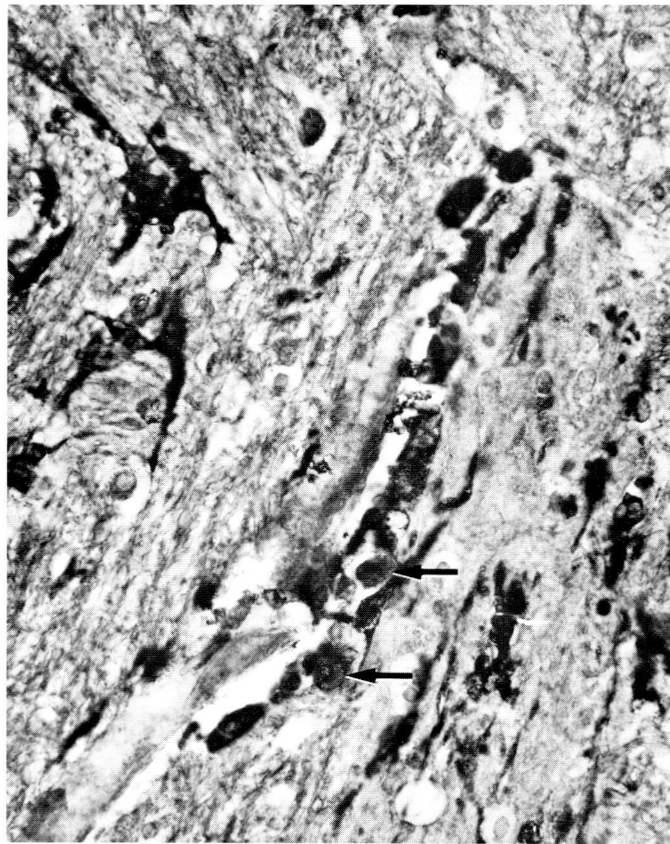

Figure 4. A small blood vessel with prominent endothelial cells near the field shown in Fig. 3 is seen here. A few foamy macrophages (arrows) with low levels of immunoreactivity for HIV and many heavily immunoreactive cells of uncertain type are in close proximity to the vascular wall. Nearby immunoreactive cells appear to be white-matter glial cells. The presence of the small foamy macrophages constitutes the only structural abnormality that would be appreciated on a routinely-stained slide. (Original magnification ×400. FRE-3, 1 : 150. Blue filter.)

tion by AZT allows damaged glial cells to be replaced in these patients. Wernicke's encephalopathy[46] and central pontine myelinolysis are examples of other diseases with glial cell degeneration and neuronal preservation in which the involved tissue is grossly shrunken, clinical deficits are evident, and improvement can be seen with therapy.[47]

Some of the histopathologic findings in AIDS encephalitis are the same as those in Wernicke's encephalopathy. Reports of Wernicke's encephalopathy in the absence of any history or symptoms consistent with this disease in two AIDS patients bring into question the diagnosis of the structural lesions in those cases.[48,49] Can AIDS encephalitis affecting certain areas of the CNS mimic other diseases? HIV myelitis in our patients clinically mimics tabes dorsalis, and pathologically, it mimics avitaminosis B_{12}.[32,50]

HYPOTHESIS OF THE PATHOGENESIS OF AIDS ENCEPHALOMYELITIS

The cells of the immune system share a variety of glycoproteins with the nervous system.[51] T-cell surfaces contain some epi-

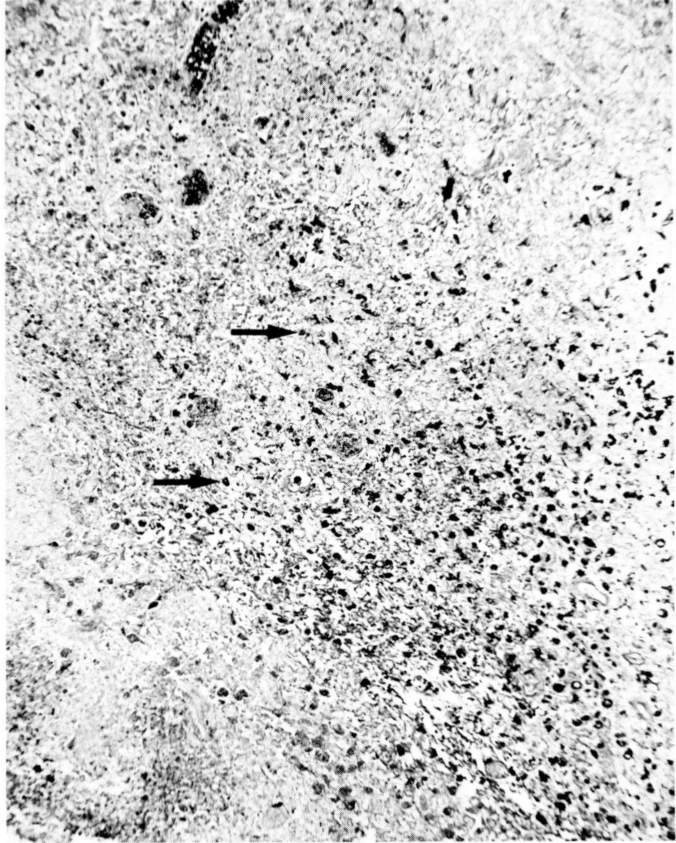

Figure 5. Necrotic primary cerebral lymphoma in an AIDS patient following radiotherapy is infiltrated with numerous foamy macrophages (arrows) that are heavily immunostained for HIV antigens. (Original magnification ×80. FRE-3. 1:150. Blue filter.)

topes also recognized as structural components of myelin.[43,52] Together, such epitopes and retroviral proteins on T-cell surface receptors may provide an immunogen against which monocytes respond by recognizing normal myelin, or perhaps even cell-surface viral protein, as part of the immune target in the CNS.[8,24,51] Early and advanced destruction of deep cerebral white matter and of spinal cord long tracts in AIDS may be the subsequent step following a T-cell and monocyte-macrophage autoaggressive response.

Figure 8 is a schematic diagram depicting a possible series of events by which HIV and hypersensitivity responses might lead to CNS damage. HIV, once it has infected T cells and monocytes, provides cell-surface antigens on circulating white blood cells. The expression of CD4 protein on endothelial cells may be normal. CNS endothelial cell infection by HIV may be directly related to CD4 protein expression. Routinely-stained sections, HIV immunostained preparations,[6,7] and CD4 immunostaining show thickening of endothelial cells in the CNS in AIDS, but endothelial cell syncytial formation is not found. This lack of vascular syncytial formation could be due to the low surface density of CD4 molecules that are important in the fusion process.[15] CNS endothelial cells can express major histocompatibility complex (MHC) antigens when stimulated,[53,54] and the presence of MHC and HIV antigens on endothelial cells could

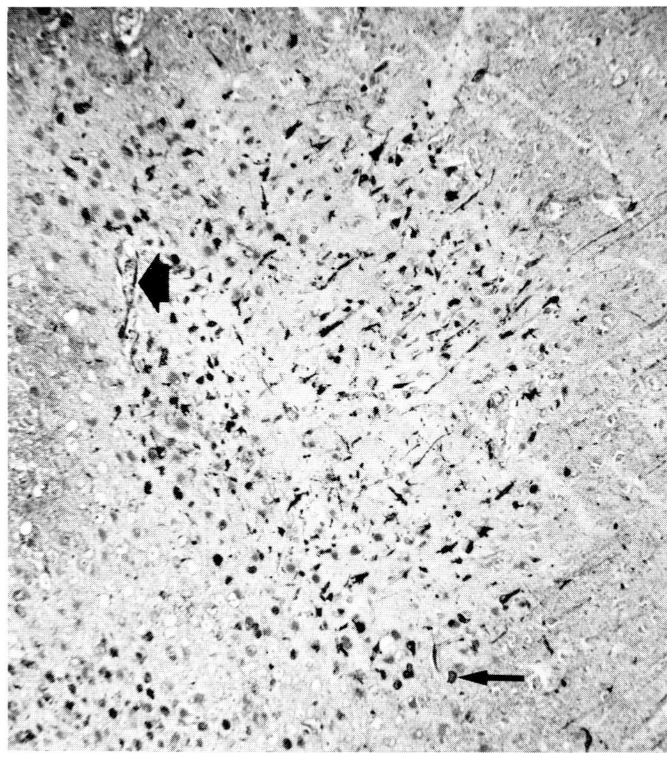

Figure 6. The inner half of the neocortex overlying a white-matter lesion of progressive multifocal leukoencephalopathy is seen not far from the area shown in Fig. 5. There is a slight pallor in the neocortex, probably indicative of focal edema. Vascular endothelial cells (arrowhead), astrocytes with long processes, possibly other glial cells and foamy macrophages (arrow) are immunoreactive for HIV antigens. (Original magnification ×80. FRE-3, 1:150. Blue filter.)

be one cause for an immune attack on the endothelial cells with subsequent breakdown of the blood-brain barrier, hemorrhage, and perivascular demyelination. CD4 protein interacts directly with MHC class II antigens,[35] and this interaction enhances the cell's immune responsiveness.[35,36] Thus, CD4 protein expression by endothelial cells may be enhanced in the presence of a CNS related immune response. HIV presumably enters perivascular astrocytes across extracellular spaces or by cell-cell transfer from vascular endothelium. Monocyte-macrophages responding to HIV antigens on degenerating perivascular astrocytes might take up virions to perpetuate an intraparenchymal reservoir, or the hematogenous cells

might be infected with HIV before they entered the CNS.

Viral infections can stimulate increased expression of MHC antigens (Ia and H-2) on the surface of astrocytes and oligodendrocytes.[55,56] Coexpression of MHC antigens and HIV antigens on glial cell surfaces would make these cells vulnerable to immune attack. The sum of the immune processes would very likely lower the blood-brain barrier even when the endothelial cells are not infected. Lymphokines, as products of cellular inflammatory activity, can recruit glial cells into an immune response through the induction of MHC antigens,[57-61] and endothelial cells may be similarly affected.[53,54,62] Cerebral endothelial cells are

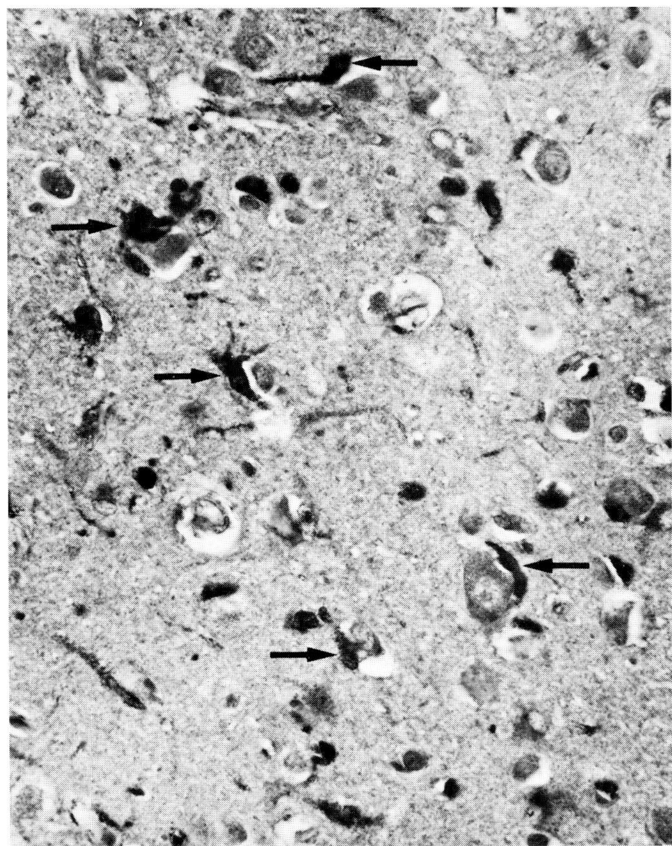

Figure 7. The middle of the neocortical strip not far from the area seen in Fig. 6 shows many cells heavily immunostained for HIV antigens. Several of these cells appear to be perineuronal glial cells (arrows). (Original magnification ×400. FRE-3, 1:150. Blue filter.)

part of an antigen-presenting system operating in conjunction with astrocytes and the immune system,[37,38,57,58,63-65] and it is possible that once some CNS immune activity begins, the endothelium-astrocyte immune control system[37] is recruited into further activity.

Primed T cells, immunoglobulin (Ig) and complement components (C') crossing the blood-brain barrier would interact not only with HIV on cellular surfaces, but myelin and other self-antigens in the nervous system would also be involved in immune reactivity. Once myelin or other self-antigens are sampled by the immune system, T cells might be primed directly against the ner-

vous system in the presence of a leaky blood-brain barrier and MHC antigens.[66] T cells, primed to neural antigens, could act in concert with macrophages, Ig and C' to attack the brain and spinal cord directly, whether HIV is present within the neural parenchyma or not. B cells receiving appropriately processed antigen might then provide further immune attack on neural self-antigens. Once an immunodeficient state is established, an infection with any of a variety of common viruses potentially could provide the patient with viral sequence homologies similar to normal myelin or other CNS molecules, and enough immune activity may be present for an immune attack on

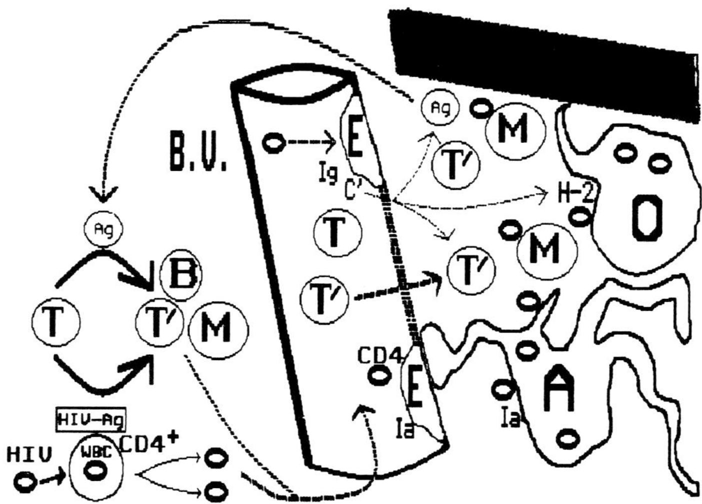

Figure 8. Schematic diagram showing possible mode of histopathogenesis of AIDS encephalomyelitis. The broken double-line wall of the blood vessel (B.V.) represents a leaky blood-brain barrier. Myelin is represented by a hatched bar. A, astrocyte; Ag, antigen; B, B lymphocyte; C', complement component; CD4, cell-surface receptor protein for HIV; E, endothelial cell; H-2, class I major histocompatibility complex antigen; HIV-Ag, HIV cell-surface antigen; Ia, class II major histocompatibility complex antigen; Ig, immunoglobulin; M, monocyte-macrophage; O, oligodendrocyte; T, T lymphocyte; T', primed T lymphocyte; and WBC, white blood cell. (Reproduced with permission of IVF/Andrology International, Inc.)

the CNS, possibly completely independent of any other CNS lesions.[41,42,67] The blood-brain barrier is apparently bypassed by T cells sensitized to myelin basic protein[65,68] or by a strong systemic immune response,[69] so prior CNS structural lesions might not be necessary for demyelination to occur in AIDS.

SUMMARY

Early events of HIV infection of the CNS are not yet clear. HIV infection in most recent cases, generally shows a prolonged interval between diagnosis and death. HIV infection, months to years before the patient's death, may or may not result in early neurologic symptoms. AIDS patients with spinal cord symptoms often show a sudden onset of long tract signs and a temporally related altered mental status indicating the appearance of both myelitis and encephalitis. Immunohistochemical localization of the HIV cell-surface receptor protein, CD4, and of

HIV antigens in cerebral and lymph node venular endothelial cells suggests that a natural occurrence or induction of CD4 protein in some endothelial cells allows transmission of HIV from circulating infected white blood cells preferentially to certain tissues through endothelial cell infection.

HIV immunolocalization is present in perivascular astrocytes, particularly in long white matter tracts, and on the surface of oligodendrocytes. HIV immunoreactivity is mostly in macrophages and multinucleated cells in a typical autopsy case, but this may be due to the clearing of HIV antigen from early sites of infection by the hematogenous cells. Not all immunoreactivity for HIV antigens is necessarily due to HIV gene products. Cross reacting epitopes, such as that of HIV envelope glycoprotein gp120 and neuroleukin, may be "seen" not only by antibodies on tissue sections, but by an AIDS patient's immune system, thus targeting a CNS antigen for immune-complex formation.

Evidence for hypersensitivity disease in the CNS in AIDS includes the frequent findings of demyelination, perivenous chronic inflammation, chronic vasculitis, and perivenous hemorrhages. The white matter demyelination so frequently reported in all areas of the CNS in AIDS could be the result of a combination of factors that include direct HIV vasculitis, opportunistic infections, and hypersensitivity responses. The blood-brain barrier is breached when immune-related antigens interact on CNS vascular endothelial cells. Perhaps the CD4 antigen, which responds to interaction with antigen-presenting cells and enhances cellular immune activity, is induced or increased in the CNS in association with immune activity and in the presence of a leaky blood-brain barrier. Therefore, with or without HIV in the CNS, hypersensitivity disease, including demyelination, may be the result of long-standing activity of the immune system in AIDS patients.

ACKNOWLEDGMENTS

Immunostaining was performed by Mrs. Cynthia A. Thompson and Mr. Karim Damji. Mr. Andy Gero, Chief Medical Photographer at the Los Angeles County University of Southern California Medical Center, provided the excellent photomicrographs.

REFERENCES

1. Gabuzda DH, Ho DD, de la Monte SM, et al: Immunohistochemical identification of HTLV-III antigen in brains of patients with AIDS. Ann Neurol 1986; 20:289–295
2. Gyorkey F, Melnick JL, Gyorkey P: Human immunodeficiency virus in brain biopsies of patients with AIDS and progressive encephalopathy. J Infect Dis 1987; 155:870–876
3. Pumarola-Sune T, Navia BA, Cordon-Cardo C, et al: HIV antigen in the brains of patients with the AIDS dementia complex. Ann Neurol 1987; 21:490–496
4. Stoler MH, Eskin TA, Benn S, et al: Human T-cell lymphotropic virus type III infection of the central nervous system: A preliminary in situ analysis. JAMA 1986; 256;2360–2364
5. Vazeux R, Brousse N, Jarry A, et al: AIDS subacute encephalitis: Identification of HIV-infected cells. Am J Pathol 1987; 126:403–410
6. Ward JM, O'Leary TJ, Baskin GB, et al: Immunohistochemical localization of human and simian immunodeficiency viral antigens in fixed tissue sections. Am J Pathol 1987; 127:199–205
7. Wiley CA, Schrier RD, Nelson JA, et al: Cellular localization of human immunodeficiency virus infection within the brains of acquired immune deficiency syndrome patients. Proc Natl Acad Sci USA 1986; 83:7089–7093
8. Rhodes RH: Histopathology of the central nervous system in the acquired immunodeficiency syndrome. Hum Pathol 1987; 18:636–643
9. Rhodes RH: Neuropathology of AIDS. (Abstract) Arch AIDS Res 1987; 1:184–187
10. Gartner S, Markovits P, Markovitz DM, et al: The role of mononuclear phagocytes in HTLV-III/LAV infection. Science 1986; 233:215–219
11. Koenig S, Gendelman HE, Orenstein JM, et al: Detection of AIDS virus in macrophages in brain tissue from AIDS patients with encephalopathy. Science 1986; 233:1089–1093
12. de la Monte SM, Ho DD, Schooley RT, et al: Subacute encephalomyelitis of AIDS and its relation to HTLV-III infection. Neurology 1987; 37:562–569
13. Navia BA, Cho E-S, Petito CK, Price RW: The AIDS dementia complex: II. Neuropathology. Ann Neurol 1986; 19:525–535
14. Gabuzda DH, Hirsch MS: Neurologic manifestations of infection with human immunodeficiency virus: Clinical features and pathogenesis. Ann Intern Med 1987; 107:383–391
15. Ho DD, Pomerantz RJ, Kaplan JC: Pathogenesis of infection with human immunodeficiency virus. N Engl J Med 1987; 317:278–286
16. Lee MR, Ho DD, Gurney ME: Functional interaction and partial homology between human immunodeficiency virus and neuroleukin. Science 1987; 237:1047–1051
17. Rhodes RH, Novak R, Beattie JF, et al: Immunoperoxidase demonstration of herpes simplex virus type 1 in the brain of a psychotic patient without history of encephalitis. Clin Neuropathol 1984; 3:59–67
18. Young PR, Zygas AP: Secretion of lactic acid by peritoneal macrophages during extracellular phagocytosis: The possible role of local hyperacidity in inflammatory demyelination. J Neuroimmunol 1987; 15:295–308
19. Naylor PH, Naylor CW, Badamchian M, et al: Human immunodeficiency virus contains an epitope immunoreactive with thymosin α_1 and the 30-amino acid synthetic p17 group-specific antigen peptide HGP-30. Proc Natl Acad Sci USA 1987; 84:2951–2955
20. Sarin PS, Sun DK, Thornton AH, et al: Neutralization of HTLV-III/LAV replication by antiserum to thymosin α_1. Science 1986; 232:1135–1137
21. Reiher WE III, Blalock JE, Brunck TK: Sequence homology between acquired immunodeficiency

syndrome virus envelope protein and interleukin 2. Proc Natl Acad Sci USA 1986; 83:9188–9192

22. Weigent DA, Hoeprich PD, Bost KL, et al: The HTLV-III envelope protein contains a hexapeptide homologous to a region of interleukin-2 that binds to the interleukin-2 receptor. Biochem Biophys Res Commun 1986; 139:367–374

23. Klatzmann D, Montagnier L: Approaches to AIDS therapy. (Editorial) Nature 1986; 319:10–11

24. Lyerly HK, Matthews TJ, Langlois AJ, et al: Human T-cell lymphotropic virus III$_B$ glycoprotein (gp120) bound to CD4 determinants on normal lymphocytes and expressed by infected cells serves as target for immune attack. Proc Natl Acad Sci USA 1987; 84:4601–4605

25. Kowalski M, Potz J, Basiripour L, et al: Functional regions of the envelope glycoprotein of human immunodeficiency virus type 1. Science 1987; 237:1351–1355

26. Lifson JD, Feinberg MB, Reyes GR, et al: Induction of CD4 dependent cell fusion by the HTLV-III/LAV envelope glycoprotein. Nature 1986; 323:725–728

27. Matthews TJ, Weinhold KJ, Lyerly HK, et al: Interaction between the human T-cell lymphotropic virus type III$_B$, envelope glycoprotein gp120 and the surface antigen CD4: Role of carbohydrate in binding and cell fusion. Proc Natl Acad Sci USA 1987; 84:5424–5428

28. Pert CB, Hill JM, Ruff MR, et al: Octapeptides deduced from the neuropeptide receptor-like pattern of antigen T4 in brain potently inhibit human immunodeficiency virus receptor binding and T-cell infectivity. Proc Natl Acad Sci USA 1986; 83:9254–9258

29. Sattentau QJ, Dalgleish AG, Weiss RA, Beverley PCL: Epitopes of the CD4 antigen and HIV infection. Science 1986; 234:1120–1123

30. Hoxie JA, Alpers JD, Rackowski JL, et al: Alterations in T4 (CD4) protein and mRNA synthesis in cells infected with HIV. Science 1986; 234:1123–1127

31. Hill JM, Farrar WL, Pert CB: Autoradiographic localization of T4 antigen, the HIV receptor, in human brain. Int J Neurosci 1987; 32:687–693

32. Petito CK, Navia BA, Cho E-S, et al: Vacuolar myelopathy pathologically resembling subacute combined degeneration in patients with the acquired immunodeficiency syndrome. N Engl J Med 1985; 312:874–879

33. Rhodes RH, Ross AA, Damji K, et al: HIV encephalitis and opportunistic brain infections: Papovaviral-retroviral and fungal encephalitis as examples. (Abstract) Arch AIDS Res 1987; 1:187

34. Kupfer A, Singer SJ, Janeway CA Jr, Swain SL: Coclustering of CD4 (L3T4) molecule with the T-cell receptor is induced by specific direct interaction of helper T cells and antigen-presenting cells. Proc Natl Acad Sci USA 1987; 84:5888–5892

35. Gay D, Maddon P, Sekaly R, et al: Functional interaction between human T-cell protein CD4 and the major histocompatibility complex HLA-DR antigen. Nature 1987; 328:626–629

36. Sleckman BP, Peterson A, Jones WK, et al: Expression and function of CD4 in a murine T-cell hybridoma. Nature 1987; 328:351–353

37. Fontana A, Fierz W: The endothelium-astrocyte immune control system of the brain. Springer Sem Immunopathol 1985; 8:57–70

38. Duijvestijn AM, Schreiber AB, Butcher EC: Interferon-γ regulates an antigen specific for endothelial cells involved in lymphocyte traffic. Proc Natl Acad Sci USA 1986; 83:9114–9118

39. Malone JD, Richards M, Kahn AJ: Human peripheral monocytes express putative receptors for neuroexcitatory amino acids. Proc Natl Acad Sci USA 1986; 83:3307–3310

40. Pert CB, Ruff MR, Weber RJ, Herkenham M: Neuropeptides and their receptors: A psychosomatic network. J Immunol 1985; 135:820S–826S

41. Fujinami RS, Oldstone MBA: Amnio acid homology between the encephalitogenic site of myelin basic protein and virus: Mechanism for autoimmunity. Science 1985; 230:1043–1045

42. Jahnke U, Fischer EH, Alvord EC Jr: Sequence homology between certain viral proteins and proteins related to encephalomyelitis and neuritis. Science 1985; 229:282–284

43. Murray N, Page N, Steck AJ: The human anti-myelin-associated glycoprotein IgM system. Ann Neurol 1986; 19:473–478

44. Reichert CM, O'Leary TJ, Levens DL, et al: Autopsy pathology in the acquired immune deficiency syndrome. Am J Pathol 1983; 112:357–382

45. Yarchoan R, Berg G, Brouwers P, et al: Response of human immunodeficiency virus-associated neurological disease to 3′-azido-3′-deoxythymidine. Lancet 1987; 1:132–135

46. Cravioto H, Korein J, Silberman J: Wernicke's encephalopathy: A clinical and pathological study of 28 autopsied cases. Arch Neurol 1961; 4:510–519

47. Norenberg MD, Gregorios JB: Central nervous system manifestations of systemic disease. In: Davis RL, Robertson DM, eds., Textbook of Neuropathology. Baltimore, Williams & Wilkins, 1985; 403–467

48. Davtyan DG, Vinters HW: Wernicke's encephalopathy in AIDS patient treated with zidovudine. Lancet 1987; 1:919–920

49. Foresti V, Confalonieri F: Wernicke's encephalopathy in AIDS. Lancet 1987; 1:1499

50. Duchen LW, Jacobs JM: Nutritional deficiencies and metabolic disorders. In: Adams JH, Corsellis JAN, Duchen LW, eds, Greenfield's Neuropathology, 4th ed. New York, John Wiley & Sons, 1984; 573–626

51. Rhodes RH: Diagnostic immunostaining of the nervous system. In: Taylor CR, ed., Immunomicroscopy: A Diagnostic Tool for the Surgical Pathologist. Philadelphia, WB Saunders 1986; 334–362

52. Peault B, Chen CH, Cooper MD, et al: Phylogenetically conserved antigen on nerve cells and lymphocytes resembles myelin-associated glycoprotein. Proc Natl Acad Sci USA 1987; 84:814–818

53. Frank E, Pulver M, de Tribolet N: Expression of class II major histocompatibility antigens on reactive astrocytes and endothelial cells within the gliosis surrounding metastases and abscesses. J Neuroimmunol 1986; 12:29–36

54. Traugott U, Scheinberg LC, Raine CS: On the presence of Ia-positive endothelial cells and astro-

cytes in multiple sclerosis lesions and its relevance to antigen presentation. J Neuroimmunol 1985; 8:1–14

55. Massa PT, Dorries R, ter Meulen V: Viral particles induce Ia antigen expression on astrocytes. Nature 1986; 320:543–546

56. Suzumura A, Lavi E, Weiss SR, Silberberg DH: Coronavirus infection induces H-2 antigen expression on oligodendrocytes and astrocytes. Science 1986; 232:991–993

57. Hirsch M-R, Wietzerbin J, Pierres M, Goridis C: Expression of Ia antigens by cultured astrocytes treated with gamma-interferon. Neurosci Lett 1983; 41:199–204

58. Pulver M, Carrel S, Mach JP, de Tribolet N: Cultured human fetal astrocytes can be induced by interferon-γ to express HLA-DR. J Neuroimmunol 1987; 14:123–133

59. Suzumura A, Silberberg DH: Expression of H-2 antigen on oligodendrocytes is induced by soluble factors frcm concanavalin A activated T cells. Brain Res 1985; 336:171–175

60. Suzumura A, Silberberg DH, Lisak RP: The expression of MHC antigens on oligodendrocytes: Induction of polymorphic H-2 expression by lymphokines. J Neuroimmunol 1986; 11:179–190

61. Wong GHW, Bartlett PF, Clark-Lewis I, et al: Interferon-γ induces the expression of H-2 and Ia antigens cn brain cells. J Neuroimmunol 1985; 7:255–278

62. Matsumoto Y, Fujiwara M: In situ detection of class I and II major histocompatibility complex antigens in the rat central nervous system during experimental allergic encephalomyelitis: An immunohistochemical study. J Neuroimmunol 1986; 12:265–277

63. Fontana A, Fierz W, Wekerle H: Astrocytes present myelin basic protein to encephalitogenic T-cell lines. Nature 1984: 307:273–276

64. Kraal G, Duijvestijn AM, Hendriks HH: The endothelium of the high endothelial venule: A specialized endothelium with unique properties. Exp Cell Biol 1987; 55:1–10

65. McCarron RM, Spatz M, Kempski O, et al: Interaction between myelin basic protein-sensitized T lymphocytes and murine cerebral vascular endothelial cells. J Immunol 1986; 137:3428–3435

66. Birnbaum G, Clinchy B, Widmer MB: Recognition of major histocompatibility complex antigens on murine glial cells. J Neuroimmunol 1986; 12:225–233

67. Khalili-Shirazi A, Gregson N, Webb HE: Immunological relationship between a demyelinating RNA enveloped budding virus (Semliki Forest) and brain glycolipids. J Neurol Sci 1986; 76:91–103

68. Meyermann R, Korr J, Wekerle H: Specific target retrieval by encephalitogenic T line cells. (Abstract) Clin Neuropathol 1986; 5:101

69. Hickey WF, Kimura H: Graft-vs.-host disease elicits expression of class I and class II histocompatibility antigens and the presence of scattered T lymphocytes in rat central nervous system. Proc Natl Acad Sci USA 1987; 84:2082–2086

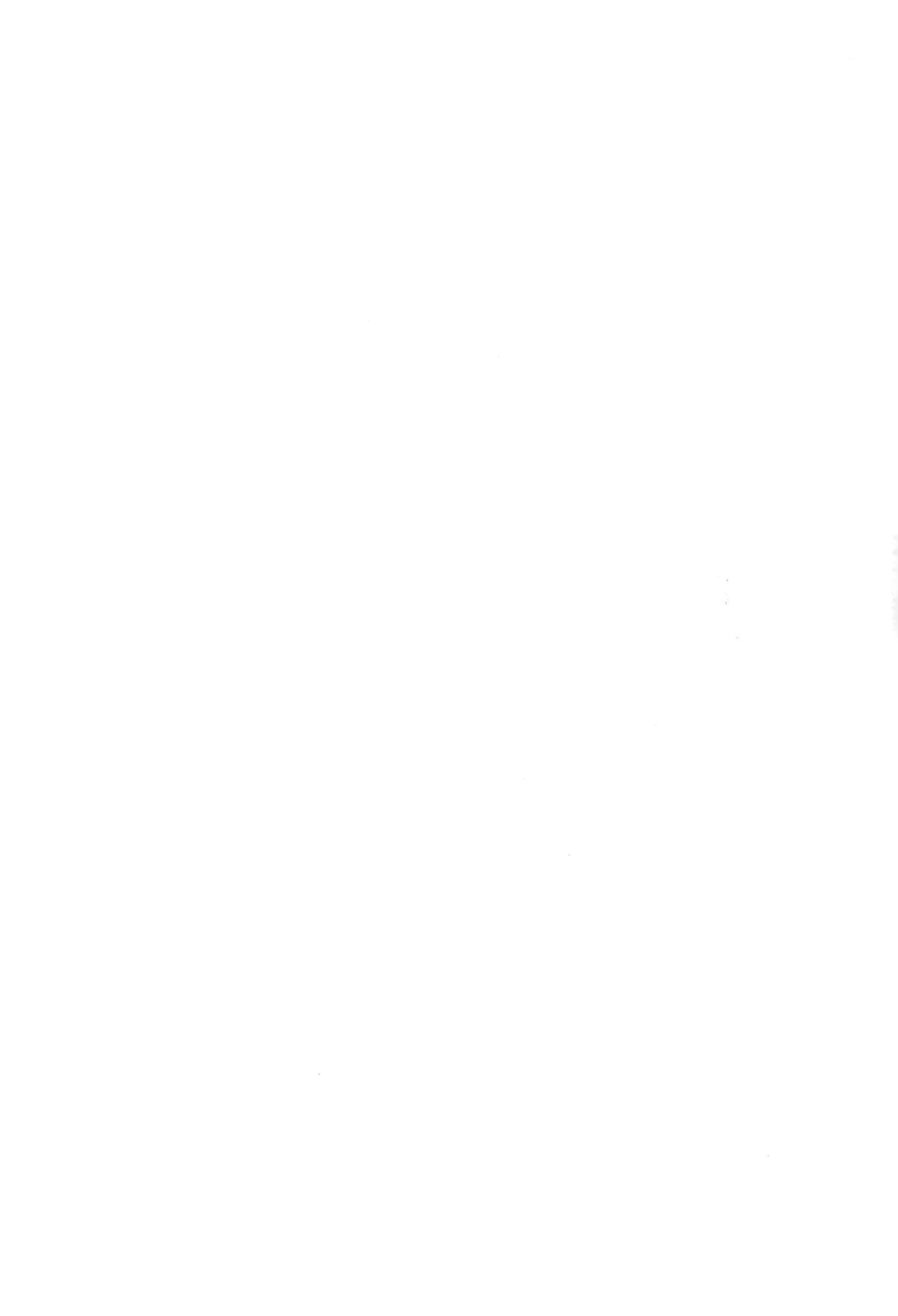

12

Specific Immunity to HIV and Other Retroviral Infections

Miroslaw K. Gorny
Abraham Pinter
Susan Zolla-Pazner

HUMAN IMMUNODEFICIENCY VIRUS type 1 (HIV-1) primarily infects a subset of lymphocytes carrying the CD4 marker (cells known as T4 cells or helper T lymphocytes) and cells of the monocyte/ macrophage lineage. The infection causes impairment of immune functions resulting in severe immunosuppression and culminating in the disease entity known as AIDS. The disease develops at a variable pace and can appear within one year of infection or, more commonly, after several years of infection. The mechanism by which this infectious agent circumvents the immune system is only partially understood. The virus is known to mutate with relatively high frequency, resulting in the generation of variants. The presence of many conserved immunogenic regions, however, makes it unlikely that the variants in a single individual would totally escape the host's immune response. The virus can also infect monocytes that are not destroyed by the virus and that apparently serve as a reservoir of infection.[1,2] Most importantly, the virus ultimately destroys the T4 lymphocytes that it infects, depriving the body of this critical cell, which orchestrates much of the immune response. These and other pathogenic mechanisms allow the virus to escape immunologic attack.

Despite the long latent period between infection and disease development, however, a detectable immune response to the virus, marked by the appearance of specific antibodies, usually occurs within a few weeks of infection.[3,4] This long period between seroconversion and onset of disease indicates that the specific immune response to the virus may play an important role in controlling the infection. Thus, studies of various types of immune reactions against the virus should reveal various mechanisms that protect against disease progression. Means to augment these particular types of immune responses would appear to be critical as modalities for the prevention and treatment of HIV infection. Therefore, the study of specific immunity to HIV is critical in the design of methods to prevent and treat HIV infection. This article presents a summary of our current understanding of the humoral and cellular responses to HIV. In addition, we present a brief review of studies of specific immunity to animal retroviruses, so that the studies of immunity to HIV can be seen in a broader biological context.

181

HUMORAL IMMUNITY TO HIV

Primary infection with HIV (also known as human lymphotropic virus III, HTLV-III, and lymphodenopathy-associated virus, [LAV]) often induces an acute disease with the clinical manifestations of a mononucleosis-like illness.[3] The incubation period ranges from a few days up to 3 months.[3,5] In one study the pattern of antibody response to HIV primary infection was examined in eight homosexual men.[6] An initial IgM response, measured by immunofluorescence, appeared within a mean of five days after the onset of the acute illness and disappeared at a mean of 81 days. IgG antibodies, demonstrated by immunofluorescence, were first detected at a mean of 11 days after the onset of acute infection and did not disappear during the study. The immunofluorescence technique was more sensitive than ELISA and Western immunoblot methods, which only detected antibodies at a mean of 20–30 days after onset. Western immunoblot used by this group identified several IgG antibodies to several HIV proteins; antibodies to p24, gp41, and p55 appeared first, followed by antibodies to the reverse transcriptase proteins. Antibodies to the higher and lower molecular weight components (gp160, gp120, and p17) could not be detected by the technique used by this group. (The definitions of these viral proteins are listed in Table 1.)

Seroconversion has been carefully studied in several instances where the exact date of infection could be identified. For example, in the instance where a nurse was accidentally infected by a deep needlestick, the acute illness appeared 2 weeks after injury and the subject's serum was positive for anti-HTLV-III on week five.[7] In two other cases, where HIV-infection was due to transfusion of anti-HTLV-III/LAV-positive blood, antibodies to p24 by Western blot analysis appeared 6–8 weeks post transfusion and antibodies against gp41 and p64 appeared at weeks 14 and 10, respectively.[4]

In sexually transmitted HIV infections, the progression of infection appears to be much slower than in diseases transmitted by transfused blood or blood products. The dif-

TABLE I

Immunogenic Proteins of HIV-1 Recognized by Sera of HIV-infected Individuals

Viral Proteins	Gene	Description
gp160	env	envelope and transmembrane glycoprotein precursor
gp120(110)*	env	envelope glycoprotein
gp41	env	transmembrane glycoprotein
p55	gag	core protein precursor
p41	gag	core protein precursor
p24(p25)	gag	core protein
p17(p15,p19)	gag	core protein
p65(p64,p66,p68)	pol	reverse transcriptase
p51	pol	reverse transcriptase
p31(p34)	pol	integrase
p23	sor	?
p14	tat-III	trans-activator
p18	art/trs	anti-repressor/trans-activator
p27	3'orf	negative regulatory element
p15	R	?

*Different scientific groups refer to the same component by slightly different designations, which are shown here in parentheses.

ference in rate of seroconversion with different modes of transmission may result from variations in the infectious dose, from the differential susceptibility of the hosts, and from the different sensitivities of the assays being used for antibody detection in the different studies. Antibodies to HIV-1, detectable by commercial ELISA may not appear until 6–14 months after initial signs of virus infection.[8] The confirmation of this long latent HIV infection was based on detection of core antigen, p24, in the serum by the antigen capture assay and detection of low titre antibodies by Western blot to recombinant structural (*gag, env*) or nonstructural (*3′orf, sor, tat-III*) proteins.[8] In these subjects, during the early months of infection, reciprocal antibody titres by Western blot ranged from 50–200, whereas overtly positive serum titres usually range from 200 to over 12,800.

The viral proteins are coded for by three structural genes, *gag, env* and, *pol,* whose expressed proteins are present both in extracellular virions and virus-infected cells, and by five additional genes, *3′orf, tat-III, sor, art/trs* and *R* (see Table 1).[9–12] All the HIV-1 gene products are immunogenic *in vivo,* and antibodies have been detected in the sera of HIV-infected subjects. The most immunogenic proteins appear to be the *env* and *gag* proteins. Antibodies to *env* proteins, detected by radioimmunoprecipitation and Western blot, were present in 97–100% of patients with AIDS and ARC. Antibodies to the *gag* protein p24 were found in 90–100% of asymptomatic HIV-seropositive individuals and in 50% of patients with AIDS; the percentage of seropositivity was similar in individuals with respect to the *pol* gene products p65/p51 (reverse transcriptase). Antibodies to products of *3′orf, sor, tat-III,* and *R* were detected in 30–65% of patients depending on the antigen.[11,13,14] The spectrum of antibodies to core protein p24 and the reverse transcriptase enzyme p65/p51 and R protein p15 seems to correlate with disease stage. In contrast, no significant difference in anti-

body prevalence to the transmembrane protein gp41 and to the *3′orf, sor,* and *tat-III* proteins appeared with regard to progression to disease.[11,13,14]

Isotype analysis of HIV antibody indicates that all immunoglobulin classes and subclasses participate in the response. The isotype and antibody levels generally are affected by changes in clinical status and may be useful in predicting the outcome of HIV infection.[13,15] Almost all sera from asymptomatic HIV-seropositive individuals and AIDS patients have IgG_1 and IgG_2 antibody demonstrated by Western blot analysis directed to all of the major *gag, pol* and, *env* gene products. IgG_3 responses were found less frequently than IgG_1 and IgG_2 and were mostly confined to *gag* antigens. Some authors did not detect an IgG_3 response in AIDS patients,[13] while others did not find any significant differences in the proportion of IgG_3 antibodies between AIDS patients and asymptomatic men.[15] IgG_4 antibodies were found to be relatively rare in both groups examined, but were not restricted to any HIV proteins. IgM and IgA responses were generally weaker than the IgG responses and were directed predominantly against *gag,* more than against *pol* and *env* proteins. IgA antibody was only found in subjects in the presence of an IgM response. In most cases, the primary response against HIV is the IgM antibody that switches to an IgG response. In some instances, however, IgM antibody persists in the absence of IgG and may be the only antibody marker of HIV infection. The IgM-positive, IgG-negative phase may last for several weeks or several months.[16,17]

Several reports have shown that the antibody to *gag*-encoded core protein p24 is reduced or absent in AIDS patients, while the antibody to the *env*-encoded transmembrane protein gp41 is consistently present in patients with AIDS, as well as in asymptomatic HIV-seropositive subjects.[13,18–21] Using titration of sera in Western blot, McDougal et al.[13] found that in AIDS patients there was a generalized decrease in antibody titre to *gag* proteins (p17, p24), *pol* proteins (p31, p51, p65) and the *env* protein gp110. Antibody titres to *env* protein gp41 were an exception because they were preserved and similar in AIDS patients and in asymptomatic men. Similar results were obtained with progressors (asymptomatic men and patients with persistent generalized lymphadenopathy who progressed to AIDS) in comparison to nonprogressors. Thus, the former had significantly lower antibody titres to most viral proteins except gp41. Study of the correlation between clinical status and immunological parameters have shown a significant association of progression with lower numbers of CD4 cells, a lower absolute lymphocyte count, a lower CD3 cell count, and a lower CD4/CD8 ratio. The next strongest correlation with clinical status was with lower antibody titres to the envelope protein gp110, the core protein p24, and the reverse transcriptase enzyme p65/p51.[13]

Weber et al.[21] have studied the incidence of anti-p24 and anti-gp41 antibodies in HIV-infected subjects who remained symptom-free and in those who manifested AIDS or ARC. Individuals who presented with a sequential decrease or lack of anti-p24 antibodies had a worse prognosis during the 4 years of the study than those who did not. This observation was relevant up to 27 months before the diagnosis of AIDS, even when the clinical status was normal. These results indicate that changes in antibody levels might signify loss of control of infection and could be a useful predictor.

The study of *in vitro* production of anti-HIV antibodies by circulating B lymphocytes sheds some light on the problem of the apparent discrepancy between different antibody titres to p24 and gp41 in subjects developing AIDS.[22,23] In most patients infected with HIV-1, peripheral blood B lymphocytes spontaneously secrete, *in vitro*, anti-HIV antibodies. Secreted antibodies to HIV were exclusively of the IgG isotype despite the fact that circulating B cells from the same patients spontaneously secreted IgG,

IgM, and IgD of unknown specificity. In some patients in which antibody to p24 was detectable in the serum, it was apparent from the analysis of cellular supernatants, that cultured antibody-producing cells made antibody to gp41, p66, p51, gp120 but little detectable antibody to p24 (Fig. 1). Thus, the frequency of cells making antibody to p24 was proportionately low. Knowing that the frequency of antibody-producing cells decreases with progression of HIV infection,[22,24] it follows that cells producing antibody to p24 might be first affected by the progressive lymphopenia of AIDS. Furthermore, increased expression of HIV antigen in serum might be an additional factor for declining anti-p24 antibodies by trapping them into immune complexes.[20]

Generation of human monoclonal antibodies to HIV antigens should permit the analysis of the specificity of the human humoral response to HIV infection and also provide an immunotherapeutic potential. Three conference abstracts have reported on human monoclonal antibodies directed against HIV viral antigens.[25-27] Stabilized lymphoblastoid cell lines have been produced by Epstein-Barr virus transformation of peripheral blood, tonsillar, and splenic B cells derived from HIV-seropositive individuals. McClure et al.[25] were the first to describe a human monoclonal antibody made from peripheral blood cells that had specificity for gp41. Banapour et al.[26] also described a cell line secreting monoclonal antibody made from spleen cells fused with a heteromyeloma partner; the antibody was reactive with an epitope of 11 amino acids in gp41. This monoclonal antibody recognized a largely conserved epitope among multiple distinct HIV isolates, but a high concentration of this antibody failed to interfere with HIV envelope/CD4 interactions. Another human monoclonal antibody was derived from the tonsils of an HIV-infected individual by Evans et al.[27] and was reactive to the *gag* precursor (p55), intermediate (p41), and core protein (p25); however, no neutralizing capacity or cytotoxicity was reported.

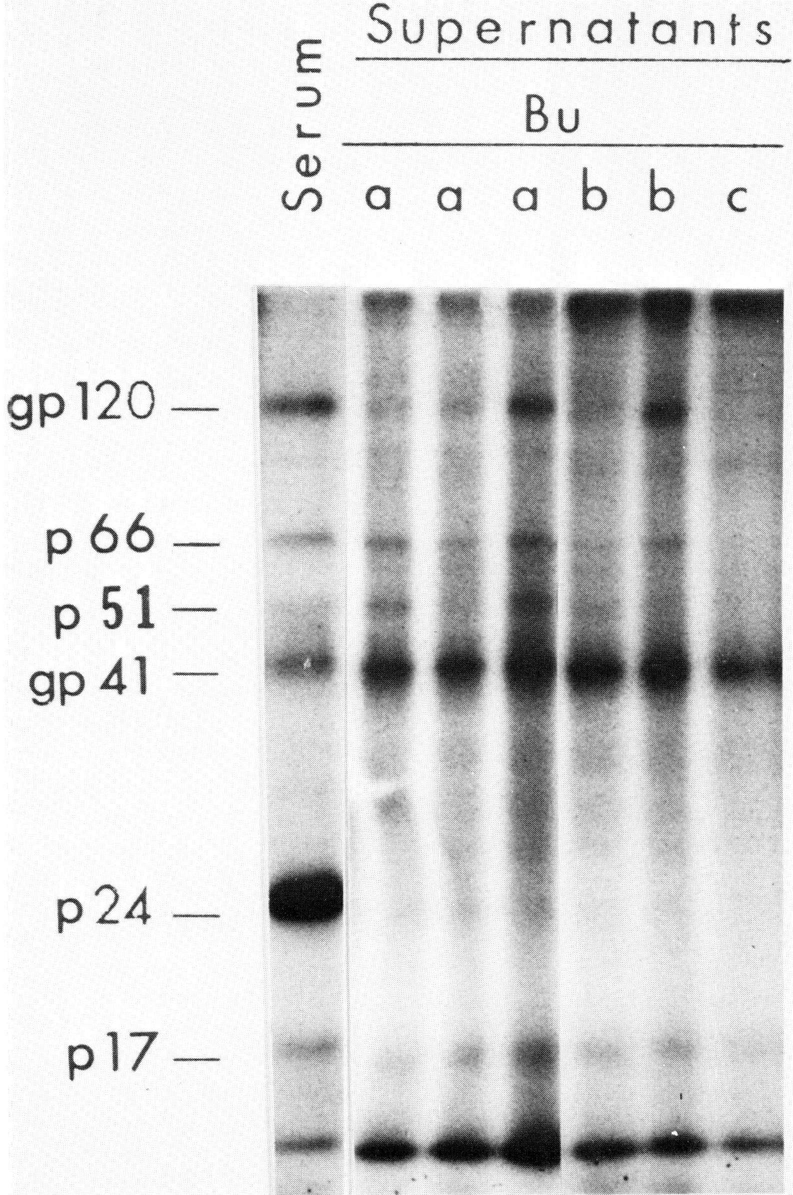

Figure 1. Radioimmunoprecipitation assay of serum and culture supernatants from peripheral blood mononuclear cells from patient Bu. Cells were cultured overnight in medium lacking mitogenic stimulation at concentrations of (a) 500,000 cells/well, (b) 250,000 cells/well and (c) 100,000 cells/well. Antibodies secreted into the supernatants were radioimmunoprecipitated and electrophoresed on SDS gels. When cells are plated at differing concentrations, the predominant reactivity is seen to reflect the higher frequency of cells making antibody to a particular viral component. In this patient, cells making antibody to gp41 and p17 are present at the highest frequency. While antibody to p24 is present in the patient's serum, cells making antibody to p24 are present at a low frequency (i.e., at a level undetectable by this assay in a population at a density of 500,000 cells per well).

Anti-HIV reverse transcriptase (RT) antibody has attracted interest because it is readily detectable and is present at a high titre in the majority of HIV-seropositive individuals. IgG derived from HIV-infected individuals has inhibitory activity for HIV RT. The level of this inhibitory antibody did not correlate with the anti-RT antibody measured by radioimmunoprecipitation[28] or with HIV antibody titres as determined by ELISA.[29] Antibody inhibitory to HIV RT activity was specific without cross-reaction with bacterial, avian, and other mammalian DNA polymerases, and its activity was confined to the F(ab')$_2$ fragment. This antibody may be related to the clinical status because the loss of RT inhibitory activity in asymptomatic HIV-seropositive individuals appeared prior to development of clinical ARC or AIDS.[28]

Protective humoral immunity toward a variety of viruses is mediated by antibodies that (1) prevent the binding to cellular receptors and subsequent internalization; (2) induce antibody-dependent complement-mediated cytotoxicity that results in virolysis; or (3) lyse those cells that are infected with the infectious agent. Discrepancies have arisen, however, in results concerning the ability of a neutralizing antibody to prevent disease progression. These discrepancies may depend on the different assays utilized as well as on various criteria used for neutralizing activity and on the particular viral isolates used in the assays. Several methods have been used to determine neutralizing antibody such as: (1) reduction of infectivity of HIV-1 for permissive cell lines;[30-33] (2) inhibition of syncytium induction;[31,34] (3) neutralization of envelope pseudotypes of vesicular stomatitis virus;[21,31] (4) inhibition of reverse transcriptase activity in culture supernatants;[34,35] (5) and reduction of cytopathic effects.[36] Neutralizing antibody to HIV-1 has been observed in the serum of most infected individuals, both asymptomatic men and patients with AIDS. The titres of neutralizing antibodies in HIV-infected subjects were generally low compared to high titres of neutralizing antibodies in sera of subjects infected with HTLV-I and HTLV-II.[31] Weber et al.[21] suggest that neutralizing antibodies may play a significant role if levels of viremia are low (in early stages of infection) and may therefore have a biological role. This is consistent with the findings of some authors who report a correlation between advanced disease and low or absent neutralizing antibody titre.[34,37] Other authors, however, found a trend but no statistically significant correlation between titres of neutralizing antibody and the clinical stage of disease.[21,31,35,36]

Neutralizing activity of serum did not correlate significantly with ELISA or Western blot antibody titres.[21,35,36] This may suggest that these different tests measure different antibodies. A four-year study in a cohort of asymptomatic individuals has shown that the neutralizing titre was not significantly different between those who remained asymptomatic and those whose disease progressed, while anti-p24 antibodies in the latter group were significantly lower. Thus, a stronger case has been made for the correlation of anti-p24 antibody decrease and disease progression than for neutralizing antibody decrease and disease progression. However, the mechanism of protection rendered by anti-p24 antibody has not been defined and may be due to a mechanism other than neutralization.[21]

Neutralizing antibodies have activity against different HIV isolates suggesting that antibodies are directed toward conserved viral regions.[34,35] The major target for antibody is gp120 with four regions relevant to neutralization. Three of these four sites overlap significantly with conserved domains.[34] Experiments with rabbits immunized with two synthetic peptides corresponding to HIV-1 proteins indicated that there are at least two neutralizing epitopes on the envelope associated with gp41 and gp120 subunits.[38] However, Matthews et al.[32] have shown that molecules other than gp120 may serve as targets for neutralizing antibody. Thus, anti-gp120 antibody isolated by specific immunoadsorption from an HIV-infected individual neutralized only one type-specific HIV isolate, but the nonbiding fraction (effluent) of the same serum contained neutralizing activity against two different virus isolates. In addition, Sarin et al.[39] suggested that antibodies against p17, a product of the *gag* gene, may also have neutralizing activity for HIV replication. Antiserum against thymosin alpha-1, which has 44–50% homology with *gag* p17, effectively neutralized HIV-1 and blocked its replication in H9 cells.

Immunization of chimpanzees with recombinant vaccinia virus expressing the envelope glycoproteins of HIV resulted in neutralizing antibodies and T-cell responses. However, all challenged chimpanzees replicated the virus in their lymphocytes. This indicates that envelope antigens as presented in this vaccinia vector are not sufficient for inducing neutralizing antibodies which prevent HIV infections.[40]

Cytotoxic antibodies might also have protective effects on viral infection. Chimpanzees and goats immunized with the viral gp120 protein of HTLV-III$_B$ produced cytotoxic antibodies that lysed target cells infected with homologous virus.[41] Similar assays with human sera, however, did not display cytotoxic antibodies with activity against virus. This qualitative difference in the type of antibody produced by HIV-infected animals and HIV-seropositive subjects may partially explain the difference in the pathogenic potential of HIV in chimpanzees and man.

CELL-MEDIATED IMMUNITY TO HIV

Cell-mediated immune reactions are known to be critical in host resistance to, and defense against, viral infections. Lysis of infected cells is the main process by which virus-infected cells are eliminated. There are three distinct mechanisms that contribute to the cytolysis of these cells: antigen-specific T cell-mediated cytotoxicity, natural cytotoxicity, and antibody dependent cell-mediated cytotoxicity.[42]

Cytotoxic and Suppressor T Cells

Cytotoxic T lymphocytes (CTL) appear early in virus infection and require HLA class I compatibility between effector and target cells for cytolysis. Human CTLs belong to the suppressor-cytotoxic subset and bear the phenotypic marker CD8 as defined by monoclonal antibodies OKT8 or Leu2. Several groups have reported increases in the percentage and absolute number of CD8 cells[43,44,45] in HIV-infected patients. Giorgi et al.[46] using monoclonal antibody to Leu8, which defines two subsets within both the CD4 and the CD8 populations, have shown a selective threefold elevation in the number of Leu8⁻CD8⁺, but not Leu8⁺CD8⁺ cells in early HIV infection, as well as in ARC and AIDS, compared to controls. Some preliminary experiments suggest that the Leu8⁻CD8⁺ cells represent cytotoxic T cells[46]; their increased number in AIDS patients could contribute to lysis of HIV-infected cells. Similarly, Nicholson et al.[47] reported the elevation of cytotoxic T lymphocytes in homosexual men infected with HIV. They identified phenotypically, by two-color immunofluorescence, cytotoxic cells as CD8⁺Leu15⁻ and suppressor cells as CD8⁺Leu15⁺. There was, however, no significant difference in the number of CD8⁺Leu15⁻ cells between asymptomatic HIV-seropositive individuals who progressed to AIDS and those who did not progress. This indicates that the level of cytotoxic cells, believed to be cytotoxic against HIV-1, cannot predict the immunologic status of HIV-seropositive subjects or their eventual progression to AIDS.

The function of cytotoxic T cells in virus infections has been well delineated. Infection with influenza virus provides a particularly useful model of CTL-mediated viral immunity (for reviews, see Lamb et al.[48], and Wraith.[49]) Although there are substantial differences in the biology of HIV infection and influenza infection, some features of influenza-specific CTL immunity seem to be shared with immunity to HIV. For example, influenza-specific CTL exhibited full cross-reactivity among the three subtypes of influenza A virus that infect man: thus, specific murine CTL clones each lysed target cells infected with different strains of influenza A virus. A small proportion of the cytotoxic T cell response was subtype specific against the hemagglutinin antigen of the virus, but only soon after immunization. On secondary *in vitro* expansion, the reactivity was entirely cross-reactive between strains. Similar cross-reactive recognition of different retroviruses has been demonstrated between T cells specific for HTLV-III/LAV and HTLV-I. Thus, both HTLV-III/LAV-specific cytotoxic T lymphocytes from the blood of seropositive individuals and a long-term cultured HTLV-I-specific line from an individual with adult T cell leukemia lysed, in an HLA-restricted way, T cells infected with either of the two retroviruses. Therefore, retrovirus-specific cytotoxic T cells recognize retrovirus-associated common antigenic determinants on cells infected with different T lymphotropic retroviruses.[50]

Influenza A-specific CTL recognize various target antigens such as surface hemagglutinin glycoproteins and internal proteins such as a nucleoprotein, polymerases, and nonstructural proteins. Another internal matrix glycoprotein has been detected as a target antigen for CTL in humans but not in mice. CTL from HIV-seropositive individuals primarily recognize surface *env*-coded proteins, but also, more rarely, *gag*-coded proteins.[51,52]

Recently, several reports described the presence of HIV-specific CTL in healthy HIV-seropositive homosexuals and in AIDS patients, but not in seronegative controls. The effector cells consisted of CD8 cells and were isolated from peripheral blood[51-53] or were obtained by broncho-alveolar lavage (BAL) from the lungs of seropositive patients with lymphocytic alveolitis.[54] Their specific lysis was inhibited by addition of monoclonal antibodies against CD3 and CD8 or by depletion of cytotoxic effector cells through the cytotoxic effect of the same monoclonal antibodies and complement. Various HIV-infected target cells have been used, including autologous EBV-immortalized B cell lines, phytohemagglutinin-stimulated peripheral blood lymphocytes, human skin fibroblasts, and alveolar macrophages. All target cells, except macrophages, were infected with recombinant vaccinia virus expressing HIV-1 *env* and *gag* genes and the bacterial *lac Z* gene as a control. The macrophages were infected with HIV. HIV-specific cytotoxicity was detected in all seropositive subjects tested including ARC and AIDS patients. Cytotoxicity was directed against the *env* region. In some patients, activity was detected against the *gag* coded protein p55.[51,52] In one study the HIV envelope-specific cytotoxic activity was detected only after five days of stimulation of peripheral lymphocytes with autologous, irridiated HIV-infected T lymphoblasts.[53] The beneficial effect of HIV-specific cytotoxicity is unclear because no correlation with disease was found.[51] Plata et al.[54] suggest that HIV-specific CD8-positive T lymphocytes may induce local inflammation in the lungs as lymphocytic alveolitis by their interactions with HIV-infected alveolar macrophages. Thus, macrophages infected with HIV-1 can be both a reservoir for the virus and an inflammatory stimulus in the lungs.

CTL activities against HIV are generally restricted by Class I molecules and maximum lysis of target cells has been observed in autologous systems. However, some cytotoxicity was also reported in heterologous systems where at least one serologically defined HLA antigen was shared between effector and target cells.[51] Similar cytotoxic effects were displayed in a xenogenic system when mouse target cells were transfected with plasmid DNA containing the HLA-A2 gene and the HIV *env* gene, and when effector cells expressed HLA-A2.[54] Taking into account the very high genetic variability of HIV isolates,[55] it is likely that the patients tested were infected with heterologous HIV genotypes. Despite this, CTL specifically lysed target cells expressing HIV envelope proteins suggesting that effector cells recognize conserved cross-reactive epitopes.

HIV-specific CTL clones were also obtained from chimpanzees and in murine experimental systems. Chimpanzees were immunized with recombinant vaccinia virus expressing HIV-1 *env* glycoproteins gp41 and gp110, and CTL clones were isolated following stimulation of lymphocytes with *env* glycoproteins.[56] In the murine system, CTL were generated by immunization with syngeneic fibroblasts expressing the HIV-1 *env* gene. The murine cytotoxic activity of Thy 1^+, Lyt 2^+ lymphocytes was clearly restricted by the Class I H-$2D^d$ antigen of BALB/c mice.[57]

All of these studies indicate the presence of HIV-1-specific cytotoxic T cells in HIV-seropositive subjects and in AIDS patients as well as in appropriately immunized chimpanzees and mice. The cytotoxic effects on target cells were observed *in vitro*. It is still unclear, however, to what extent cytotoxic T cells contribute to the elimination of virus-infected cells *in vivo*.

Recently, suppression of HIV-1 replication in peripheral blood lymphocytes by $CD8^+$ cells has also been demonstrated *in vitro*.[58] The presence of HIV-1, measured by reverse transcriptase activity in supernatants of cultures, was substantially increased in $CD8^+$-depleted peripheral blood cells compared to unseparated cells from HIV-seropositive individuals. The suppression was dependent on the relative number of $CD8^+$ lymphocytes in culture and was most apparent with autologous lymphocytes. It was suggested that HIV-specific $CD8^+$ cells produce antiviral lymphokines, most likely γ-interferon, which inhibit HIV replication. However, the role of $CD8^+$ cells *in vivo* in preventing HIV replication is still unclear, especially since the absolute number of

$CD4^+$, but not $CD8^+$ lymphocytes correlates with disease progression.[13]

Natural Killer Cells

Another feature of depressed cellular immunity in patients with AIDS is the impaired function of natural killer (NK) cells,[59,60] although the number of circulating NK cells in HIV-infected individuals is normal or increased. NK cells are known to play an important role in the control of viral infections, and their impaired activity in AIDS patients might have an impact on the progression of this disease.

NK cells are found in normal individuals not previously exposed to relevant antigens and have cytotoxic activity against transformed and virally-infected cells in a non-MHC-restricted way. The structure of target cells recognized by NK cells has not been defined. NK cells are heterogeneous and most of them belong to a class of large granular lymphocytes (LGL). Some human cells with NK activity display markers shared by T lymphocytes (CD2, CD3, CD7, CD8, CD25, OKT10), macrophages (CD11), and B cells, although the major NK effector cell is a non-T/non-B $CD3^-$, $CD16^+$, Leu 19^+ lymphocyte.[61-63]

The percentage and absolute number of NK cells in peripheral blood of AIDS patients is normal or increased in comparison to healthy individuals. Differences noted in the literature reflect the use of different NK markers and the study of patients at various stages of disease. Thus, for example, two groups[47,64] found that the number of NK cells estimated by expression of Leu11 (CD16) was not significantly different between AIDS, ARC, and healthy seropositive individuals, but a third group[65] found a significant increase in Leu11-positive cells in AIDS patients. When, however, NK cells were enumerated with Leu7[66] or Leu2a and Leu7, the percentage of NK cells was again found to vary, being significantly elevated in AIDS and ARC patients (20% vs 10% in normals) according to one group[67] and normal by others.[47,68] The absolute number of Leu7 cells was increased in non-AIDS seropositive patients, but changed with progression of disease and was significantly lower in AIDS patients, probably due to the lymphopenia in these patients.[66]

NK cytotoxicity occurs after conjugate formation between the NK cell and the target; subsequent killing is mediated by NK cytotoxic factor (NKCF), which is capable of lysing NK-sensitive cells in the absence of effector cells. NK cells might be stimulated to release NKCF by the target cells. The frequency of formation of NK cell-target cell conjugates measured at the single cell level is the same for cells from AIDS patients and normal controls.[69] NK cells derived from AIDS and ARC patients, however, could not release active NKCF *in vitro* during culture with NK-sensitive target cells (U937). NK cells from patients did release NKCF when stimulated with Concanavilin A or a mixture of 12-0-tetradecanoyl-phorbo-13-acetate and ionophore, but to a lesser extent than controls. It was postulated that the receptor on NK cells for recognition of target cells and conjugate formation is different than the receptor, which mediates the trigger signal for release of NKCF. Thus, NK cells from AIDS or ARC patients appear to recognize properly the target cells, but have some defects in the trigger involved in the release of NKCF.[69]

NK cells can also mediate antibody-dependent cellular cytotoxicity (ADCC) through their Fcγ receptors and can release NKCF when stimulated by antibody-coated target cells. ADCC activity in peripheral blood from AIDS patients was within the normal range when tested at the population level and at the single cell level.[70] When mixtures of NK-sensitive U937 cells and antibody-coated NK-nonsensitive Raji cells were used as targets, peripheral blood cells from AIDS patients were capable of killing only the coated Raji cells. As in the case above, the effector cells from AIDS patients were unable to lyse uncoated NK targets but were capable of mediating ADCC activity.[70] Thus, NK cells in AIDS patients appear to express the receptor for conjugate formation and Fcγ receptor at normal levels and NKCF release is triggered normally via the Fcγ receptor, but triggering NKCF release after conjugate formation with NK-sensitive cells is inhibited.

NK activity is positively and negatively regulated by various immunomodulators. Interferons (IFN) induce expression of IL-2 receptors on the NK progenitor and markedly augment NK lysis of sensitive targets. IL-2 may induce proliferation and stimulate NK activity. Suppression of NK activity is mediated by prostaglandin PGE$_2$ produced mostly by macrophages and certain tumor cells. When NK cells are activated by IFN or IL-2, they become resistant to suppression mediated by PGE$_2$.

Defective NK cell cytotoxicity in AIDS patients may be the consequence of diminished levels of IL-2 in these patients.[71,72] The incubation of AIDS or ARC lymphocytes with recombinant IL-2 leads to augmentation of NK activity but not to the level of activity from healthy controls.[63,74,75] NK cytotoxicity was augmented among cells from controls after 1 and 12 hours of incubation with IL-2, while among cells from AIDS patients, activity was augmented after 12 hours, but not after 1 hour of incubation with recombinant IL-2, suggesting that the cells from AIDS patients are responsive to IL-2, but that the mechanism underlying the response is at least partially impaired.[74] IL-2-activated AIDS lymphocytes, unlike similarly-derived nonactivated cells, release NKCF after stimulation with the NK-sensitive targets.[69] IL-2 also generates lymphokine-activated killer cells (LAK). In AIDS there is a strong correlation between the augmentation of NK cytotoxicity and generation of LAK cells.[75] The biological response modifier, OK-432 (a low virulent strain of Group A *Streptococus pyogenes*) also augments NK cytotoxicity and increases secretion of NKCF by NK cells in AIDS patients.[73] The OK-432 activation is independent of IL-2. IFN-α and -β increase NK cytotoxicity in controls, but have no effect on NK cells in AIDS patients.[74.] Thus, IL-2 and OK-432, but not IFNs, partially restore the cytotoxic function of NK cells from AIDS and ARC patients.

Antibody-Dependent Cellular Cytotoxicity (ADCC)

A third element of cell-mediated immunity is ADCC. ADCC is mediated by peripheral blood cells that bear receptors for the Fc fragment of IgG but do not bear surface immunoglobulins. Lysis results from the attachment of the effector cells, frequently designated as "K cells", to the Fc portion of the IgG bound to the target cell surface antigens. The specificity of the reaction depends exclusively on the specificity of the antibody; cytotoxicity is not HLA-restricted.

ADCC has been demonstrated *in vitro* to be an efficient means of lysis of cells infected with various viruses. For example, cells from human blood lyse herpes simplex virus (HSV)-infected cells in the presence of IgG antibody to HSV as early as three hours after infection of cells. The target cell damage appears prior to the release of infectious virus; thus ADCC can inhibit the spread of virus.[76] In retrovirus infection, sera from HTLV-I seropositive subjects have been shown to mediate lysis of virus-infected cells by ADCC.[77] It is believed that this immune mechanism has an important role in limiting the spread of the virus.

Recently, ADCC has been demonstrated using serum from asymptomatic individuals and from AIDS patients. Sera at dilutions between 10^{-1} to 10^{-5} in the presence of normal peripheral blood leukocytes, caused lysis of HIV-infected target cells. Antibody to the HIV envelope proteins gp160, gp120, gp41, to *gag* protein p24 and to *pol* protein p55 were present in reactive sera. In one study, antibodies reactive with the p24 protein correlated with higher levels of ADCC activity than did antibodies reactive with gp120/160.[78] In another study, sera that lacked antibodies to p19, p24, and p55, but that were still positive for gp120/160 and gp41, could mediate ADCC.[79] In a third study, cytotoxic activity mediated by an "NK-like cell" appeared to be directed specifically against gp120-coated CD4 cells. The apparent antigenic specificity of this reaction suggests it may involve antibody to gp120 and cells capable of ADCC.[80]

STUDIES OF SPECIFIC IMMUNITY TO ANIMAL RETROVIRUSES

The epidemic of HIV infection began at a time when a great deal was known about retroviral infections in animals, but relatively little was known about retroviral diseases in man. The studies of human immunity to HIV summarized above need to be viewed in the context of a broader picture that has been painted by workers studying immunity to retroviruses in animal models, especially since these model systems provide important insights concerning various approaches to immunotherapeutic intervention against viral pathogenesis.

Humoral Responses to Murine Leukemia Virus (MuLV) Infection

Like the *env* gene of HIV, the *env* gene of MuLV codes for two surface proteins, an external glycoprotein, gp70, which bears the receptor specificity of the virus,[81] and p15(E), a transmembrane protein[82] that anchors the gp70 by both covalent and noncovalent interactions.[83,84] Evidence has been presented suggesting that in addition to its role as a virion structural protein, p15(E) possesses inhibitory activity for a broad range of humoral and cellular immune functions in mice, cats, and humans.[85-88] This may account in part for the observed defect in immune functions associated with MuLV leukemogenesis, and may contribute to the leukemogenicity of these viruses.

The MuLV *env* components represent major targets of the immune response in animals infected with these viruses. However, inbred mouse strains differ in their natural immune response towards MuLVs. For example, high leukemic strains of mice such as AKR, which express high levels of virus at an early age, do not display significant levels of circulating anti-viral antibodies. If however these mice are treated neonatally with high-titred antisera against MuLV, viremia is prevented, and the mice subsequently mount an immune response against viral antigens.[89-95] Low leukemic strains of mice, on the other hand, generally do exhibit an immune response against endogenously expressed gp70 and p15(E).[96-99] These antibodies recognize endogenous as well as exogenous virus isolates,[100,101] however they specifically neutralize only the endogenous, AKR-type viruses.[102] Other studies have shown that 13–18-month-old BALB/c mice spontaneously develop virus-specific antibodies against ecotropic, amphotropic, and xenotropic classes of MuLV[103] which result in complement-mediated killing of infected cells. These antibodies appear to be directed against gp70 as well as *gag* gene-coded components. In addition to these studies showing anti-*env* antibodies in mice with naturally occurring retroviral infection, other studies have shown the production of antibodies against the *env* protein after immunization of mice with MuLV-expressing tumors. Frequently, these antibodies are type-specific for the immunizing virus.[104-106]

MuLV gene products other than the *env* proteins can also act as targets of the immune system. Thus, immunization of many mouse strains with MuLV-infected tumors or with the purified *gag* gene product, p30, results in the formation of broadly cross-reacting, group-specific and interspecies-specific antibodies against p30.[107-109] For example, hyperimmunization of C57BL/6 with an AKR spontaneous leukemia cell line, K36, produces a type-specific antibody

that is cytotoxic for Gross virus-infected lymphoid cells.[110] The antigen responsible for this activity is referred to as Gross Cell Surface Antigen (GCSA) and has been shown to consist of determinants present on the *gag* gene products p30 (the major capsid protein) and p15 (the N-terminal *gag* protein) which are expressed on the cell surface in the form of glycosylated polyproteins with molecular weights of 85 and 95 KDa.[111-114] These components are not incorporated into virions, but are found on the membranes of infected cells and are released into the culture medium. The function of these gene products is not known; mutants which cannot produce them remain replication-competent. Similar molecules have been found on Friend leukemia cells and on fibroblasts infected with isolates of the Friend, Moloney, and Rauscher class of MuLV,[115-117] and related products are also made by feline leukemia virus,[118] avian retroviruses[119] and gibbon ape retroviruses.[120] In view of the common occurrence of antibodies against *gag* products in humans infected with HIV, the possibility of a similar, highly immunogenic glycosylated *gag* polyprotein as an antigenic stimulus in these patients should be considered.

In addition to *env* and *gag* gene products, evidence exists that the MuLV *pol* products can also act as targets for the immune system. Aaronson et al.[121] have found that sera of rats bearing transplanted tumors induced by MuLV contain antibodies that inhibit the reverse transcriptase activity of virions. Hollis et al.[122] have found immune complexes containing naturally occurring antibodies that inhibit MuLV reverse transcriptase activity in kidney eluates of AKR mice. Antibodies to reverse transcriptase have also been found in other species including cats infected with FeLV,[123] gibbons infected with GaLV,[124] and cows infected with BLV.[125] These examples represent precedents for the common detection of antibodies to *pol* gene products of HIV in sera of infected individuals.

Immunization Studies with MuLV

Several groups have reported results of active immunization of different strains of mice with either inactivated viruses or purified gp70. Treatment of STU mice (a low leukemic strain) with purified Friend gp70 protected these mice from subsequent exogenous infection with Friend virus complex.[126,127] The protective mechanism appeared to involve repression of viremia, with only marginal levels of cell-mediated immunity detected. Immunization of BALB/c and C57BL/6 mice with Friend gp70 resulted in the production of both humoral and cell-mediated responses, including the development of cytotoxic antibodies and lymphocytes in BALB/c mice.[128,129]

In contrast to these results, immunization of AKR mice with Friend virus gp70 did not result in protection against the spontaneous disease that occurs in this strain. Whereas these mice mounted a type-specific immune response against the gp70 of Friend virus used as the immunogen, these antibodies were not cross-reactive with Akv gp70, and the immunization protocol resulted in an increased rate of mortality.[130] Immunization of mice with AKR type-specific vaccines did produce more effective protective responses. Treatment of both NIH Swiss and SWR/J mice with formalin-inactivated AKR MuLV resulted in the production of neutralizing and cytotoxic antibodies type-specific for the endogenous AKR-Gross viruses.[131] The predominant antibodies in these mice were directed against gp70 and p15(E). The antibodies against gp70 were primarily type-specific, while those against p15(E) were group-specific. Similar immunization of F_1 progeny of AKR and several low leukemic mouse strains resulted in up to 10,000-fold suppression of expression of endogenous virus.[132] These studies demonstrate the potential of vaccination against retroviruses, and stress the importance of proper serotype in the development of an effective protective response.

A number of studies have demonstrated that the spontaneous progression towards leukemia in AKR mice can be effectively prevented by passive immunotherapy. Treatment of neonatal mice with high titered goat antibodies against either AKR or Friend MuLV gp70 resulted in a marked suppression of viremia and leukemia.[90-92] Intact antibodies were required, and $F(ab')_2$ fragments were not effective,[93] suggesting that Fc-mediated events are responsible. The animals protected in this manner produced neutralizing antibodies later in life, demonstrating that AKR mice are genetically capable of producing antibodies against their endogenous virus if the viremia that normally occurs is prevented. Similar studies have shown protection of STU and BALB/Mo mice against disease induced by Friend and Moloney MuLV in these strains.[94,95]

In order for passive immunotherapy with anti-gp70 sera to be effective in the AKR system, the treatment has to be initiated at a very early age, during the first three days after birth. Administration of antiserum after the first week of life is not effective. Recently it was shown that this window of treatment could be significantly extended by including a high-titred antiserum against p15(E) in the protocol.[133] The combination of antibodies to both gp70 and p15(E) resulted in a clear suppression of leukemia when applied as late as five months of age, or shortly before the natural onset of leukemia. Similar, though less dramatic, results were obtained by foster nursing on mice possessing high anti-p15(E) titres. These antibodies may be blocking an immunosuppressive activity of p15(E), they may be inhibiting the surface expression of the viral *env* proteins, or they may be facilitating a cytolytic response. This latter hypothesis is consistent with studies showing that monoclonal antibodies to p15(E), but not to gp70 are virolytic for MuLV in the presence of complement.[134] In any case, these studies suggest that the development of antibodies against both gp41 and gp120 may be beneficial in any immunization protocol designed against HIV.

Cell-mediated Immunological Response to MuLV Infection

In addition to the humoral response to MuLV infection, mice often mount a cellular immune response against retrovirus-infected cells, a response that plays an important role in protection *in vivo*. Cytotoxic T lymphocytes, generated by immunization of mice with virus-producing tumors, show specificity for both viral antigens and products of the major histocompatibility complex.

Both viral *env* and *gag* antigens can serve as targets for CTL. This has been shown by studies utilizing cells coexpressing appropriate H-2 molecules and cloned MuLV genes.[135-138] Recently, it has been shown that the intensity of the CTL response against specific Gross-MuLV antigens varies according to the H-2 antigens with which the viral proteins are associated.[139] Thus, the bulk population of CTL from BALB/c mice (H-2^d haplotype) recognize an *env* gene product, whereas BALB.B mice (H-2^b haplotype) preferentially recognize a *gag* gene product, and C57BL/6 mice (H-2^b) recognize both *gag* and *env* gene products with equal intensities. These data suggest that the antigenicity of the different viral proteins may be affected by the specific H-2 molecule with which they are associated.

An approach towards generating an effective cellular immune response against the Friend virus *env* gene product using a recombinant vaccinia virus vector was recently reported.[140] Whereas unimmunized and control animals did not develop any CTL, mice inoculated with the vaccinia recombinant exhibited an *env*-specific T-cell proliferative response, and after challenge with Friend virus, developed neutralizing antibodies and cytotoxic T cells and were protected against leukemia. The vaccinia vector was not, however, as effective as an attenuated N-tropic Friend virus. This may be an indication that either the vaccinia virus did not replicate as efficiently in mice as the attenuated Friend virus, or that expression of additional antigens such as *gag* may enhance the protective response. This study also indicates that vaccinia immunization leads to a priming effect, and only after exposure to the challenge virus did the mice develop neutralizing antibodies and CTL.

SPECULATION ON VIRAL ESCAPE FROM IMMUNITY

HIV-1 infection clearly induces a broad spectrum of specific humoral and cellular immunity in its hosts. The fact that the disease eventually progresses in individuals with active anti-HIV immune responses does not indicate that the immunity has been ineffective in initially controlling and slowing the disease. Indeed, some studies, summarized above, indicate that certain types of antibodies and cell-mediated immune reactions are found early in infection but decrease with disease progression. These studies suggest that the response of the immune system, when it is still fully functional, does impart protection and that disease progression occurs when immunity has been compromised.

The reason that the virus cannot be cleared from the body during the early stages of infection most probably lies in the fact that the infectious agent is a retrovirus that irreversibly infects cells, integrates into the cellular genome, and lies dormant until the cell is further stimulated. It has been suggested, but not yet proven, that the mere presence of the provirus in a T4 lymphocyte is sufficient to alter or impair its function. Thus, as more and more cells become infected by periodic bursts of virus replication or repeated exposure to the virus, more and more functional impairment might be noted, even before a significant drop in T4 lymphocyte numbers occurs. Other functional impairments of antigen-presentation, phagocytosis, and chemotaxis apparently occur as the result of the infection of cells of the monocyte/macrophage lineage, cells that are not lysed by this infection but that harbor and replicate the organism. Thus, in a healthy individual, in the early stages of infection, which may in fact last for many years, the virus may remain relatively quiescent, and virus production may be negatively regulated by both humoral and cellular immune mechanisms.

The events that precipitate the progression of disease are not yet defined. *In vitro*, it has been shown that viral replication in latently infected cells can be initiated by antigenic or mitogenic stimulation. Thus, exposure to infectious agents and/or to allogeneic products could begin to shift the balance from viral regulation to viral growth. Alternatively, this balance could gradually shift within the host with each round of viral replication and/or with repeated exposure to the virus. Whatever the mechanism, the balance does shift from one of immunologic containment to viral growth and destruction of the immune system.

It is the purpose of the studies summarized above and of the continuing studies of immunity to HIV to understand how this relationship between HIV and the immune response can be altered so that the host, rather than the virus, will be favored.

Supported in part by funding from the National Institute of Health (AI72658 and AI62542), by a grant from the New York State AIDS Institute and by research funds from the Veterans Administration.

REFERENCES

1. Gyorkey F, Melnick JL, Sinkovics JG, Gyorkey P: Retrovirus resembling HTLV in macrophages of patients with AIDS. Lancet 1985; 1:160
2. Popovic M Gartner S: Isolation of HIV-1 from monocytes but not T lymphocytes. Lancet 1987; 2:916
3. Cooper DA, Maclean P, Finlayson R, et al: Acute AIDS retrovirus infection. Definition of a clinical illness associated with seroconversion. Lancet 1985; 1:537
4. Esteban J, Shih JW-K, Tai C-C, et al: Importance of Western blot analysis in predicting infectivity of anti-HTLV-III/LAV positive blood. Lancet 1985; 1:1083
5. Piette A, Tusseau F, Vignon F, et al: Acute neuropathy coincident with seroconversion for anti-LAV/HTLV-III. Lancet 1986; 1:852
6. Cooper D, Imrie A, Penny R: Antibody response to human immunodeficiency virus after primary infection. J Inf Dis 1987; 155:1113
7. Anonymous: Needlestick transmission of HTLV-III from a patient infected in Africa. Lancet 1984; 2:1376
8. Ranki A, Valle S-L, Krohn M, et al: Long latency overt seroconversion in sexually transmitted human-immunodeficiency-virus infection. Lancet 1987; 2:589
9. Essex M, Allan J, Kanki P, et al: Antigens of human T-lymphotropic virus type III/lymphadenopathy associated virus. Ann Intern Med 1985; 103:700
10. Kan N, Franchini G, Wong-Staal F, et al: A novel protein (sor) of HTLV-III expressed in bacteria is immunoreactive with sera from infected individuals. Science 1986; 231:1553
11. Wong-Staal F, Chanda P, Ghrayeb J: Human immunodeficiency virus type III: The eighth gene. AIDS Res Hum Retroviruses 1987; 3:33
12. Feinberg M, Jarret R, Aldovini A, et al: HTLV-III expression and production involve complex regulation at the levels of splicing and translation of viral RNA. Cell 1986; 46:807
13. McDougal J, Kennedy M, Nicholson J, et al: Antibody response to human immunodeficiency virus in homosexual men. Relation of antibody specificity, titer, and isotype to clinical status, severity of immunodeficiency, and disease progression. J Clin Invest 1987; 80:316
14. Franchini G, Robert-Guroff M, Aldovini A, et al: Spectrum of natural antibodies against five HTLV-III antigens in infected individuals: Correlation of antibody prevalence with clinical status. Blood 1987; 69:437
15. Hendry R, Judkins K, Wittek A, et al: Subclass and isotope specific antibody responses to HIV infection analyzed by Western blotting: Correlation with clinical status. III International Conference on AIDS 1987; 31
16. Parry J, Mortimer P: Place of IgM antibody testing in HIV serology. Lancet 1986; 2:979
17. Bedorida G, Cambie G, D'Agostino F, et al: HIV IgM antibodies in risk groups who are seronegative on ELISA testing. Lancet 1986; 2:570
18. Schupback J, Haller O, Vogt M, et al: Antibodies to HTLV-III in Swiss patients with AIDS and pre-AIDS and in groups at risk for AIDS. N Engl J Med 1985; 312:265
19. Biggar R, Melbye M, Ebbesen P, et al: Variation in human T lymphotropic virus type III (HTLV-III) antibodies in homosexual men: Decline before onset of illness related to acquired immune deficiency syndrome (AIDS). Br Med J 1985; 291:997

20. Lange J, Goudsmit J: Decline of antibody reactivity to HIV core protein secondary to increased production of HIV antigen. Lancet 1987 1:190
21. Weber J, Clapham P, Weiss R, et al: Human immunodeficiency virus in two cohorts of homosexual men: Neutralizing sera and association of anti-gag antibody with prognosis. Lancet 1987; 1:119
22. Zolla-Pazner S, Mizuma H, Gianakakos V, et al: Production of antibody by circulating B cells of HIV-seropositive subjects. III International Conference on AIDS 1987; 80
23. Amadori R, De Rossi A, Faulkner-Valle G, et al: In vitro synthesis of antibodies against HIV-1 components. III Intl Conference on AIDS 1987; 79
24. Yarchoan R, Redfield R, Broder S: Mechanisms of B cell activation in patients with AIDS and related disorders: Contribution of antibody-producing cells, of Epstein-Barr Virus-infected B cells, and of immunoglobulin production induced by HTLV-III/LAV. J Clin Inv 1986; 78:439
25. McClure J: Human monoclonal antibodies of LAV/HTLV-III. International Conference on AIDS 1986; 13
26. Banapour B, Rosenthal K, Rabin L, et al: Production, characterization and epitope mapping of a human monoclonal antibody reactive with the envelope glycoprotein of HIV. III International Conference on AIDS 1987; 81
27. Evans L, Homsy J, Gaston I, et al: Human monoclonal antibodies directed against gag gene products of the human immunodeficiency virus (HIV). III International Conference on AIDS 1987; 84
28. Laurence J, Saunders A, Kulkosky J: Characterization and clinical association of antibody inhibitory to HIV reverse transcriptase activity. Science 1987; 235:1502
29. Chatterjee R, Rinaldo C, Jr, Gupta R: Immunogenicity of Human immunodeficiency virus (HIV) reverse transcriptase: Detection of high levels of antibodies to HIV reverse transcriptase in sera of homosexual men. J Clin Immunol 1987; 7:218
30. Robert-Guroff M, Brown M, Gallo RC: HTLV-III neutralizing antibodies in patients with AIDS and AIDS-related complex. Nature 1985; 316:72
31. Weiss RA, Clapham PR, Cheingsong-Popov R, et al: Neutralization of human T-lymphotropic virus type III by sera of AIDS and AIDS-risk patients. Nature 1985; 316:69
32. Matthews T, Langlois A, Robey W, et al: Restricted neutralization of divergent human T-lymphotropic virus type III isolates by antibodies to the major envelope glycoprotein. Proc Natl Acad Sci USA 1986; 83:9709
33. Krohn K, Robey W, Putney S, et al: Specific cellular immune response and neutralizing antibodies in goats immunized with native or recombinant envelope proteins derived from human T-lymphotropic virus type IIIB and in human immunodeficiency virus-infected men. Proc Natl Acad Sci USA 1987; 84:4994
34. Ho D, Sarngadharan M, Hirsch M, et al: Human immunodeficiency virus neutralizing antibodies recognize several conserved domains on the envelope glycoproteins. J Virology 1987; 61:2024
35. Prince A, Pascual D, Kosolapov L, et al: Prevalence, clinical significance, and strain specificity of neutralizing antibody to the human immunodeficiency virus. J Inf Dis 1987; 156:268
36. Wendler I, Bienzle U, Hunsmann G: Neutralizing antibodies and the course of HIV-induced disease. AIDS Res Human Retroviruses 1987; 3:157
37. Robert-Guroff M, Goedert J, Jennings A, et al: High HTLV-III/LAV neutralizing antibody titers correlate with better clinical outcome. III International Conference on AIDS 1987; 53
38. Chanh T, Dreesman G, Kanda P, et al: Induction of anti-HIV neutralizing antibodies by synthetic peptides. EMBO J 1986; 5:3065
39. Sarin PS, Sun DK, Thornton AH, et al: Neutralization of HTLV-III/LAV replication by antiserum to thymosin alpha-1. Science 1986; 232:1135
40. Hu S-L, Fultz P, McClure H, et al: Effect of immunization with a vaccinia-HIV env recombinant on HIV infection of chimpanzees. Nature 1987; 328:721
41. Nara P, Robey W, Gonda M, et al: Absence of cytotoxic antibody to human immunodeficiency virus-infected cells in humans and its induction in animals after infection or immunization with purified envelope glycoprotein gp120. Proc Natl Acad Sci USA 1987; 84:3797
42. Sissons J, Oldstone M: Killing of virus-infected cells by cytotoxic lymphocytes. J Inf Dis 1980; 142:114
43. Fahey JL, Prince H, Weaver M, et al: Quantitative changes in T helper or T suppressor/cytotoxic lymphocyte subsets that distinguish acquired immune deficiency syndrome from other immune subset disorders. Am J Med 1984; 76:95
44. Seligmann M, Chess L, Fahey JL, et al: AIDS —an immunologic reevaluation. N Engl J Med 1984; 311:1286
45. Zolla-Pazner S, Des Jarlais DC, Friedman SR, et al: Nonrandom development of immunologic abnormalities after infection with human immunodeficiency virus: Implications for immunologic classification of the disease. Proc Natl Acad Sci USA 1987; 84:5404
46. Giorgi J, Nishanian P, Schmid I, et al: Selective alterations in immunoregulatory lymphocyte subsets in early HIV (human T-lymphotropic virus type III/lymphadenopathy-associated virus) infection. J Clin Immunol 1987; 7:140
47. Nicholson J, Echenberg D, Jones B, et al: T-cytotoxic/suppressor cell phenotypes in a group of asymptomatic homosexual men with and without exposure to HTLV-III/LAV. Clin Immunol Immunopath 1986; 40:505
48. Lamb J, McMichael J, Rothbard J: T-cell recognition of influenza viral antigens. Hum Immunol 1987; 19:79
49. Wraith D: The recognition of influenza A virus-infected cells by cytotoxic T lymphocytes. Immunol Today 1987; 8:239
50. Rook A, Koenig S, Mitsuya, H, et al: Cross reac-

tive recognition of different human T lymphotropic retroviruses by HTLV-I and HTLV-III/LAV specific cytotoxic T lymphocytes (CTL). III International Conference on AIDS 1987; 27

51. Walker B, Chakrabarti S, Moss B, et al: HIV-specific cytotoxic T lymphocytes in seropositive individuals. Nature 1987; 328:345

52. Koenig S, Earl P, Powell D, et al: Cytotoxic T Cells directed against target cells expressing HIV-1 proteins. III International Conference on AIDS 1987; 59

53. Shepp D, Mann D, Chakrarti S, et al: Detection of HLA restricted human immunodeficiency virus (HIV) envelope antigen-specific cytotoxic lymphocytes. III International Conference on AIDS 1987; 59

54. Plata F, Autran B, Martins L, et al: AIDS virus-specific cytotoxic T lymphocytes in lung disorders. Nature 1987; 328:348

55. Wong-Staal F, Gallo R: Human T-lymphotropic retroviruses. Nature 1985; 317:395

56. Zarling J, Eichberg J, Moran P, et al: Proliferative and cytotoxic T cells to AIDS virus glycoproteins in chimpanzees immunized with a recombinant vaccinina virus expressing AIDS virus envelope glycoproteins. J Immunol 1987; 139:988

57. Langlade-Demoyen P, Michel F, Garcia-Pons F, et al: Generation of HIV-1-specific cytotoxic T lymphocytes in a genetically-defined murine experimental system. III International Conference on AIDS 1987; 131

58. Walker C, Moody D, Stites D, Levy J: CD8+ lymphocytes can control HIV infection in vitro by suppressing virus replication. Science 1986; 234:1563

59. Rook A, Masur H, Lane HC, et al: Interleukin-2 enhances the depressed natural killer and CMV-specific cytotoxic activities of lymphocytes from patients with AIDS. J Clin Invest 1983; 72:398

60. Gold JWM, Weike CS, Godbold J, et al: Unexplained persistent lymphadenopathy in homosexual men and the acquired immune deficiency syndrome. Medicine 1985; 64:203

61. Herberman R: Natural cell-mediated immunity against tumors. Orlando FL, Academic Press 1980

62. Lanier L, Le A, Civin C, et al: The relationship of CD15 (Leu-11) and Leu-19 (NKH-1) antigen expression on human peripheral blood NK cells and cytotoxic T lymphocytes. J Immunol 136:4480–4486

63. Ortaldo J, Herberman R,: Heterogeneity of natural killer cells. Ann Rev Immunol 1984; 2:359

64. Rappocciolo G, Piazza P, Cai Q, et al: Natural killer cell activity against HIV infected U937 cells in homosexual men. III International Conference on AIDS 1987; 128

65. Lewis DL, Puck JM, Babcock GF, Rich RR: Disproportionate expansion of a minor T cell subset in patients with lymphodenopathy syndrome and acquired immunodeficiency syndrome. J Inf Dis 1985; 151:555

66. Amiel C, May T, Bene MC, et al: Leu 7 (HNK-1) cells in AIDS and related syndromes. III International Conference on AIDS 1987; 29

67. Reuben J, Gschwind C, Hersh E: Expansion of a subset of T lymphocytes capable of natural killer activity in individuals infected with the human immunodeficiency virus (HIV). III International Conference on AIDS 1987; 132

68. Plaeger-Marshall S, Spina C, Giorgi J, et al: Alterations in cytotoxic and phenotypic subsets of natural killer cells in acquired immune deficiency syndrome (AIDS). J Clin Immunol 1987; 7:16

69. Bonavida BT, Katz J, Gottlieb M: Mechanism of defective NK cell activity in patients with acquired immunodeficiency syndrome (AIDS) and AIDS-related complex. J Immunol 1986; 137:1157

70. Katz J, Mitsuyasu R, Gottlieb M, et al: Mechanism of defective NK cell activity in patients with acquired immunodefiency syndrome (AIDS) and AIDS-related complex. II. Normal antibody-dependent cellular cytotoxicity (ADCC) mediated by effector cells defective in natural killer (NK) cytotoxicity. J Immunol 1987; 139:55

71. Alcocer J, Alarcon-Segovia D, Abud-Mendoza C: Immunoregulatory circuits in the acquired immunodeficiency syndrome and related complex. Production of and response to interleukins 1 and 2, NK function and its enhancement by interleukin-2 and kinetics of the autologous mixed lymphocyte reaction. Clin Exp Immunol 1985; 60:31

72. Gluckman J-C, Klatzmann D, Cavaille-Coll M, et al: Is there correlation of T cell proliferative functions and surface marker phenotypes in patients with acquired immune deficiency syndrome or lymphadenopathy syndrome? Clin Exp Immunol 1985; 60:8

73. Bonavida B, Katz J, Haddadian A, et al: Restoration of AIDS defective natural killer (NK) function by OK-423. III International Conference on AIDS 1987; 127

74. Ramsey K, Tran C, Patten C, et al: Kinetics of interleukin-2 augmentation of natural killer cell cytotoxicity in the acquired immunodeficiency syndrome. III International Conference on AIDS 1987; 131

75. Reuben J, Rios A, Brewton G, Mansell P: The generation of natural killer and lymphokine activated killer cells in HIV-infected individuals. III International Conference on AIDS 1987; 186

76. Shore S, Cromeans T, Romano TJ: Immune destruction of virus-infected cells early in the infectious cycle. Nature 1976; 262:685

77. Miyakoshi H, Koide H, Aoki T: In vitro antibody-dependent cellular cytotoxicity against human T-cell leukemia/lymphoma virus (HTLV)-producing cells. Int J Cancer 1984; 33:267

78. Rook A, Lane H, Folks T, et al: Sera from HTLV-III/LAV antibody-positive individuals mediate antibody-dependent cellular cytotoxicity against HTLV-III/LAV-infected T cells. J Immunol 1987; 138:1064

79. Ljunggren K, Fenyo E-M, Bottiger B, et al: Antibody-dependent cellular cytotoxicity (ADCC)-inducing antibodies against human immunodeficiency virus (HIV). III International Conference on AIDS 1987; 8

80. Weinhold K, Lyerly H, Matthews T, et al: Gp 120-specific cell-mediated cytotoxicity in patients exposed to HIV. III International Conference on AIDS 1987; 59

81. DeLarco J, Todaro GJ: Membrane receptors for murine leukemia viruses: Characterization using the purified viral envelope glycoprotein gp71. Cell 1976; 8:365–371

82. Pinter A, Honnen WJ: Topography of murine leukemia virus envelope proteins: Characterization of transmembrane components. J Virol 1983; 46:1056–1060

83. Pinter A, Lieman-Hurwitz J, Fleissner E: The nature of the association between the murine leukemia virus envelope proteins. Virology 1978; 91:345–351

84. Montelaro, RC, Sullivan SJ, Bolognesi DP: An analysis of type-C retrovirus polypeptides and their associations in the virion. Virology 1978; 84:19–31

85. Cianciolo GJ, Copeland TD, Oroszlan S, Synderman R: Inhibition of lymphocyte proliferation by a synthetic peptide homologous to retroviral envelope proteins. Science 1985; 230:453–455

86. Schmidt DM, Sidhu NK, Cianciolo GJ, Syndermann R: Recombinant hydrophilic region of murine retroviral p15E inhibits stimulated T-lymphocyte proliferation. Proc Natl Acad Sci 1987; 84:7290–7294

87. Mathes, LE, Olsen RG, Hebebrand LG, et al: Immunosuppressive properties of a virion polypeptide, a 15,000-dalton protein, from feline leukemia virus. Cancer Res 1979; 39:950–955

88. Lafrado LJ, Lewis MG, Mathes LE, Olsen RG: Suppression of in vitro neutrophil function by feline leukaemia virus (FeLV) and purified FeLV-p15E. J Gen Virol 1987; 68:507–513

89. Nowinski RC: Genetic control of natural immunity to ecotropic mouse leukemia viruses: Immune response genes. Infect and Immunol 1976; 13:1098–1102

90. Huebner RJ, Gilden RV, Toni R, et al: Prevention of spontaneous leukemia in AKR mice by type-specific immunosuppression of endogenous ecotropic virogenes. Proc Natl Acad Sci 1976; 73:4633–4635

91. Schafer W, Schwarz H, Thiel HJ, et al: Properties of mouse leukemia viruses. XIV. Prevention of spontaneous AKR leukemia by treatment with group-specific antibody against the major virus gp71 glycoprotein. Virology 1977; 83:207–210

92. Schwarz H, Fischinger PJ, Ihle JN, et al: Properties of mouse leukemia viruses. XVI. Suppression of spontaneous fetal leukemias in AKR mice by treatment with broadly reacting antibody against the viral glycoprotein gp71. Virology 1979; 93:159–174

93. Schwarz H, Thiel HJ, Weinhold K, et al: Properties of mouse leukemia viruses: XX. Variation of AKR substrains in response to antibody therapy. Virology 1986; 150:247–251

94. Hunsmann G, Moennig V, Schafer W: Properties of mouse leukemia viruses. IX. Active and passive immunization of mice against Friend leukemia with isolated viral GP71 glycoprotein and its corresponding antiserum. Virology 1975; 66:327–329

95. Nobis P, Jaenisch R: Passive immunotherapy prevents expression of endogenous Moloney virus and amplification of proviral DNA in BALB/Mo mice. Proc Natl Acad Sci 1980; 77:3677–3681

96. Ihle JN, Yurconic M, Hanna MG: Autogenous immunity to endogenous RNA tumor virus. Radioimmune precipitation assay of mouse serum antibody levels. J Exp Med 1973; 138:194–208

97. Nowinski RC, Kaehler SL: Antibody to leukemia virus: Widespread occurrence in inbred mice. Science 1974; 185:869–871

98. Ihle JN, Hanna MG, Schafer W, et al: Polypeptides of mammalian oncornaviruses. III. Localization of p15 and reactivity with natural antibody. Virology 1975; 63:60–67

99. Pierotti MA, Colnaghi MI: Natural antibodies directed against murine lymphosarcoma cells: variability of level in individual mice. Int J Cancer 1976; 18:223–229

100. Ihle JN, Domotor Jr JJ, Bengali KM: Characterization of the type and group specificities of the immune response in mice to murine leukemia viruses. J Virol 1976; 18:124–131

101. Hanna MG, Jr, Ihle JN, Lee JC: Autogenous immunity to endogenous RNA tumor virus: Humoral immune response to virus envelope antigens. Cancer Res 1976; 36:608–614

102. Ihle JN, Lazar B: Natural immunity in mice to the envelope glycoprotein of endogenous ecotropic type C viruses: Neutralization of virus infectivity. J Virol 1977; 21:974–980

103. Kende M, Veronese F, Hill DW, et al: Naturally occurring humoral immunity to endogenous xenotropic and amphotropic type-C virus in the mouse. Int J Cancer 1981; 27:235–242

104. Stockert E, Old LJ, Boyse EA: The G_{IX} system. A cell surface allo-antigen associated with murine leukemia virus; implications regarding chromosomal integration of the viral genome. J Exp Med 1971; 133:1334–1355

105. Tung JS, Vitetta ES, Fleissner E, Boyse EA: Biochemical evidence linking the G_{IX} thymocyte surface antigen to the gp69/71 envelope glycoprotein of murine leukemia virus. J Exp Med 1975; 141:198–205

106. Tung JS, Shen FW, Fleissner E, Boyse EA: X-gp70: A third molecular species of the envelope protein gp70 of murine leukemia virus, expressed on mouse lymphoid cells. J Exp Med 1976; 143:696–974

107. Geering G, Old LJ, Boyse EA: Antigens of leukemias induced by naturally occurring murine leukemia virus: Their relation to the antigens of Gross virus and other murine leukemia viruses. J Exp Med 1966; 124:753–772

108. Gilden RV, Oroszlan S: Group-specific antigens of RNA tumor viruses as markers for subinfectious expression of the RNA virus genome. Proc Natl Acad Sci 1972; 69:1021–1025

109. Strand M, August JT: Structural proteins of mammalian oncogenic RNA viruses: Multiple antigenic determinants of the major internal protein and envelope. J Virol 1974; 13:171–180

110. Old LJ, Boyse EA, Stockert E: The G (Gross) leukemia antigen. Cancer Res 1965; 25:813–819

111. Snyder H, Stockert E, Fleissner E: Characterization of molecular species carrying gross cell surface antigen. J Virol 1977; 23:302–314

112. Ledbetter J, Nowinski RC: Identification of the Gross cell surface antigen associated with murine leukemia virus-infected cells. J Virol 1977; 23:315–322

113. Tung JS, Yoshiki T, Fleissner E: A core polyprotein of murine leukemia virus on the surface of mouse leukemia cells. Cell 1976; 9:573–578

114. Tung JS, Pinter A, Fleissner E: Two species of type-C core polyprotein on AKR mouse leukemia cells. J Virol 1977; 23:430

115. Evans LH, Dresler S, Kabat D: Synthesis and glycosylation of polyprotein precursors to the internal core proteins of Friend murine leukemia virus. J Virol 1977; 24:856–874

116. Edwards SA, Fan H: Gag-Related polyproteins of Moloney murine leukemia virus: Evidence for independent synthesis of glycosylated and unglycosylated forms. J Virol 1979; 30:551–563

117. Ruta M, Kabat D: Plasma membrane glycoproteins encoded by cloned Rauscher and Friend spleen focus-forming viruses. J Virol 1980; 35:844–853

118. Neil JC, Smart JE, Hayman MG, Jarrett O: Polypeptides of feline leukemia virus: a glycosylated gag-related protein is released into culture fluids. Virology 1980; 105:250–253

119. Buetti E, Diggelman H: Avian oncovirus proteins expressed on the surface of infected cells. Virology 1980; 102:251–261

120. Thiel HG, Iglehart D, Mattheus TJ, Broughton EM: Preparation of autologous antiserum against SSV nonproducer cells and its partial characterization. Virology 1981; 112:634–641

121. Aaronson SA, Parks WP, Scolnick EM, Todaro GJ: Antibody to the RNA-dependent DNA polymerase of mammalian C-type RNA tumor viruses. Proc Natl Acad Sci 1971; 68:920–924

122. Hollis VW Jr, Aoki T, Barrera O, et al: Detection of naturally occurring antibodies to RNA-dependent DNA polymerase of murine leukemia virus in kidney eluates of AKR mice. J Virol 1974; 13:448–454

123. Jacquemin PC, Saxinger C, Gallo RC: Surface antibodies of human myelogenous leukaemia leukocytes reactive with specific type-C viral reverse transcriptases. Nature 1978; 276:230–236

124. Gallagher RE, Schrecker AW, Walter CA, Gallo RC: Oncornavirus lytic activity in the serum of gibbon apes. J Natl Canc Inst 1978; 60:677–682

125. Wuu KD, Graves DC, Ferrer JR: Inhibition of the reverse transcriptase of bovine leukemia virus by antibody in sera from leukemic cattle and immunological characterization of the enzyme. Cancer Res 1977; 37:1438

126. Hunsmann G, Moennig V, Schafer W: Properties of mouse leukemia virus. IX. Active and passive immunization of mice against Friend leukemia with isolated viral gp71 glycoprotein and its corresponding antiserum. Virology 1975; 66:327–329

127. Hunsmann G, Schneider J, Schultz A: Immunoprevention of Friend virus-induced erythroleukemia by vaccination with viral envelope glycoprotein complexes. Virology 1981; 113:602–612

128. Ihle JN, Collins JJ, Lee JC, et al: Characterization of the immune response to the major glycoprotein (gp71) of Friend leukemia virus. I. Response in BALB/c mice. Virology 1976; 75:74–87

129. Ihle JN, Lee JC, Collins JJ, et al: Characterization of the immune response to the major glycoprotein (gp71) of Friend leukemia virus. II. Response in C57B1/6 mice. Virology 1976; 75:88–101

130. Ihle JN, Collins JJ, Lee JC, et al: Characterization of the immune response to the major glycoprotein (gp71) of Friend leukemia virus. III. Influence on endogenous MuLV-mediated pathogenesis. J Virol 1976; 102–112

131. Lee JC, Ihle JN, Huebner R: The humoral immune response of NIH Swiss and SWR/J mice to vaccination with formalinized AKR or Gross leukemia virus. Proc Natl Acad Sci 1977; 74:343–347

132. Huebner RJ, Gilden RV, Lane WT, et al: Suppression of murine type-C RNA virogenes by type-specific oncornavirus vaccines: Prospects for prevention of cancer. Proc Natl Acad Sci 1976; 73:620–624

133. Thiel HJ, Schwarz H, Fischinger P, et al: Role of antibodies to murine leukemia virus p15E transmembrane protein in immunotherapy against AKR leukemia: A model for studies in human acquired immunodeficiency syndrome. Proc Natl Acad Sci-USA 1987; 84:5893–5897

134. Oroszlan S, Nowinski RC: Lysis of retroviruses with monoclonal antibodies against viral envelope proteins. Virology 1980; 101:296–299

135. Flyer DC, Burakoff SJ, Faller DV: The immune response to Moloney murine leukemia virus-induced tumors: Induction of cytolytic T lymphocytes specific for both viral and tumor-associated antigens. Nature 1983; 305:815–817

136. Abastado JP, Plata F, Morello D, et al: H-2-restricted cytolysis of L cells doubly transformed with a cloned H-2Kb gene and cloned retroviral DNA. J Immunol 1985; 135:3512–3519

137. Holt CA, Osorio K, Lilly F: Friend virus-specific cytotoxic T lymphocytes recognize both gag and env gene-encoded specificities. J Exp Med 1986; 211–226

138. Plata F, Langlade-Demoyen P, Abastado JP, et al: Molecular definition of retrovirus-induced antigens recognized by tumour-specific H-2-restricted cytolytic T lmyphocytes. J Immunogenet 1986; 13:263–268

139. Plata F, Langlade-Demoyen P, Abastado JP, et al: Retrovirus antigens recognized by cytolytic T lymphocytes activate tumor rejection in vivo. Cell 1987; 48:231–240

140. Earl PL, Moss B, Morrison RP, et al: T-lymphocyte priming and protection against Friend leukemia by vaccinia-retrovirus env gene recombinant. Science 1986; 234:728–731

13

The Acquired Immunodeficiency Syndrome (AIDS) and Neoplasia

Jay H. Beckstead

IMMUNODEFICIENCY SYNDROMES AND NEOPLASIA—GENERAL

Numerous studies have clearly established that an immunodeficiency state predisposes humans to the development of neoplasms.[1-6] Although it is clear that the primary immunodeficiencies are associated with an increased incidence of neoplasia, specific figures are difficult to establish and vary with the type of immunodeficiency. Figures reported in the literature range from 1% up to 15%. The primary immunodeficiency states most clearly associated with an increased incidence of malignancy are ataxia-telangiectasia, Wiskott-Aldrich syndrome, common variable immunodeficiency, and severe combined immunodeficiency. The neoplasms most increased in these patients are primarily non-Hodgkin's lymphomas. The incidence of leukemias, Hodgkin's disease, and some cancers may also be increased in these disorders, but the evidence in the available literature is less definitive and more controversial.

Other naturally occurring immunodeficiency states that predispose to the development of neoplasms are the chronic autoimmune disorders. Since many of these conditions are treated with a variety of immunosuppressive regimens, the contribution of therapy versus that of natural history may be difficult to establish. Despite this, it appears that these disorders are associated with an increased incidence of neoplasia, primarily non-Hodgkin's lymphomas, independent of therapy. On the other hand, the increase in acute nonlymphoid leukemias seems primarily a result of therapy with radiation and radiomimetic drugs. An increase in other neoplasms is much more difficult to establish.

Modern medicine can also produce significant secondary immunodeficiency states independently. This is most clearly documented in studies of patients purposely immunosuppressed for organ transplantation. The tumors that develop in these patients are primarily high-grade non-Hodgkin's lymphomas, which frequently present extranodally, especially in the central nervous system. These patients also show a distinct increase in the incidence of Kaposi's sarcoma. Increases in the incidence of other tumors have been less clear. Some studies have reported an increase in the incidence of squamous cell carcinoma in the skin and oral tissues, gastric carcinoma, and uterine cervical carcinoma in situ (CIS). The incidence of Hodgkin's disease is not felt to be increased. Cancer chemotherapy itself is also somewhat immunosuppressive, but most authors have not identified a significant increase in neoplasia with the exception of that seen with radiation and radiomimetic drugs. The increase in acute nonlymphoid leukemias associated with these agents appears to be largely independent of immunosuppressive effects.

AIDS-ASSOCIATED NEOPLASIA — GENERAL

The acquired immunodeficiency syndrome (AIDS) was originally identified in a large part due to an unusual incidence of Kaposi's sarcoma in young homosexual males.[7] Thus, from its earliest descriptions, an increased incidence of neoplasia has been associated with AIDS. Shortly after the initial descriptions of AIDS, Ziegler et al.,[8] in San Francisco, noted a remarkable increase in the incidence of high-grade non-Hodgkin's lymphomas in patients with AIDS as well as those with the AIDS-Related Complex (ARC). Subsequent studies clearly established an increased incidence of these neoplasms in patients infected with the Human Immunodeficiency Virus (HIV).

An increased incidence of other neoplasms has also been suggested, but has been difficult to establish. Virus-associated hyperplasias/neoplasias are increased in this population, and a unique lesion, "hairy leukoplakia," which is apparently associated with AIDS exclusively, has been described. An increase in squamous cell carcinomas in the anal/genital and oral tissues has also been suggested, but this remains somewhat controversial. Also controversial is the incidence of Hodgkin's disease in this population. It has also been suggested that these patients might be at risk for developing hepatocellular carcinoma because of the high incidence of hepatitis B-virus infection.[6,9] Scattered reports of other unusual tumors raise the possibility that the list of AIDS-associated neoplasia cannot yet be closed.

AIDS-ASSOCIATED NON-HODGKIN'S LYMPHOMAS

The first report of a high-grade malignant lymphoma in a probable AIDS/ARC patient was a single case from Arizona in May, 1982.[10] One month later, workers in San Francisco briefly reported four similar cases in the MMWR.[8] These same four patients, all with undifferentiated Burkitt's-like lymphomas, were subsequently described in detail.[11] All of them presented with extranodal disease, including one in the central nervous system (CNS), and had aggressive clinical courses. Parallels were drawn to malignant lymphomas described in other immunodeficiency states.

These initial reports were followed by a number of additional contributions that generally confirmed the clinicopathologic pattern, but broadened the spectrum to include large cell and immunoblastic lymphomas and possibly other hematopoietic malignancies.[12-17] In 1983, workers in Japan reported a Burkitt's lymphoma in an AIDS patient with hemophilia,[18] expanding the risk groups involved. Ziegler and colleagues clarified the increased risk of lymphoma suggested by these reports in a case-controlled study of single men living in the San Francisco Bay Area.[19] Using cancer registry data, they found a highly significant ($p < 0.001$ by Chi-square) increase in the incidence of undifferentiated non-Hodgkin's lymphomas in single men aged 20 – 25 in the four-year period 1979 – 1982 when compared to the previous four-year period 1974 – 1978. Examination of the data for this group of the five-year period 1979 – 1983 showed 18 patients with lymphoma (with an expected incidence of two patients for this group over that time period). All but one of the identified patients were homosexuals with ARC. In this larger group, 11 of the patients had Burkitt's-like lymphoma, 4 had immunoblastic lymphoma, 2 had large cell lymphoma, and 1 had diffuse mixed lymphoma. Response to therapy was also examined in the 11 patients with Burkitt's-like tumors and results were compared to a National Cancer Institute control group with similar tumor histologies. At one year, there was a striking difference in survival (13% vs. 48%), suggesting that the anecdotal expression of poor prognosis was very real.

In 1984, Ziegler and coworkers[20] reported on a study of 90 homosexual patients with non-Hodgkin's lymphomas, which combined data from Univ. of Calif., San Francisco (UCSF), Univ. of Southern Calif. (USC), Cornell, Univ. of Texas, Houston, New York University, and Memorial-Sloan Kettering. These data firmly established an increased incidence of non-Hodgkin's lymphomas with a preponderance of high-grade extranodal lymphomas and a uniformly poor prognosis. These authors strongly suggested that the occurrence of a high-grade extranodal non-Hodgkin's lymphoma in a patient with an AIDS risk group should be considered evidence of AIDS. Subsequent studies[21-37] have generally confirmed the overall findings of this large study.

Overlapping reports from many institutions and morphologic imprecision make estimates of relative percentages of histologic lymphoma types somewhat imprecise. Despite this, it is clear that small noncleaved cell lymphomas (Fig. 1), immunoblastic lymphomas, and diffuse large cell lymphomas account for the overwhelming majority of the lymphomas seen in these patients. Some observers have suggested that the low grade lymphomas may not be related to AIDS/ARC.[26] Lymphomas in these patients may be difficult to classify precisely and a number of reports list "unclassified" malignant lymphoma as a diagnostic group.

The morphologic appearance of the majority of these lymphomas is compatible with a B-cell origin but confirmatory immunologic data have been rather limited. Three of the four patients in Ziegler's first study[11]

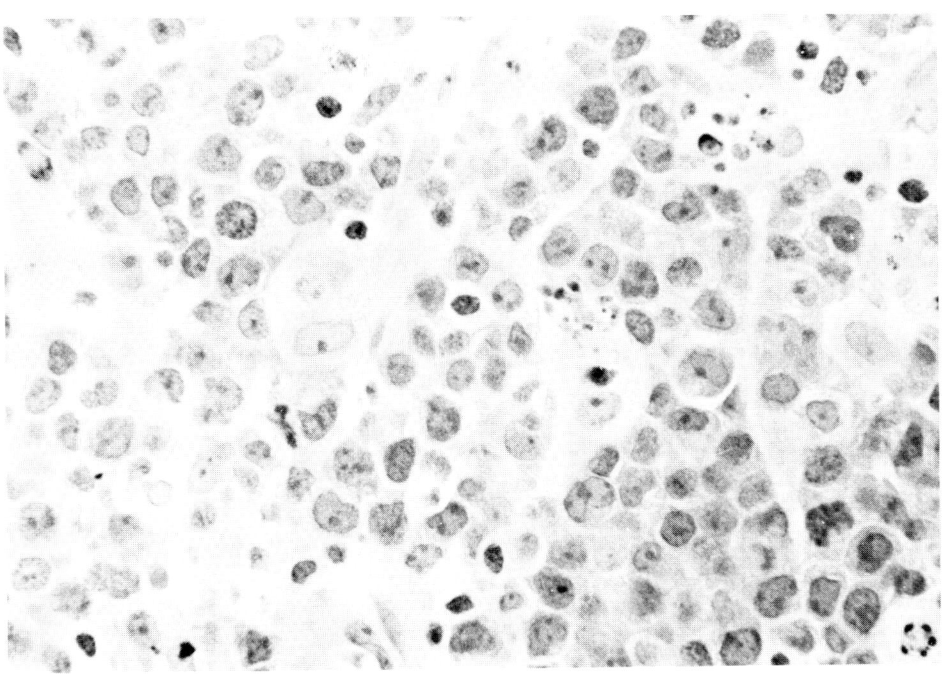

Figure 1. A typical extranodal, small, noncleaved cell lymphoma in a patient with AIDS. The nuclei have open chromatin and are approximately the same size as those of the intermixed macrophages. (Plastic section, H&E, original magnification ×640.)

showed monoclonal IgM-κ staining. Ciobanu et al.[12] demonstrated Tdt positivity in their case of probable acute lymphocytic leukemia (ALL). Two cases of Burkitt's-like lymphoma described by Chaganti et al.[13] demonstrated light chain restriction, as did a plasmacytoma described by Israel et al.[15] Levine et al.[21] demonstrated light chain restriction in five out of six lymphomas.

The large combined institution study of Ziegler et al.,[20] which included all of the above cases and some of the following cases, noted monoclonal surface immunoglobulin in 32 cases plus two cases positive for another B-cell marker, but the results were not presented in detail. Petersen et al.[22] thoroughly phenotyped a single case of Burkitt's-like lymphoma and found it to be of B-cell origin. Gill et al.,[24] in a study of CNS lymphomas, found light chain restriction in three out of six lymphomas, and LN-1 (a B-cell marker) in another. Kalter et al.,[25] using frozen sections, found B-cell markers (details not given) in four cases. In a large study (27 cases) from USC,[26] 19 cases were found with light chain restriction, plus one case that was positive for IgG and two positive for LN-1.

Ioachim et al.[27] studied eight cases using frozen sections and found four with light chain restriction and four without T or B cell markers (Ig, OKT3, OKT4, OKT8, OKT11). Groopman et al.[28] studied a single case using frozen sections and DNA analysis and found light chain restriction and a corresponding gene rearrangement. So et al.[31] used a wide range of markers (αNAE, ATP, I$_2$, PanB, Leu12, Leu14, Leu4, Leu9, LeuM1, IgM) on plastic sections to study five cases of CNS lymphoma. All five cases showed a phenotype consistent with a B-cell origin. DiCarlo et al.[32] studied eight cases using frozen sections and found seven positive for Leu-14 (B-cell marker); three of the seven also showed light chain restriction. Gaurner et al.[33] studied two cases and found probable light chain restriction in one; other markers in both cases were negative.

At the recent meeting of the United States–Canadian Division of the International Academy of Pathology, Knowles et al.[35] reported immunophenotype studies on 16 lymphomas, all with B-cell markers, and confirmed this with molecular genetic data on 10.[36] We have examined a series of 31 lymphomas from AIDS/ARC patients using a spectrum of markers[37] and found that all 31 had one or more markers of B-cell origin (Fig. 2). No cases expressed T-cell markers (Fig. 3) or mononuclear phagocyte origin. The data can be briefly summarized as follows: αNAE, 0/31; ATP 8/31; Ia, 25/31; PanB, 24/31; Leu-12, 20/31; Leu-14, 11/31; IgM, 25/31; Leu 4, 0/31; Leu-M1, 0/31. This author believes there is overwhelming evidence that the vast majority of these tumors are monoclonal B-cell proliferations.

T-cell tumors are extremely rare in AIDS/ARC patients and of uncertain significance. Ziegler's study listed two "lymphoblastic" lymphomas, but one of these was the case of probably early ALL. The presence of Tdt positivity in such a lesion is not evidence of a T-cell origin since Tdt positivity is a common finding in virtually all ALLs, the majority of which are now known to be of early B-cell lineage. The other listed case had no marker data. Abrams et al.[34] noted a single case of mycosis fungoides in one of their patients, but a relationship to AIDS/ARC was not proven. Knowles et al.[35] reported two cases of chronic lymphocytic leukemia (CLL) with a suppressor phenotype and clonal T-cell gene rearrangements. Kaplan[17] reported a similar case. The relationship between these case reports and patients with T8 lymphocytosis and visceral lymphocytic infiltration[38] is uncertain.

The etiology of the lymphomas in AIDS is still unclear, but most workers have suggested that a diffuse polyclonal expansion of EBV-infected/transformed B cells may be the starting point for these tumors. It has been suggested that the immunodeficient status of these patients leaves them unable to control such proliferations and that continued proliferation allows the emergence of a malignant clone. A similar hypothesis has been raised in other immunodeficiency

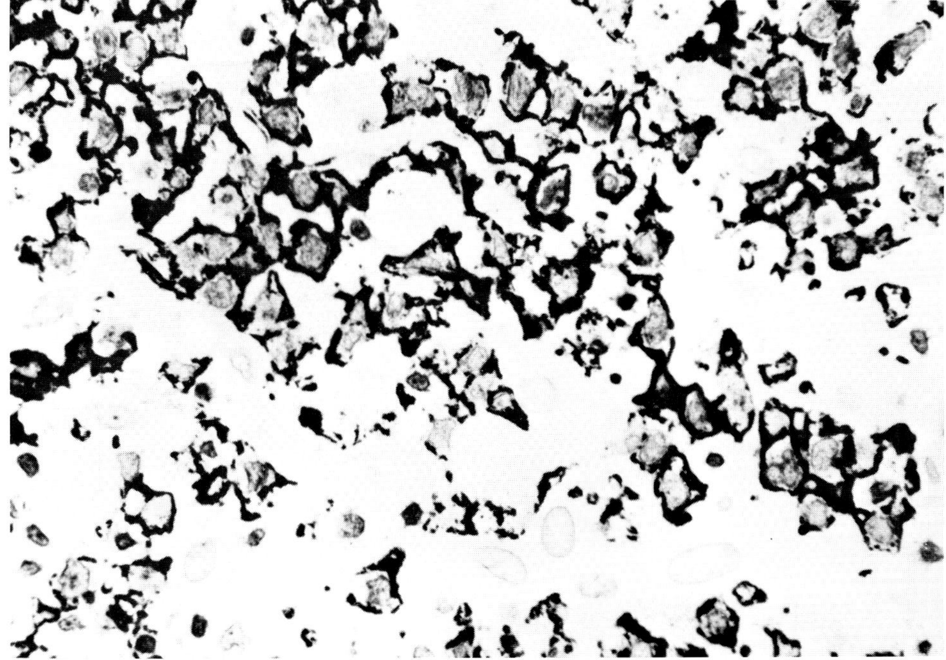

Figure 2. AIDS-associated malignant lymphoma stained for a B-lymphocyte antigen using an immunoperoxidase technique. Black reaction product is present on the plasma membranes of the neoplastic cells. (Plastic section, Pan B (Dako), original magnification ×640.)

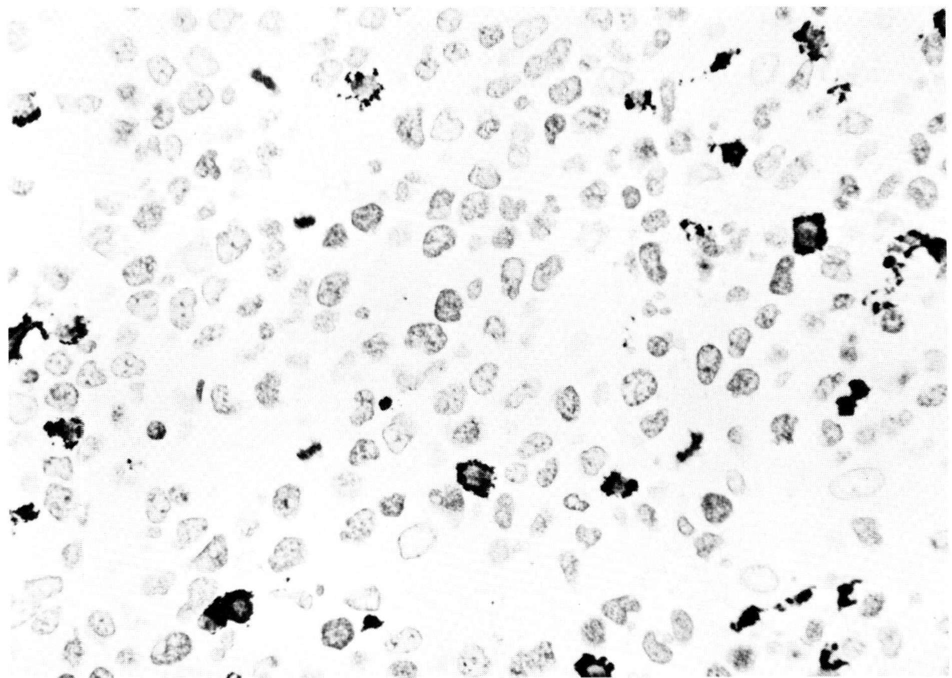

Figure 3. Same case as Figure 2 stained for a T-lymphocyte antigen. Only scattered small lymphocytes infiltrating the tumor show black reaction product. (Plastic section, Leu 4 (B-D), original magnification ×640.)

states and at least some of the morphologically and clinically malignant proliferations in those patients appeared to be polyclonal.[5] As noted above, most of the lymphomas in AIDS/ARC have shown a more uniform morphologic phenotype and monoclonality, suggesting that the parallels are not exact. Recently, however, five patients with polymorphous proliferations similar to those described in transplant patients have been reported.[39,40]

AIDS-ASSOCIATED KAPOSI'S SARCOMA

Kaposi's sarcoma (KS) in this country was, until recently, a rare indolent skin lesion presenting primarily in the lower extremities of elderly men. A much more aggressive, lymphadenopathic form of the disease was described in sub-Saharan Africa. In addition, an increased incidence of relatively indolent KS had been well described in the iatrogenic immunosuppression of organ transplantation. This picture changed dramatically in the United States beginning in 1979. A marked increase in aggressive KS in young homosexual men was noted by groups in New York and California.[7,41-43] It is now clear that this represented one of the first manifestations of AIDS. Epidemiologic studies have shown that KS is strongly associated with the homosexual lifestyle and is seen much less frequently in other groups with AIDS. Interestingly, recent data in California show a distinct decrease in the incidence of KS in the homosexual population, probably part of a general decline in the incidence of venereal disease in this population.* These data strongly suggest a sexually transmitted cofactor. Cytomegalovirus (CMV) has been frequently suggested,[44] but definitive evidence for an etiologic role is still lacking.

Pathologically, most authors have found little or no difference between the KS lesions occurring in association with AIDS and

those previously described. The histologic diagnosis of KS and differential diagnostic problems have been described in the skin,[45] oral mucosa,[46] and lymph nodes.[47] We have found that the presence of atypical, angulated, vascular channels is the most helpful feature in the recognition of the earliest lesions (Fig. 4). In more advanced cases these may be absent or present only at the periphery of the lesion, apparently crowded out by the proliferating spindle cells. In advanced lesions, the presence of eosinophilic bodies can be extremely helpful. Although their origin is unknown, they are almost uniformly present in KS. They can be stained with PTAH, PAS, or Mallory's trichrome.

Although numerous papers have been published on the subject, the histogenesis of KS remains controversial. Modern observers have been convinced that the lesion is of endothelial origin, but the question of vascular versus lymphatic origin remains a subject of debate. Data from our laboratory and from others[48,49] have strongly suggested that the lesion is of lymphatic endothelial origin, but other laboratories remain convinced that the lesion is of blood vascular origin.[50]

The other interesting question regarding KS is whether or not the lesion is truly neoplastic. Although historically most observers have considered it a neoplasm, a number of observers have suggested that the lesion is non-neoplastic.[51] Certainly, its behavior is unusual. Spontaneous regressions are frequently observed, multifocality is common (clearly metastatic lesions are difficult to prove), and the symmetry of lesions in some patients is exceedingly unusual for a neoplastic process. Unfortunately, definitive data to resolve this interesting question remain unavailable.

AIDS-ASSOCIATED HODGKIN'S DISEASE: INCREASED INCIDENCE?

As noted above, an increase in the incidence of Hodgkin's disease has not been

---

*D. Abrams, personal communication

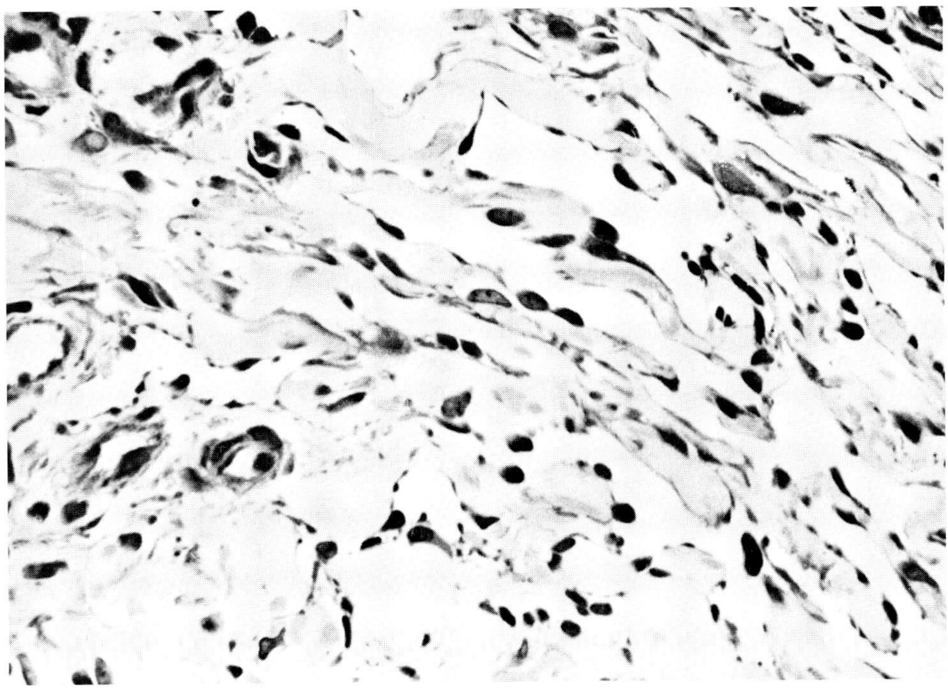

Figure 4. Early lesion of Kaposi's sarcoma in the skin of a man with AIDS. The irregular vascular channels dissect through bundles of collagen. (Plastic section, H&E, original magnification ×640.)

generally accepted as a consequence of either primary or secondary immunodeficiency. It has been suggested by some authors, however, that there may be an increase in the incidence of Hodgkin's disease in AIDS.[52-60] In addition to these reports, several authors reporting on lymphomas in AIDS have included cases of Hodgkin's disease.[27,32,34] It is clear from these reports and from our own experience at UCSF that Hodgkin's disease must be considered in the evaluation of patients with AIDS/ARC and that those AIDS/ARC patients with Hodgkin's disease frequently have atypical presentations, unusually aggressive courses, and an extremely poor prognosis. These observations, however, fail to answer the question of an increased incidence of Hodgkin's disease in ARC and AIDS. Incidence figures for Hodgkin's disease have recently been carefully examined by the group at UCSF[61] and no evidence for an increase in incidence has been shown.

ORAL LESIONS

Unusual oral infections, especially oral candidiasis, were some of the first well described problems in AIDS patients. Subsequent studies have also revealed that oral and adjacent tissues are frequent sites for a variety of neoplastic and other unusual growths that have increasingly been seen in AIDS and ARC patients.[62] Although not widely noted in the literature, oral warts have been seen with increased frequency in this patient population at UCSF. Besides these relatively common papillomavirus-associated lesions, Greenspan et al.[63] described an extremely unusual lesion, hairy leukoplakia, that may be exclusively associated with AIDS.[64]

Hairy leukoplakia presents clinically as a painless, slightly raised, irregular, white patch with a corrugated or "hairy" surface. Microscopically, this lesion shows hyperkeratosis with surface projections, parakeratosis, acanthosis, and koilocytic changes (Fig. 5A & B). Atypia, if present, is minimal and inflammation is generally absent. A variety of techniques have been utilized to show that the lesion is uniquely associated with human papillomavirus (HPV) and the Epstein-Barr virus (EBV).[63,65] Evidence for infection of neoplastic epithelium with EBV is generally accepted in nasopharyngeal carcinoma, some carcinomas of the tonsil and supraglottic larynx, and in thymic carcinoma; however, these infections are non-

productive and viral particles are not generally demonstrated. In contrast, large numbers of complete viral particles, as well as large amounts of EBV-DNA can be demonstrated within the cells of the hairy leukoplakia lesions, strongly suggesting that the virus is actively replicating in these same cells. Additional studies have shown that the same lesion can occur in nonhomosexual HIV-positive patients[66] and that the lesions appear to be restricted to oral epithelium.[67]

An association of oral squamous cell car-

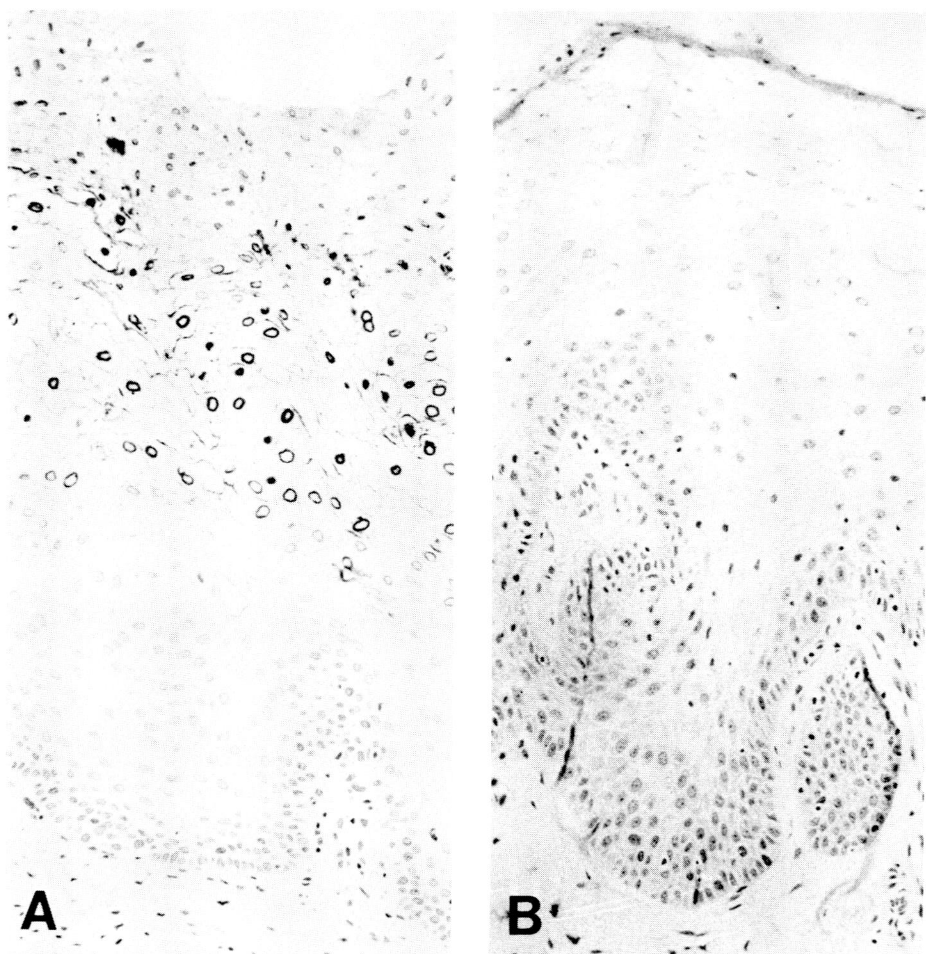

Figure 5. Oral hairy leukoplakia lesion in a patient with AIDS. (A) shows the lesion stained for Epstein-Barr virus using an immunoperoxidase technique. The nuclei of the cells in the mid and upper portion of the epithelium show strong ring-like nuclear staining. (B) is a negative control section. (Plastic section, EBV-VCA (NEN), original magnification ×160.)

cinoma with AIDS remains highly speculative and controversial. In 1981 and 1982, the workers at UCSF described several cases;[62,68] subsequently, the same group collected additional, anecdotal cases. Unfortunately, these patients have not been well characterized. There are several reasons for expecting a possible increase in oral epithelial malignancies despite the current limited clinical evidence. First, as noted above, the incidence of oral papillomavirus infection is high and there is strong evidence of an association with malignancy in the cervix and other sites.[69] Second, the association of EBV with nasopharyngeal and other oral region carcinomas is clear.[65] Finally, at least some studies of immunosuppressed transplant patients show an increased incidence of oral carcinomas.[3]

Before leaving the subject of oral neoplasms in AIDS, it should be mentioned that the oral cavity is a frequent site of presentation and involvement of Kaposi's sarcoma.[46] A number of patients have presented with high grade lymphomas in oral and nasopharyngeal tissues, as well as in the salivary glands.

ANAL/GENITAL EPITHELIAL LESIONS

It has been known for some time that venereal transmission of HPV is a frequent problem in male homosexuals and that the lesions frequently involve not only the penile mucous membrane, but also the perineum, perianal area, and anorectal junction. The spectrum of lesions includes small papules and flat warts as well as condylomata acuminata. Recent studies have clearly shown a role for HPV in the development of intraepithelial neoplasia in the genital tract. Some studies have suggested a synergistic role for herpes simplex virus infection, another common sexually transmitted disease in the homosexual population. Furthermore, an increase in the incidence of HPV infection and cervical intraepithelial neo-

plasia has been shown in immunosuppressed patients.[69] These observations suggest that an increase in the incidence of epithelial neoplasia of the anal/genital region could be expected in the homosexual population with AIDS/ARC.

The first report to draw attention to epithelial malignancies in the anal/genital tract was a paper from Philadelphia describing four cases of cloacogenic carcinoma in homosexual men.[70] These observations predated the recognition of AIDS. In the past decade, two separate epidemiological studies in Washington[71] and California[72] have shown an association between anal intercourse and anal carcinoma. These findings suggest an increase in the incidence of these malignancies dependent on lifestyle but independent of AIDS/ARC; however, data from studies of other immunodeficiency states suggest that this increased incidence may be further augmented by the immunodeficiency associated with HIV infection. Scattered reports of carcinoma in this patient population can be found in the literature.[73,74]

More recently, three studies have identified a surprisingly high incidence of intraepithelial neoplasia in the anal mucosa in homosexual males.[75-77] These reports suggest the possibility that the real increase in the incidence of anal/genital carcinomas associated with AIDS/ARC is yet to come.

OTHER NEOPLASMS

There is little evidence of an increased incidence in neoplasms other than those noted above. However, the few scattered case reports in the literature of other neoplasms will be briefly reviewed here. There have been three case reports of embryonal carcinoma of the testes. Two of the patients had clinical and laboratory findings consistent with ARC prior to the discovery of the testicular tumors.[78] The third patient developed AIDS shortly after diagnosis and chemotherapy for his testicular tumor.[79] A

Jay H. Beckstead

possible relationship with AIDS was suggested by Logothetis et al.,[78] but this remains speculative. A single patient with a seminoma has been reported.[17] Cheeseman and Gang[80] reported a rhabdomyosarcoma of the gallbladder in a child with AIDS. Chandrasoma et al.[81] reported a malignant peripheral nerve sheath tumor arising in the adrenal gland in a patient with ARC. Both of these are unusual neoplasms, but their relationship, if any, to AIDS is unclear. Other, more common neoplasms have been reported in patients with AIDS,[17,82-87] but these probably are coincidental in nature. Although it is not a neoplasm, peliosis hepatis has been reported to be a frequent finding in AIDS[88] and should be considered as a differential diagnosis in mass lesions of the liver in these patients.

Despite the suggestion that myelodysplasia is a frequent finding in AIDS,[89] there have been almost no reports of acute non-lymphoid leukemias in these patients. Napoli et al.[90] have reported a single case that evolved out of a myelodysplastic process. Our own experience has been that the dysplastic features are minimal and not likely to progress to leukemia. We have not identified any definitive lymphoid leukemias, although an occasional patient with high grade lymphoma and bone marrow involvement has also had small numbers of circulating lymphoma cells.

REFERENCES

1. Rosenblatt HM, Shearer WT: Immunodeficiency and cancer. In: Finegold ed, Pathology of Neoplasia in Children and Adolescents. Philadelphia, W.B. Saunders, 1986, pp 31-45
2. Filipovich AH, Spector BD, Kersey J: Immunodeficiency in humans as a risk factor in the development of malignancy. Prev Med 1980; 9:252-259
3. Penn I: Depressed immunity and the development of cancer. Clin Exp Immunol 1981; 46:459-474
4. Gatti RA, Good RA: Occurrence of malignancy in immunodeficiency diseases. A literature review. Cancer 1971; 28:89-98
5. Frizzera G, Rosai J, Dehner LP, et al: Lymphoreticular disorders in primary immunodeficiencies: New findings based on an up-to-date histologic classification of 35 cases. Cancer 1980; 46:692-699
6. Puntilo DT, Manolov G, Manolov Y, et al: Squamous carcinoma, Kaposi's sarcoma, and Burkitt's lymphoma are consequences of impaired immune surveillance of ubiquitous viruses in acquired immunodeficiency syndrome, allograft recipients, and tropical African patients. IARC Sci Publ 1984; 63:749-770
7. Friedman-Kien AE: Disseminated Kaposi's sarcoma syndrome in young homosexual men. J Am Acad Dermatol 1981; 5:468-471
8. Ziegler JL, Wagner G, Greenspan JS, et al: Diffuse, undifferentiated non-Hodgkin's lymphoma among homosexual males—United States. MMWR 1982; 31:277-279
9. Sonnabend J, Witkin SS, Purtilo DR: Acquired immunodeficiency syndrome, opportunistic infections, and malignancies in male homosexuals. A hypothesis of etiologic factors in pathogenesis. JAMA 1983; 249:2370-2374
10. Doll DC, List AF: Burkitt's lymphoma in a homosexual (Letter). Lancet 1982; 1:1026-1027
11. Ziegler JL, Drew WL, Miner RC, et al: Outbreak of Burkitt's-like lymphoma in homosexual men. Lancet 1982; 2:631-633
12. Ciobanu N, Andreeff M, Safai B, et al: Lymphoblastic neoplasia in a homosexual patient with Kaposi's sarcoma. Ann Intern Med 98:151-155
13. Chaganti RSK, Suresh SC, Koziner B, et al: Specific translocations characterize Burkitt's-like lymphoma of homosexual men with the acquired immunodeficiency syndrome. Blood 1983; 61:1269-1272
14. Snider WD, Simpson DM, Aronyk KE, et al: Primary lymphoma of the central nervous system associated with the acquired immunodeficiency syndrome (Letter). N Engl J Med 1983; 308:45
15. Israel AM, Koziner B, Straus J: Plasmacytoma and the acquired immunodeficiency syndrome. Ann Intern Med 1983; 99:635-636
16. Case Records of the Massachusetts General Hospital. No 32-1983. N Engl J Med 1983; 309:359-369
17. Kaplan MH, Susin M, Pahwa SG, et al: Neoplastic complications of HTLV-III infection. Lymphomas and solid tumors. Am J Med 1987; 82:389-396
18. Shibuya A, Saitoh K, Tsuneyoshi H, et al: Burkitt's lymphoma in a haemophiliac. (Letter) Lancet 1983; 2:1432
19. Ziegler JL, Bragg K, Abrams D, et al: High-grade non-Hodgkin's lymphoma in patients with AIDS. Ann NY Acad Sci 1985; 437:412-419
20. Ziegler JL, Beckstead JH, Volberding PA, et al: Non-Hodgkin's lymphoma in 90 homosexual men. N Engl J Med 1984; 311:565-570
21. Levine AM, Meyer PR, Begandy MK, et al: Development of B-cell lymphoma in homosexual men. Ann Intern Med 1984; 100:7-13
22. Petersen JM, Tubbs, RR, Savage RA, et al: Small noncleaved B cell Burkitt-like lymphoma with chromosome +(8; 14) translocation and Epstein-Barr virus nuclear-associated antigen in a homosexual man with acquired immunodeficiency syndrome. Am J Med 1985; 78:141-148
23. Steinberg JJ, Bridges N, Feiner HD, et al: Small intestinal lymphoma in three patients with acquired immune deficiency syndrome. Am J Gastroenterol 1985; 80:21-26

24. Gill PS, Levine AM, Meyer PR, et al: Primary central nervous system lymphoma in homosexual men. Clinical, immunologic, and pathologic features. Am J Med 1985; 78:742–748

25. Kalter SP, Riggs SA, Cabanillas F, et al: Aggressive non-Hodgkin's lymphomas in immunocompromised homosexual males. Blood 1985; 66:655–659

26. Levine AM, Gill PS, Meyer PR, et al: Retrovirus and malignant lymphoma in homosexual men. JAMA 1985; 254:1921–1925

27. Ioachim HL, Cooper MC, Hellman GC: Lymphomas in men at high risk for the acquired immunodeficiency syndrome. Cancer 1985; 56:2831–2842

28. Groopman JE, Sullivan JL, Mulder C, et al: Pathogenesis of B cell lymphoma in a patient with AIDS. Blood 1986; 67:612–615

29. Caccamo D, Pervez NF, Marchevsky A: Primary lymphoma of the liver in the acquired immunodeficiency syndrome. Arch Pathol Lab Med 1986; 100:553–555

30. Balasubramanyam A, Waxman M, Kazal HL, et al: Malignant lymphoma of the heart in acquired immunodeficiency syndrome. Chest 1986; 90:243–246

31. So YT, Beckstead JH, Davis RL: Primary central nervous system lymphoma in acquired immune deficiency syndrome: A clinical and pathological study. Ann Neurol 1986; 20:566–572

32. DiCarlo EF, Amberson JB, Metroka CE, et al: Malignant lymphomas and the acquired immunodeficiency syndrome. Evaluation of 30 cases using a working formulation. Arch Pathol Lab Med 1986; 110:1012–1016

33. Guarner J, Brynes RK, Chan WC, et al: Primary non-Hodgkin's lymphoma of the heart in two patients with the acquired immunodeficiency syndrome. Arch Pathol Lab Med 1987; 111:254–256

34. Abrams DI, Kaplan LD, McGrath MS, et al: AIDS-related benign lymphadenopathy and malignant lymphoma: Clinical aspects and virologic interactions. AIDS Res 1986; 2(Suppl 1):5131–5138

35. Knowles DM, Pelicci PG, Subar M, et al: Immunophenotypic and molecular genetic analysis of AIDS-associated lymphoid proliferations. (Abstract) Invest 1987; 56:129a

36. Pelicci P-G, Knowles DM, Arlin ZA, et al: Multiple monoclonal B cell expansions and c-*myc* oncogene rearrangements in acquired immune deficiency syndrome-related lymphoproliferative disorders. J Exp Med 1986; 164:2049–2076

37. Egerter DA, Beckstead JH: Malignant lymphomas in the acquired immunodeficiency syndrome: Additional evidence for a B-cell origin. Arch Pathol Lab Med 1988; 112:602–606

38. Guillon JM, Fouret P, Mayand C, et al: Extensive T8-positive lymphocytic visceral infiltration in a homosexual man. Am J Med 1987; 82:655–661

39. Beissner RS, Rappaport ES, Diaz JA: Fatal case of Epstein-Barr virus-induced lymphoproliferative disorder associated with a human immunodeficiency virus infection. Arch Pathol Lab Med 1987; 111:250–253

40. Joshi VV, Kauffman S, Oleske JM, et al: Polyclonal polymorphic B-cell lymphoproliferative disorder with prominent pulmonary involvement in children with acquired immunodeficiency syndrome. Cancer 1987; 59:1455–1462

41. Hymes KB, Cheung T, Green JB, et al: Kaposi's sarcoma in homosexual men—A report of eight cases. Lancet 1981; 2:598–600

42. Gottlieb GJ, Rywlin AM, Ragaz A, et al: A preliminary communication on extensively disseminated Kaposi's sarcoma in young homosexual men. Am J Dermatopathol 1981; 3:111–114

43. Friedman-Kien AE, Laubenstein LJ, Rubinstein P, et al: Disseminated Kaposi's sarcoma in homosexual men. Ann Intern Med 1982; 96:693–700

44. Drew WL, Miner RC, Ziegler JL: Cytomegalovirus and Kaposi's sarcoma in young homosexual men. Lancet 1982; 2:125–127

45. Blumenfeld W, Egbert BM, Sagebiel RW: Differential diagnosis of Kaposi's sarcoma. Arch Pathol Lab Med 1985; 109:123–127

46. Green TL, Beckstead JH, Lozada-Nur F, et al: Histopathologic spectrum of oral Kaposi's sarcoma. Oral Surg, Oral Med, Oral Pathol 1984; 58:306–314

47. Finkbeiner WE, Egbert BM, Groundwater JR, et al: Kaposi's sarcoma in young homosexual men. A histopathologic study with particular reference to lymph node involvement. Arch Pathol Lab Med 1982; 106:261–264

48. Beckstead JH, Wood GS, Fletcher V: Evidence for the origin of Kaposi's sarcoma from lymphatic endothelium. Am J Pathol 1985; 119:294–300

49. Jones R, Spaull J, Spry C, et al: Histogenesis of Kaposi's sarcoma in patients with and without acquired immunodeficiency syndrome (AIDS). J Clin Pathol 1986; 39:742–749

50. Rutgers J, Wieczorek R, Bonetti F, et al: The expression of endothelial antigens by AIDS-associated Kaposi's sarcoma. Evidence for a vascular endothelial cell origin. Am J Pathol 1986; 122:493–499

51. Brooks JJ: Kaposi's sarcoma: A reversible hyperplasia. Lancet 1986; 2:1309–1311

52. Schoeppel SL, Hoppe RT, Dorfman RF, et al: Hodgkin's disease in homosexual men with generalized lymphadenopathy. Ann Intern Med 1985; 102:68–70

53. Scheib RG, Siegel RS: Atypical Hodgkin's disease and the acquired immunodeficiency syndrome. (Letter) Ann Intern Med 1985; 102:554

54. Unger PD, Strauchen JA: Hodgkin's disease in AIDS complex patients. Report of four cases and tissue immunologic marker studies. Cancer 1986; 58:821–825

55. Robert NJ, Schneidermann H: Hodgkin's disease and the acquired immunodeficiency syndrome. (Letter) Ann Intern Med 1984; 101:142–143

56. Temple JJ, Andes WA: AIDS and Hodgkin's disease. (Letter) Lancet 1986; 2:454–455

57. Cid JAL-H, Cid JL-H, Sanndo EF, et al: AIDS and Hodgkin's disease. (Letter) Lancet 1986; 2:1104–1105

58. Baer DM, Anderson ET, Wilkinson LS: Acquired immune deficiency syndrome in homosexual men with Hodgkin's disease. Am J Med 1986; 80:738–740

59. Mitsuyasu RT, Coleman MF, Sun NCJ: Simulta-

neous occurrence of Hodgkin's disease and Kaposi's sarcoma in a patient with the acquired immune deficiency syndrome. Am J Med 1986; 80:954–958

60. Prior E, Goldberg AF, Conjalka MS, et al: Hodgkin's disease in homosexual men. An AIDS-related phenomenon? Am J Med 1986; 81:1085–1088

61. Kaplan LD, Volberding PA, Abrams DI: Clinical course and epidemiology of Hodgkin's disease in homosexual men in San Francisco (submitted).

62. Lozada F, Silverman S, Conent M: New outbreak of oral tumors, malignancies and infectious disease strikes young male homosexuals. CDA Journal 1982; 19:39–42

63. Greenspan D, Greenspan JS, Conant M, et al: Oral "hairy" leukoplakia in male homosexuals: Evidence of association with both papillomavirus and a herpes-group virus. Lancet 1984; 2:831–834

64. Greenspan D, Greenspan JH, Herst NG, et al: Relation of oral hairy leukoplakia to infection with the human immunodeficiency virus and the risk of developing AIDS. J Infect Dis 1987; 155:475–481

65. Greenspan JS, Greenspan D, Lennette ET, et al: Replication of Epstein-Barr virus within the epithelial cells of oral "hairy" leukoplakia, an AIDS-associated lesion. New Engl J Med 1985; 313:1564–1571

66. Greenspan D, Hollander H, Friedman-Klein A, et al: Oral hairy leucoplakia in two women, a hemophiliac, and a transfusion recipient. (Letter) Lancet 2:978

67. Hollander J, Greenspan D, Stringari S, et al: Hairy leukoplakia and the acquired immunodeficiency syndrome. (Letter) Ann Intern Med 1986; 104:892

68. Conant MA, Volberding P, Fletcher V, et al: Squamous cell carcinoma in sexual partners of Kaposi's sarcoma patients. (Letter) Lancet 1982; 1:286

69. Winkler B, Richart RM: Human papillomavirus and gynecologic neoplasia. Curr Prob Obstet Gynecol & Fertil 1987; 10:49–90

70. Cooper HS, Patchefsky AS, Marks G: Cloacogenic carcinoma of the anorectum in homosexual men: An observation of four cases. Dis Col Rectum 1979; 22:557–558

71. Darling JR, Weiss NS, Klopfenstein LL, et al: Correlates of homosexual behavior and the incidence of anal cancer. JAMA 1982; 247:1988–1990

72. Peters RK, Mack TM: Patterns of anal carcinoma by gender and marital status in Los Angeles County. Br J Cancer 1983; 48:629–636

73. Li FP, Osborn D, Cronin CM: Anorectal squamous carcinoma in two homosexual men. Lancet 1982; 2:391

74. Wexner SD, Smithy WB, Milsom JW, et al: The surgical management of anorectal diseases in AIDS and pre-AIDS patients. Dis Colon Rectum 1986; 29:719–723

75. Croxson T, Chabon AB, Rorat E, Barash IM: In-

traepithelial carcinoma of the anus in homosexual men. Dis Colon Rectum 1984; 27:325–330

76. Nash G, Allen W, Nash S: Atypical lesions of the anal mucosa in homosexual men. JAMA 1986; 256:873–876

77. Frazer IH, Medley G, Crapper RM, et al: Association between anorectal dysplasia, human papillomavirus, and human immunodeficiency virus infection in homosexual men. Lancet 1986; 2:657–660

78. Logothetis CJ, Newell GR, Samuels ML: Testicular cancer in homosexual men with cellular immune deficiency. Report of 2 cases. J Urol 1985; 133:484–486

79. Fenoglio CM, Oster MW, Genfo PL, et al: Kaposi's sarcoma following chemotherapy for testicular cancer in a homosexual man: Demonstration of cytomegalovirus RNA in sarcoma cells. Hum Pathol 1982; 13:955–959

80. Cheeseman SH, Gang D: Acquired immunodeficiency syndrome and rhabdomyosarcoma of probable gallbladder origin with extensive metastases. N Engl J Med 1986; 314:629–640

81. Chandrasoma P, Shibata D, Radin R, et al: Malignant peripheral nerve sheath tumor arising in an adrenal ganglioneuroma in an adult male homosexual. Cancer 1986; 57:2022–2025

82. Slazinski L, Stall JR, Mathews CR: Basal cell carcinoma in a man with acquired immunodeficiency syndrome. (Letter) J Am Acad Derm 1984; 111:140–141

83. Moore GE, Cook DD: AIDS in association with malignant melanoma and Hodgkin's disease. (Letter) J Clin Oncol 1985; 3:1437

84. Alhashimi MM, Krasnow SH, Johnston-Early A, et al: Squamous cell carcinoma of the epiglottis in a homosexual man at risk for AIDS. (Letter) 1985; 253:2366

85. Nusbaum NJ: Metastatic small-cell carcinoma of the lung in a patient with AIDS. (Letter) N Engl J Med 1985; 312:1706

86. Weitberg AB, Mayer K, Miller ME, et al: Dysplastic carcinoid tumor and AIDS-related complex. (Letter) N Engl J Med 1986; 314:1455

87. Overly WL, Jakubek DJ: Multiple squamous cell carcinomas and human immunodeficiency virus infection. (Letter) Ann Intern Med 1987; 106:334

88. Czapar CH, Weldon-Linee CM, Moore DM, et al: Peliosis hepatitis in the acquired immunodeficiency syndrome. Arch Pathol Lab Med 1986; 110:611–613

89. Schneider DR, Picker JL: Myelodysplasia in the acquired immune deficiency syndrome. Am J Clin Pathol 1985; 84:144–152

90. Napoli VM, et al: Myelodysplasia progressing to AML in an HTLV-III virus-positive homosexual man with AIDS-related complex. Am J Clin Pathol 1986; 86:788–791

14

AIDS and the Heart

Paul R. Meyer
Edward C. Klatt

AT AUTOPSY THE HEART OF AIDS patients may show evidence of myocarditis in up to 53% of the cases.[1] Opportunistic infections or neoplasms were found in up to 25% of our cases. Such infections are always a part of prolonged disseminated disease and only rarely cause clinical findings. The debilitating nature of these conditions may contribute to other findings, including pericardial effusions seen in one fourth to one half of the patients, and nonbacterial thrombotic (marantic) endocarditis found in 4% of our patients. Despite histopathologic examination and/or microbiologic cultures, an etiology of the nonspecific myocarditis remains unidentified.

CLINICAL FINDINGS

Only scattered clinical reports of cardiac lesions in AIDS have been published. Fink et al.[2] described 15 patients with AIDS, each of whom received a physical examination, chest X-ray, electrocardiogram and echocardiogram. They found no evidence of significant cardiac disease on physical examination. A mild cardiomegaly on chest X-ray was seen in only one patient. Electrocardiography demonstrated nonspecific ST segment changes in four patients. Eight patients were found to have pericardial effusions by echocardiography, while clinical evidence of tamponade developed in only three of the 15 (20%).

PATHOLOGIC FINDINGS

The heart of AIDS patients may show nonspecific, though readily identifiable, pathologic changes. We reviewed the microscopic changes of 57 AIDS cases at autopsy (Table 1). Serous atrophy of adipose tissue found in one half of the cases probably reflects the general disability and cachexia seen in patients with terminal AIDS.

Inflammatory reactions and scarring are common findings. The inflammatory infiltrate may be lymphocytic or a mixture of different elements (Fig. 1). Only occasional cases were associated with myocardial fiber necrosis. A careful search, utilizing special stains for organisms, should be undertaken in such cases, but a causative agent will often not be found. This is evidenced by our 12 cases of central nervous system toxoplasmosis with myocarditis. In only one case were toxoplasma organisms identified in the myocardium. In such cases, the organisms might not have formed cysts or might have been overlooked. Only the application of more sensitive techniques can resolve this problem.

Nonspecific myocarditis has been previously reported. Anderson et al.[1] found evi-

TABLE I
Microscopic Cardiac Findings in AIDS
(57 Patients)

Serous atrophy of adipose tissue	23
Pericardial chronic inflammation	17
Myocarditis	
Diffuse lymphocytic	11
Focal lymphocytic	14
Lymphoid nodules	3
Mixed inflammatory	10
Round cells, unspecified	4
Diffuse myocardial fibrosis	8
Focal myocardial fiber necrosis	7
Chronic myocardial perivasculitis	3
Aschoff-like nodules	1

dence of myocarditis at autopsy in 53% of 72 AIDS patients. The myocarditis was characterized by patchy, mostly mononuclear, inflammatory cell infiltrates and myocardial necrosis. There was gross biventricular dilation in seven of the 38 cases. In only eight cases were opportunistic pathogens identified. Myocarditis correlated clinically with tachyarrhythmia and left ventricular dysfunction. The myocardium may be inflamed as a result of specific agents as yet undetected. Alternatively, such inflammation may result from a myriad of different insults such as drugs or autoimmune phenomena.

High levels of IgG-anticardiolipin were identified in 40 of 52 patients with HIV infections (and 23 of 28 patients with AIDS) by Canoso et al.[3] However, the presence of anticardiolipin antibodies (ACA) in HIV infection was not associated with the thrombotic diathesis seen in autoimmune disorders. The high incidence of both ACA and myocarditis may suggest a correlation.

Cohen et al.[4] have identified a form of congestive cardiomyopathy in a subset of AIDS patients. Such patients had a recurrent history of opportunistic infection. The hearts of these patients were grossly dilated and microscopically showed myofibril loss and a focal myocarditis with infiltrates of

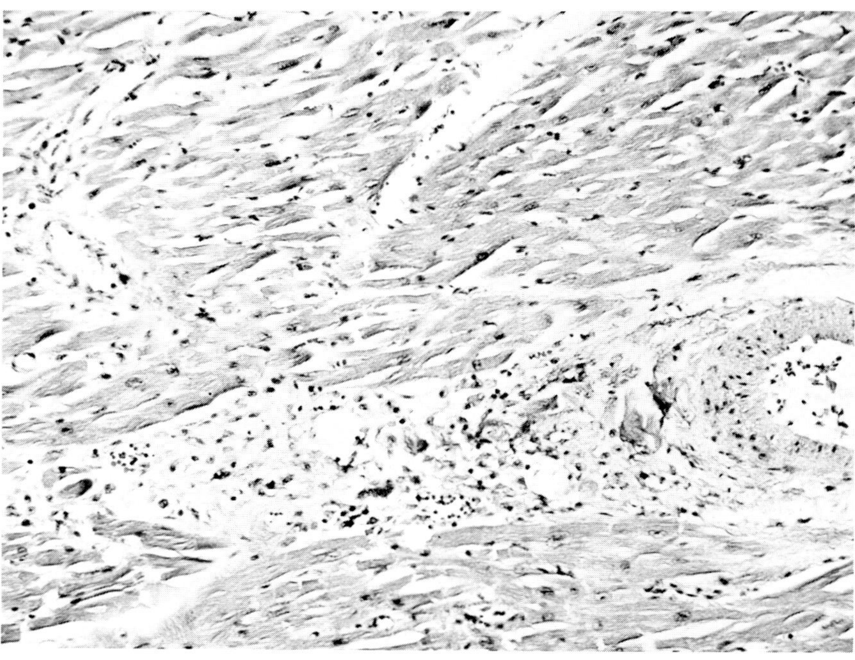

Figure 1. Nonspecific myocarditis. Mixed cell infiltrate located in a perivascular region without identifiable etiology. (H&E, original magnification ×120.)

lymphocytes, plasma cells, and eosinophils. No specific opportunistic infection or neoplasm could be identified as an etiology. A possible viral infection was postulated. Dalakas et al.[5] detected HIV in the lymphoid cells surrounding skeletal muscle fibers in cases of polymyositis associated with HIV infection. Potential prolonged survival of AIDS patients treated for HIV infection or neoplasms may increase the incidence and severity of myocardial disease.

Gross autopsy findings are given in Table 2. The general debilitation caused by AIDS may be a factor in the development of nonbacterial thrombotic endocarditis (marantic endocarditis) seen in seven cases. Small bland thrombi, usually no larger than 0.3 cm, were located on any of the four cardiac valves toward the closure line. Microscopically, these thrombi were composed of platelets and fibrin. The underlying valve showed minimal edema, without increased vascularity or inflammation. These vegetations are friable and may embolize producing infarction in organs proportionate in distribution with blood flow. Cammarosano and Lewis[6] described three cases of nonbacterial thrombotic endocarditis associated with AIDS; in two, death was attributable to embolization from these vegetations.

Pericardial effusions were seen in 28 of our cases, all less than 100 ml, with none producing clinical evidence of tamponade. The effusions were all clear, serous fluid. Localized infarcts were seen in three cases. Clinically, all three patients had profound agonal hypotension and shock, with autopsy evidence of moderate to severe coronary arteriosclerosis. Significant cardiomegaly,

TABLE II
Gross Cardiac Autopsy Findings in AIDS
(156 Patients)

Pericardial effusions	28
Cardiomegaly	15
Marantic valvular vegetations	7
Focal infarct	3

greater than 1.5 times normal weight, was seen in 15 cases with underlying renal or pulmonary disease. There were no cases of enlarged heart due solely to infectious agents. Such cases of cardiomegaly may be due to conditions preceding or coincident with HIV infection. AIDS patients in a terminal course of their disease tend to be younger than the general population of hospitalized patients. This may, in part, account for the paucity of complications from generalized arteriosclerosis observed in our series.

OPPORTUNISTIC INFECTION

In a series of 156 AIDS patients at autopsy we found only a few instances of opportunistic cardiac infection (7%) (Table 3). Death was rare from primary cardiac failure caused by these agents. In only one case, that of diffuse toxoplasma myocarditis, was the immediate cause of death attributable to an infectious myocarditis. Myocardial inflammation may be clinically suspected with the sudden onset of chest pain, arrhythmias, or acute congestive heart failure. We must admit, however, that the overwhelming nature of other organ involvement or failure may well have overshadowed the cardiac signs or symptoms of patients in our series. It seems likely that further investigation will more clearly delineate cardiac dysfunction in AIDS.

Table 3 outlines the specific infections found in the heart. *Cytomegalovirus* in three cases, *Mycobacterium avium-intracellulare* (MAI) in two cases, *Candida* in two cases, and histoplasmosis, cryptococcosis, and coccidioidomycosis in single cases involved the heart as a part of widespread disseminated disease. Often infections produced little in the way of inflammatory response. Disseminated MAI produced small clusters of pale blue histiocytes located near blood vessels. PAS, AFB, and methenamine silver stains all were useful in delineating "stacks" of bacilli within the histiocyte cytoplasm.[7] Car-

TABLE III
Specific Cardiac Opportunistic Infections
in AIDS (156 Patients)

	Heart	Elsewhere
Cytomegalovirus	3	74
Candida	2	69
Mycobacterium avium-intracellulare	2	31
Cryptococcosis	1	11
Toxoplasmosis	1	12
Histoplasmosis	1	4
Coccidioidomycosis	1	2

diac candidiasis was manifested by small microabscesses containing the budding yeasts with pseudohyphae. Coccidioidomycosis showed clusters of variably sized spherules with cardiac muscle fiber necrosis and scattered round cells. Histoplasmosis was characterized in the heart by small foci of macrophages containing multiple organisms and was only rarely accompanied by cardiac muscle fiber necrosis. In our case and in that described by Lewis et al.[8] cryptococcal organisms were seen in small clusters within myocardium or pericardium.

Toxoplasmosis can produce significant cardiac disease. In a single case, there were grossly identifiable pale tan to white irregular thin streaks throughout the myocardium alternating with normal cardiac muscle. Microscopically, these areas were composed of mixed inflammatory infiltrates of polymorphonuclear leukocytes, lymphocytes, histiocytes, and plasma cells along with localized myocardial fiber nercrosis. (Fig. 2) Even with extensive inflammation, the *Toxoplasma* cysts were difficult to find, requiring multiple sections that had to be scanned extensively. Small *Toxoplasma* cysts may resemble histocytes filled with *Histoplasma capsulatum*, but can be distinguished by electron micrsocopy. Typical *Toxoplasma*

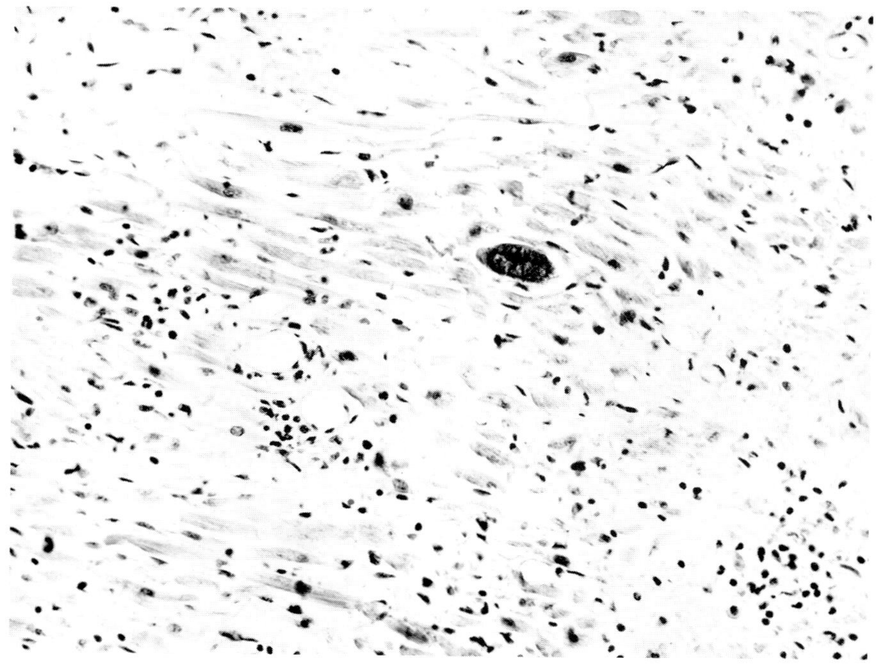

Figure 2. Myocarditis caused by *Toxoplasma gondii*. Mixed cell infiltrate with fiber necrosis. A cyst containing numerous trophozoites is present. (H&E, original magnification ×200.)

cysts have a thin wall and are filled with numerous small, dot-like organisms. The overall size of the cysts are from 10 to 30 μm.

NEOPLASMS

Neoplasms involved the heart in eight of our 156 autopsies with AIDS (Table 4). High grade malignant lymphomas in five cases were predominately of the Burkitt (small noncleaved) type. Gill et al.[9] outlined our results and the findings are presented in Table 5. Briefly, all cases occurred in male homosexuals or bisexuals in the third, fourth, or fifth decades of life. Three of the five men presented with pain mimicking an acute myocardial infarct. On chest X-ray four showed abnormalities including cardiomegaly or a left cardiac shadow. Staging revealed disseminated disease that was confirmed at autopsy. The LDH was elevated in all patients and antibodies to HIV were present in four of five. The fifth patient lacked antibodies, but virus was cultured from peripheral blood mononuclear cells. Lymphomatous infiltrates involved pericardium, myocardium, and/or endocardium. These infiltrates extended between myocardial fibers but produced little fiber necrosis.

Kaposi's sarcoma (KS), despite its vascular origin and features, appeared in the heart in only three out of 41 cases with documented KS. The distribution of KS was primarily in the perivascular region of the pericardium or myocardial interstitium, and around branches of coronary arteries. All patients were homosexual with extensive visceral and cutaneous disease.[10]

Silver et al.[10] in an autopsy study of 18 patients with AIDS, found five with KS involving the heart. In all five patients, dermatologic manifestations of KS had preceded cardiac involvement. In all cases the hearts were of normal size, and grossly, KS involvement consisted of small focal, hemorrhagic, subepicardial deposits of tumor. Microscopically, KS was seen adjacent to major coronary arteries and did not involve either myocardium or endocardium. In addition, focal deposits of KS were seen in the aortic adventitia in three cases and adjacent to a pulmonary artery in one case.

TABLE IV
Cardiac Neoplasms in AIDS (156 Patients)

Malignant lymphoma	5	18
Kaposi's sarcoma	3	41

TABLE V
AIDS-related Malignant Lymphoma Involving the Heart

Pt	Age	Race	Symptoms	X-Ray	Other Sites	HIV*	LDH (U/L)
1	37	H	pain	left cardiac shadow	renal, adrenal	−	665
2	43	W	SOB	cardiomegaly	retroperitoneum	+	494
3	39	W	pain	not done	retroperitoneum	+	3040
4	27	H	SOB	cardiomegaly	liver	+	4820
5	47	W	pain SOB	cardiomegaly	liver, adrenal	+	2295

Key: Pt-patient; W-white; H-hispanic; SOB-shortness of breath.

*HIV cultured from peripheral blood mononuclear cells.

From: Gill et al.[9]

REFERENCES

1. Anderson DW, Virmani R, Reilly J, et al: High prevalence of myocarditis in the acquired immune deficiency syndrome (AIDS). (Abstract) Lab Invest 1987; 56:1a
2. Fink L, Reichek N, Sutton MG: Cardiac abnormalities in acquired immune deficiency syndrome. Am L Cardiol 1984; 54:1161–1163
3. Conoso RT, Zon LI, Groopman JE: Anticardiolipin antibodies associated with HTLV-III infection. Br J Hematology 1987; 65:495–498
4. Cohen IS, Anderson DW, Virmani R: Cardiac Involvement by Kaposi's sarcoma in acquired immune deficiency syndrome. N Engl J Med 1986; 315:628–630
5. Dalakas MC, Pezeshkpour MD, Gravell M, Sever JL: Polymyositis associated with AIDS retrovirus. JAMA 1986; 256:2381–2383
6. Cammarosano C, Lewis W: Cardiac lesions in acquired immune deficiency syndrome (AIDS). J Am Coll Cardiol 1986; 5:703–706
7. Klatt EC, Jensen DF, Meyer PR: Pathology of *Mycobacterium avium intracellulare* infection in acquired immune deficiency syndrome. Hum Pathol 1987; 18:709–714
8. Lewis W, Lipsick J, Cammarosano C: Cryptococcal myocarditis in acquired immune deficiency syndrome. Am J Cardiol 1985; 55:1240
9. Gill PS, Chandraratna AN, Meyer PR, Levine AM: Malignant lymphoma: Cardiac involvement at initial presentation. J Clin Oncol 1987; 5:216–224
10. Silver MA, Macher AM, Reichert CM, et al: Cardiac involvement by Kaposi's sarcoma in acquired immune deficiency syndrome (AIDS). Am J Cardiol 1984; 53:983–985
11. D'Cru IA, Sengupta EE, Abrahams C, et al: Cardiac involvement, including tuberculous pericardial effusion, complicating acquired immune deficiency syndrome. Am Heart J 1986; 112:1100–1102
12. Steinherz LJ, Brochstein JA, Robins J: Cardiac involvement in congenital acquired immune deficiency syndrome. Am J Dis Child 1986; 140:1241–1246

15

The AIDS Autopsy: Comparison of Intravenous Drug Abusers with Non-Intravenous Drug Abusers

Roger Schinella
Barbara Chaitin
Elliot Gross

THERE HAVE BEEN FEW AUTOPSY studies of intravenous drug abusers (IVDA) with AIDS.[1,2] We have undertaken this analysis, which compares 18 IVDA AIDS patients with 17 non-IVDA AIDS patients and then compares them to prior autopsy studies of AIDS.

MATERIALS AND METHODS

The 18 IVDA AIDS cases included 16 men and 2 women, all Bellevue Hospital patients whose autopsies were performed at the Medical Examiners office, New York, NY, except for one New York University Hospital case. None of the IVDA cases was identified as homosexual. The 17 non-IVDA cases were patients at Bellevue and New York University Hospitals. Of the non-IVDA patients, 14 were homosexual, 2 were Haitian, and one was a woman who was infected by a bisexual ex-husband. All cases had the routine organ sections and all had fungal, acid fast, and tissue Gram stains whenever suspicious lesions were encoun-

tered, or in selected organs where prevalence of particular organisms was found to be high as determined by our prior study.[3]

RESULTS

As noted in Table 1, in most categories of disease there was no difference between IVDA and non-IVDA patients. The two notable areas of difference were in the number of fungal infections, with six (3 cryptococcal and 3 non-cryptococcal) occurring in IVDA patients and none in non-IVDA, and the number of neoplasms, with three occurring in IVDA patients and six occurring in non-IVDA.

Cytomegalovirus (CMV) was demonstrable as typical inclusions in 55% of the autopsies. There was no significant difference in incidence of disease between IVDA and non-IVDA patients. Unusual lesions associated with CMV were mycocarditis (2 cases) and one case with severe hyalinization of vessels in a colon section, suggesting chronic effects of CMV vasculitis (Fig.1). As

TABLE I
Infectious Agents and Cancers Identified in 35
Autopsies of AIDS

	IVDA (18 Patients)	Non-IVDA (17 Patients)
P. carinii	8	6
CMV	9	11
Cryptococcus	3	None
Toxoplasma	3	2
MAI	6	3
MTB	2	2
Bacterial Infections	5	8
Fungi	3*	None
Malignancies	3	6

**Candida* pneumonitis = 2; pulmonary aspergillus = 1
Abbreviations: IVDA = intravenous drug abusers;
P. carinii = *Pneumocystis carinii*;
CMV = Cytomegalovirus; MAI = *Mycobacterium avium-intracellulare*; MTB = *Mycobacterium tuberculosis*.

previously described,[3,4] lung and adrenal glands were the most commonly involved organs, in both IVDA and non-IVDA patients, but organ distribution tended to be wider and individual organ involvement more severe in non-IVDA patients. As noted previously,[3] endocrine organs, other than the adrenal glands, showed no necrosis or inflammation when involved by CMV.

Pneumocystis carinii pneumonitis (PCP) was found at autopsy in approximately half of the patients in both the IVDA and non-IVDA group. Associated reactions such as diffuse alveolar damage, organizing pneumonia, giant cell reaction, and granular calcification were common in both IVDA and non-IVDA patients. One non-IVDA patient showed clinically and at autopsy, cavitary lung lesions associated with severe PCP. In the latter part of his clinical course a spontaneous pneumothorax had developed. The infection was marked by extensive organizing pneumonia. Study of the cavitary areas revealed smaller, presumably early lesions to be dilatations of respiratory bronchiole-

alveolar duct complexes. The walls of the cysts were made up of distended alveolar ducts and respiratory bronchioles showing loss of epithelium. The edges of the cysts that formed were lined by fibrinous exudate (Fig. 2). At this point, the cysts were grossly visible. Necrosis of the edges of cysts produced larger cysts in some areas, whereas in other areas larger cysts resulted from expansion of the earlier smaller lesions.

An additional finding of interest with respect to PCP was the finding of *Pneumocystis carinii* organisms in the sinuses of a periaortic lymph node of one patient (Fig. 3).

Fungal infections were recognized in six of our 18 IVDA patients but in none of the 17 non-IVDA cases. Three of the infections were due to *cryptococcus*, presenting as cryptococcal meiningitis, and were appropriately treated, but all had widely disseminated infection at autopsy. Two patients had *Candida* pneumonitis. One of these also had *Torulopsis* demonstrated by postmortem culture. The sixth patient had focal *Aspergillus* pneumonitis.

Three cases of toxoplasmosis were found in IVDA patients and two in non-IVDA patients. One of the IVDA patients showed wide dissemination, mostly in tachyzoite form, involving heart, lung, and pancreas with clinical symptoms of pancreatitis. At autopsy, there was massive pancreatitis with numerous organisms. Interestingly, the brain was not involved by toxoplasmosis in this case. Dissemination was not suspected during life. All other patients had only central nervous system toxoplasmosis.

Mycobacterial infections were numerous in both groups. There were eight in the IVDA group, with six showing patterns typical for *Mycobacterium avium-intracellulare* (MAI) as previously described,[3] and two showing abscess-like, poorly formed granulomas in patients with *Mycobacterium tuberculosis* (MTB). All MAI infections were widely disseminated, whereas MTB infection was confined to the lung in one case and involved lung and a peritoneal lymph

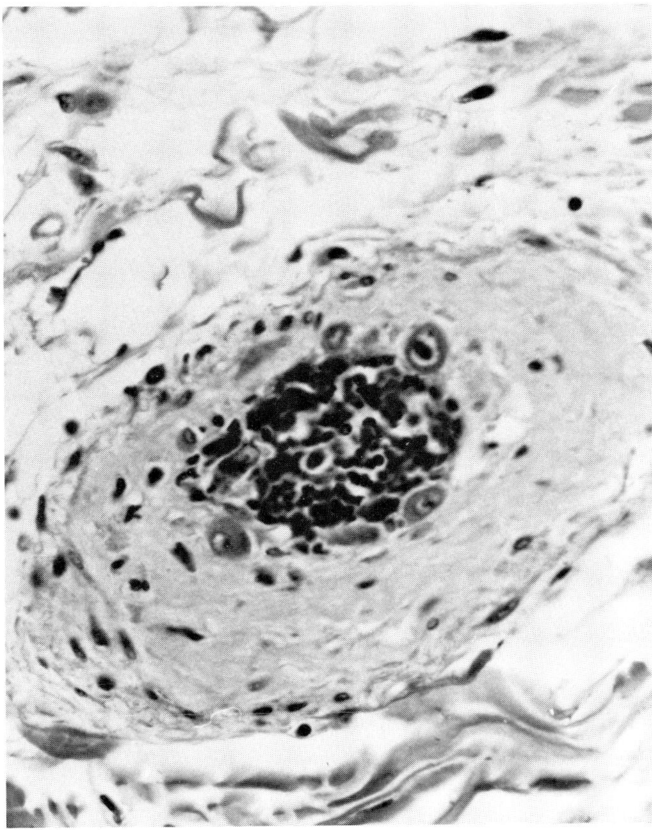

Figure 1. Hyalinizing vasculitis related to Cytomegalovirus. Note the marked hyalinization of the vessel showing intimal Cytomegalovirus involvement. (H&E, original magnification ×200)

node in the other. Both patients were diagnosed premortem and treated for MTB. One demonstrated no organisms at autopsy and the other showed sparse organisms with the acid-fast stain. There were five mycobacterial infections in non-IVDA patients; two cases of MAI infection showed widespread dissemination and one was limited to a mesenteric lymph node. One Haitian male had massive widespread MTB of typical AIDS type with abscess-like granulomas at autopsy (Fig. 4). The fifth patient had MTB in a cervical lymph node during life but none at autopsy after appropriate therapy. Of interest in the Haitian patient was the presence of intraluminal vascular granulomas in the spleen (Fig. 5).

Serious bacterial infections among AIDS patients were common. There were five among the IVDA group. Three of these were present during life but were not found at autopsy. Two were septic conditions with *Staphylococcus* and *Serratia* and with gram-negative rods, respectively, cultured from the blood. The other was a clinically proven *Pseudomonas* pneumonia. The fourth patient showed, at autopsy, a pneumonia with gram-positive cocci. The remaining patient showed a lung abscess with sparse gram-positive cocci. In neither patient was a post mortem culture performed.

There were eight cases of bacterial infections among non-IVDA patients. In seven cases the infection and organisms were de-

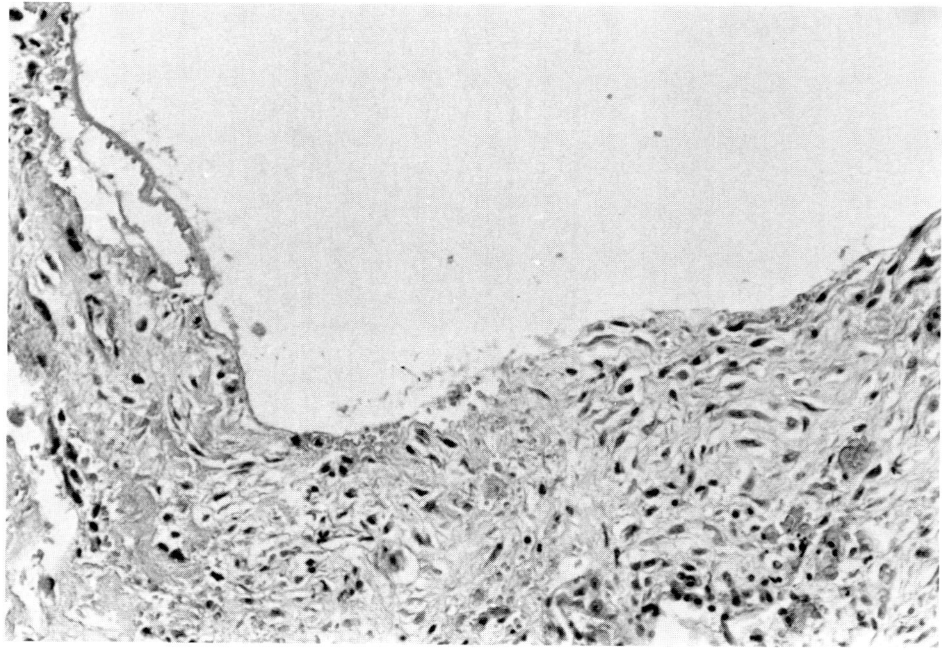

Figure 2. Adult form of bronchopulmonary dysplasia in a patient with *Pneumocystis carinii* pneumonia. Note the severe fibrosis around the cystic space and its fibrinous inner lining. (H&E, original magnification ×100)

monstrable at autopsy. Six patients had pneumonitis, one of which was secondary to aspiration. The other patient had a lung abscess. The eighth patient developed staphylococcal sepsis during life but no evidence of this was found at autopsy. A wide variety of bacterial types were found at autopsy. Two of the above patients with pneumonia were infected with *Staphylococcus* and one of these was found to have widely disseminated disease at autopsy. Another patient had pneumonitis due to gram-positive cocci but these were not cultured; nor were cultures taken from the remaining patients with bacterial infections. Two patients with pneumonitis, including one with aspiration, were infected with gram-negative rods. One patient showed gram-negative rods, gram-positive cocci, and extensive pneumonitis. The patient with the lung abscess showed gram negative rods.

Malignancies were found in three IVDA patients. One had an immunoblastic lym-phoma of the central nervous system only. One woman had visceral Kaposi's sarcoma (KS) involving lung and lymph nodes but not the skin. A third patient had a T-cell chronic lymphocytic leukemia of suppressor cell type ($T_3^+T_4^-T_8^+$). The patient's lymphocytes did not show large azurophilic granules. He was HTLV-I negative. At autopsy, no evidence of lymphoma was found despite the fact the patient received no therapy. He died with PCP and CMV infections.

Among the non-IVDA patients there were six with malignancies. Four had only KS and two patients had KS and lymphoma. All patients with KS had disseminated disease at autopsy. One of them had no skin disease, and KS was detected by lymph node biopsy. Widespread visceral disease was found at autopsy.

The lymphomas were of immunoblastic, and large, noncleaved, non-Hodgkin's type. They were both nodal with only minor extension into perinodal tissues. The immu-

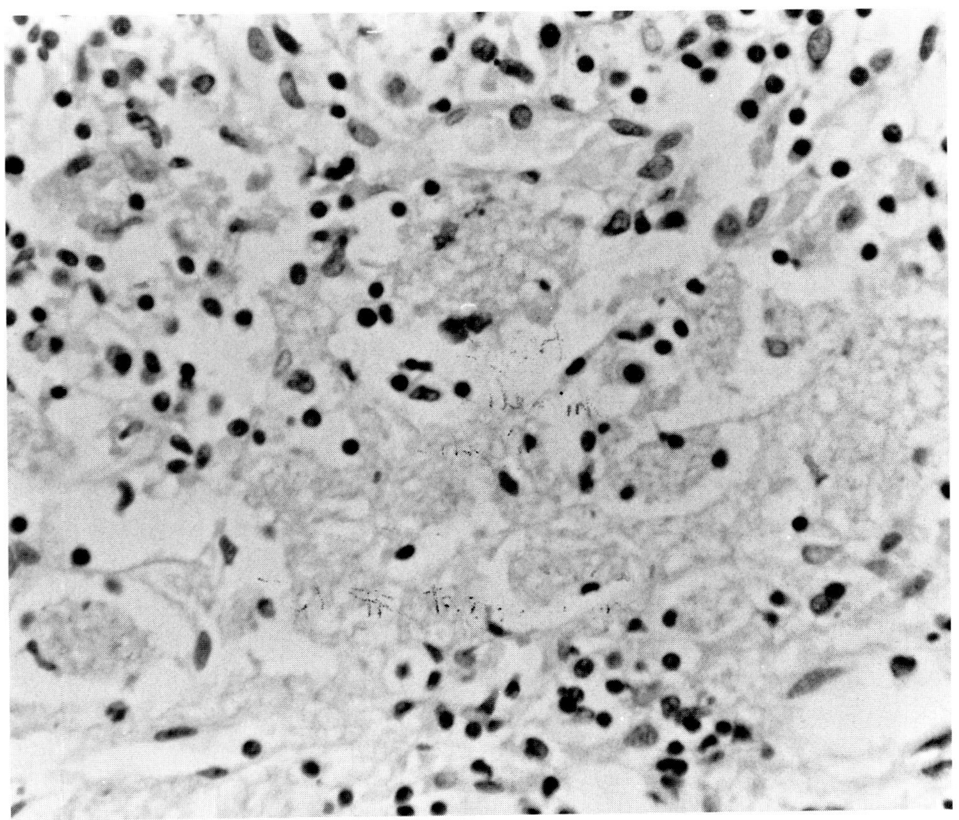

Figure 3. *Pneumocystis carinii* in a lymph node. Note the typical foamy exudate within the sinuses. (H&E, original magnification ×400)

noblastic lymphoma demonstrated extremely bizarre cells and was of B-cell origin by DNA analysis only, with all surface markers being negative.* At autopsy, the tumor was widespread and lymphoma cells were seen in vascular channels.

Also of note was the finding of large multinucleated cells with nuclei in a circle, (i.e., a Touton cell-like configuration) (Fig. 6), in two IVDA patients in the liver and brain, respectively, and in the cervix of one non-IVDA patient. Myocarditis, defined as inflammatory cells and necrosis of myocardial fibers with more than five cells per focus and

more than two foci per case, was found in two patients, both IVDA. One had associated thromboses of atria and ventricles. Similar foci of inflammation were also seen in an IVDA with healed vegetations of the mitral valve, but he was eliminated as a case of true myocarditis. There were also two cases of CMV myocarditis and one case of myocardial toxoplasmosis, as already mentioned. Nonthrombotic bacterial endocarditis was found in two patients, one IVDA and one non-IVDA.

Cirrhosis of the liver was found in three patients; all were IVDA and two of the three gave histories of alcoholism. Also of note were hemophagocytosis in reticuloendothelial tissues, serous atrophy of fat, increased

*Dr. D. Knowles, personal communication

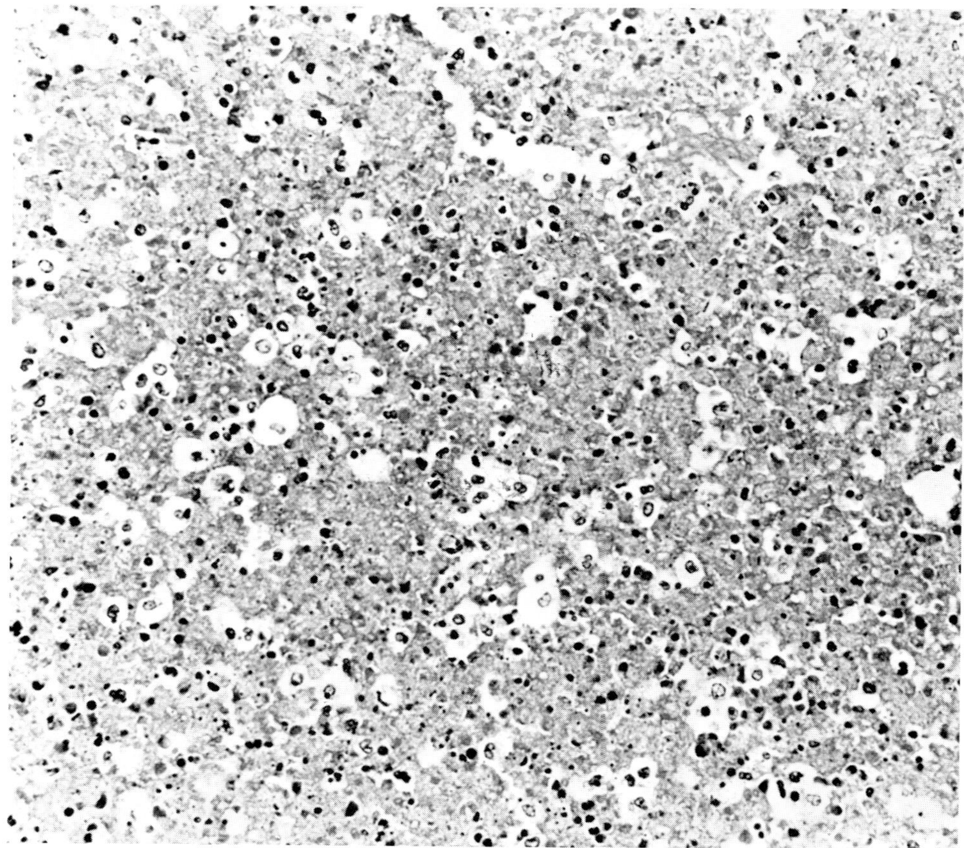

Figure 4. Abscess-like *Mycobacterium tuberculosis* infection as typically seen in AIDS. Note the necrosis with numerous necrotic leucocytes. (H&E, original magnification ×400)

tissue hemosiderin, and decreased spermatogenesis.

DISCUSSION

Few investigators have compared autopsy findings of IVDA with those of non-IVDA. A recent report by Ambros et al.[1] compared 13 IVDA with 8 non-IVDA. One of their observations was the absence of neoplasms in IVDA patients. In our series, however, we found that three of 18 IVDA patients had neoplasms. One man had a central nervous system lymphoma and one woman had KS. KS in male IVDA as well as in female IVDA, has been previously described, albeit

the incidence in IVDA patients (4%) is far less than that in homosexual patients (48%).[5] In our earlier study of AIDS autopsies, KS occurred in one IVDA.[3] In our present study there were two cases of visceral KS without skin involvement among a total of seven patients (from both groups), a higher incidence than the 5% quoted for visceral KS in the existing literature,[6] and higher than the incidence found in our previous study.[2,3,29] Guarda et al.[7] reported visceral KS, without skin involvement in two of 10 homosexual patients. These findings suggest that visceral KS without skin involvement may be more common than previously believed.

The single case of T-cell chronic lympho-

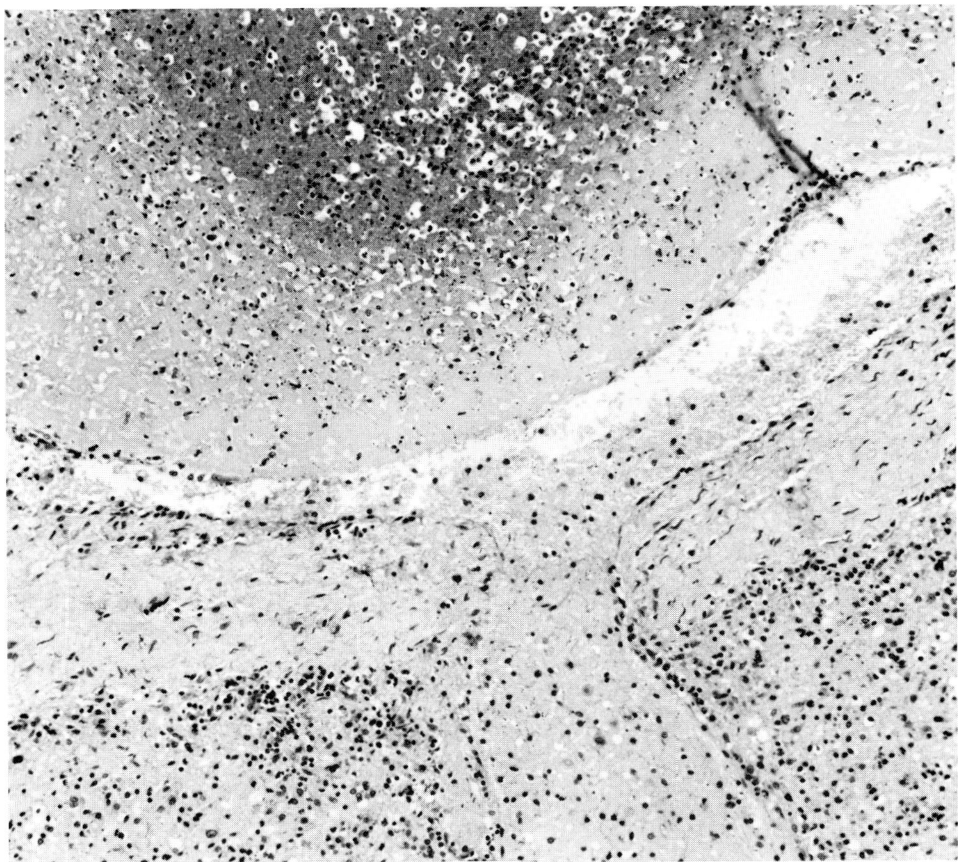

Figure 5. Intravascular granuloma seen in the spleen of an AIDS patient. Note the similarity of the granuloma to that illustrated in Figure 4. (H&E, original magnification ×200)

cytic leukemia of suppressor cell type is of considerable interest, and an extremely rare manifestation of AIDS. It is one of a large group of lymphomas occurring in AIDS and is reported in more detail elsewhere.[8]

There were six malignancies in non-IVDA patients, in concordance with prior reports that cancers are more common in non-IVDA (predominantly homosexual) than in IVDA.[6] All six patients had KS but two in addition had malignant lymphoma. Somewhat at variance with prior studies, both lymphomas were nodal rather than extranodal.[3,6-14] However, since a certain percentage of lymphomas in AIDS are nodal,[8,13,14] our findings probably represent discrepancies due to sampling. All lym-

phomas in our AIDS patients were of high grade except for the unusual T-cell chronic lymphocytic leukemia.

Ambros et al.[1] reported that CMV was more common in the IVDA group. We found nine cases with CMV inclusions in 18 IVDA patients and 11 in 17 non-IVDA patients, a non-significant difference, suggesting that CMV is equally common in non-IVDA and IVDA patients. The disease, however, appears to have a wider organ distribution in the non-IVDA than the IVDA group.

In our total series the percentage of autopsies demonstrating CMV inclusions was less than in the group of 56 autopsies we previously described (55% vs. 77%).[3] The

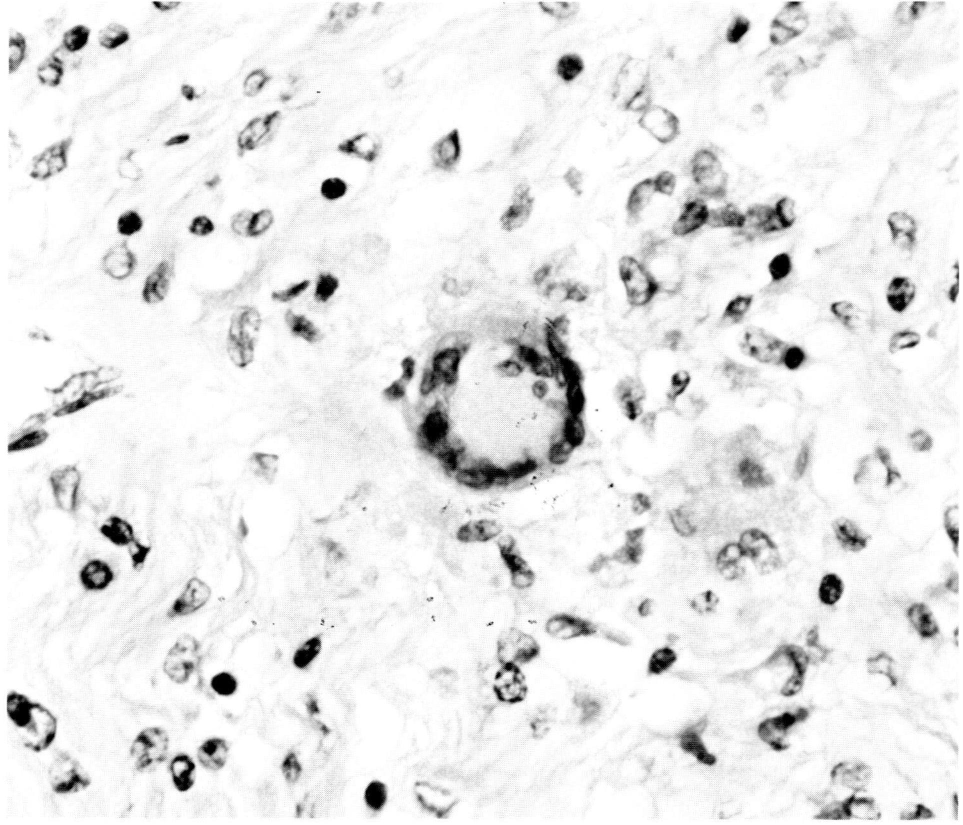

Figure 6. Touton-like cell seen in the cervix of an AIDS patient. Note the lack of significant inflammatory reaction. (H&E, original magnification ×400)

number of different organs involved and the severity of organ involvement was less in this group than in our previously reported study. The reason for this, if corroborated by further studies, is not clear. It apparently cannot be explained by earlier diagnosis or any differences in therapy of the present patients versus our earlier group.

Although we found only one case of CMV vasculitis in this series, compared to three cases in our prior study, it was of interest that instead of panarterial inflammatory infiltration of the vessel wall, as previously described,[3,7] there was a thickening and hyalinization of the vessel wall. In our previous report there was uncertainty as to whether the vasculitis was due to CMV or to circulating immune complexes. The finding in this case of highly specific vessel involvement with this unusual, histologically distinctive change, suggests that we are dealing with a true CMV vasculitis.

The incidence of toxoplasmosis was found by Ambros et al.[1] to be higher in IVDA than in non-IVDA. In the present study there were three cases in IVDA and two in non-IVDA patients. Two cases in IVDA patients were limited to the central nervous system (CNS) as were both cases in non-IVDA patients. One case in an IVDA patient showed no CNS involvement but widespread disease involved myocardium, lung, and pancreas. In the latter, there was a massive pancreatitis. Disseminated toxoplasmosis in AIDS has been previously described,[4,7,12,15] but most cases involved the

CNS and myocardium. Widespread disease such as that which occurred in our patient is distinctly unusual, especially in an adult.

Eight IVDA patients had PCP at autopsy as did six non-IVDA patients. Microscopic findings previously described in PCP such as calcifications, giant cells, and organizing pneumonia with fibrosis were again noted.[16] *P. carinii* can be a direct cause of organizing pneumonia with fibrosis.[17] At autopsy, with many other reasons for pulmonary fibrosis, the etiology of organizing pneumonia with fibrosis is probably multifactorial.

We found *P. carnii* in a periaortic lymph node of a patient who had lung involvement. Disseminated *P. carnii* has now been described in several AIDS patients[18-21] and must be accepted as an unusual finding but one that must be kept in mind and sought for. Another interesting finding was a case of PCP with pulmonary cavities. These have been described in the radiologic literature[22] and have been a cause of spontaneous pneumothorax.[23] The cysts arose as a result of severe organizing pneumonia with damage to respiratory bronchioles and alveolar ducts, which expanded to form the cystic cavities. In some areas, usually with larger cysts, necrosis of a portion of the cavity wall resulted in the formation of still larger cavities. The cavity formation, we believe, represents a phase of the evolution of honeycomb lung from diffuse alveolar damage,[24] but at a point were the extensive fibrosis associated with the honeycomb lung has not yet occurred. These changes are similar to those described as bronchopulmonary dysplasia in the adult.[25]

Mycobacterial infections occurred in about twice as many IVDA as non-IVDA patients. The MAI infections were typical of those described in AIDS patients.[26] No differences were seen in severity or patterns of distribution of MAI in IVDA versus non-IVDA patients.

Mycobacterium tuberculosis (MTB) infections manifested as large central abscess-like areas with considerable nuclear debris. At the edges of these abscess-like areas epithelioid cells and rare giant cells were inconspicuous. In untreated cases, characteristically, there are numerous organisms.[3,27] It is important to recognize this abscess-like pattern, especially since the numerous mycobacteria found in these patients may stain gram-positive,[28] leading to an erroneous diagnosis of a nonmycobacterial bacterial infection and inappropriate therapy. Of our four cases of MTB infection, one that was not suspected, and therefore not treated, appeared as described above. One patient was diagnosed during life by lymph node biopsy, treated, and at autopsy no evidence of MTB or of granulomas was found. Another patient who received a full course of antituberculous therapy during life manifested the above described lesions but had no acid-fast organisms in them. The last patient was partially treated, succumbed to a *Candida* and *Torulopsis* pneumonitis, and at autopsy showed the typical abscess-like lesions of MTB infection as seen in the immunodeficient host and only sparse acid-fast organisms. One case of MTB infection was remarkable for vascular intraluminal granulomas. This was probably responsible for rapid dissemination of the disease and for the recently described MTB bacteremia in AIDS.[29]

In conclusion, there is often a favorable response to therapy for MTB infections in AIDS patients[30] and the correct diagnosis is, therefore, important. One of our untreated patients with advanced MTB infection died of that disease alone.

As previously noted, bacterial infections are highly significant as causes of morbidity and mortality in AIDS patients.[3,31] Interestingly, bacterial infections were about twice as common (8 versus 5) in non-IVDA versus IVDA patients in the present study. Further, of the five cases in IVDA patients, three were diagnosed during life, two with sepsis (*Serratia* and *Staphylococcus* in one and gram-negative rods in the other) and the third with *Pseudomonas* pneumonia. These were successfully treated. Two showed disease at autopsy, one a pneumonia with gram-positive cocci and one a lung abscess with rare gram-positive cocci. Of the eight non-IVDA patients, seven had organisms associated with severe infections at autopsy. The eighth patient had staphylococcal sepsis, was successfully treated, but died of an unsuspected MTB infection. No traces of the sepsis were found at autopsy.

Another unexplained result in our study was the finding of six visceral fungal infections in IVDA patients and none in non-IVDA patients. This is especially puzzling, since in our earlier study visceral fungal infections were not rare in non-IVDA patients.[3] As previously described, infections with *cryptococcus*, although treated, were not only not eliminated but often disseminated.[3] Another finding that we considered of significance was the presence of large cells with peripheral, circumferentially arranged nuclei.These resemble Touton giant cells as seen in xanthomas. Similar multinucleated cells have been described in the brains of AIDS patients.[32] Warthin-Finkeldey type giant cells have been described in the lymph nodes of AIDS patients.[33] The latter differed from the herein described cells and those described in the brain.[32] Small numbers of the Touton-like cells were found in the lung and liver, respectively, of two IVDA patients, and in one non-IVDA patient a single cell was found in the cervix. The cells were not associated with necrosis and were associated with only scant inflammatory reaction. These cells resemble those described in cultures of HIV infected lymphocytes,[34] and we, therefore, believe they may be indicators of HIV infection. We have also found these Touton-like giant cells in lymph node biopsies of two AIDS patients who were not part of this autopsy study.

Recent reports[35,36] describe myocarditis in 53% and 31% of AIDS patients, respectively. Eliminating instances in which we demonstrated CMV (two cases) or toxoplasmosis (one case), we found two cases that satisfied criteria for myocarditis in which no organisms were demonstrated.[35] They both occurred in IVDA patients. Our total number

of myocarditis cases were 5/35 or 14%. We did not, however, have as many sections in our cases as in the quoted studies and more histopathologic sections may have shown more lesions. In two patients, one IVDA and one non-IVDA, we found nonbacterial thrombotic endocarditis. This is not a surprising finding in these chronically and seriously ill patients and has been previously reported.[7] No consequences of this were noted in our two patients.

Generalized organ changes, as noted previously,[3,9] were also commonly seen. These included hemophagocytosis, lymphoid depletion, increased iron stores in macrophages, and serous atrophy of fat. Decreased spermatogenesis, although again noted, was not as severe as previously described. The number of cases with total lack of spermatogenesis was smaller than in our prior study. In contrast to our prior study[3] and the studies of others,[9] we found three cases of cirrhosis in the present investigation. All three were in the IVDA group. Although the risk of cirrhosis secondary to hepatitis B is probably equally high in both the IVDA and non-IVDA group, the difference was that in two of the three IVDA patients a strong history of alcoholism was obtained. Reichert et al.[9] had pointed out that, surprisingly, evidence of chronic active hepatitis and cirrhosis was absent in AIDS patients. We did find cirrhosis in this series, but more likely due to alcoholism than to chronic hepatitis.

REFERENCES

1. Ambros RA, Lee E, Sharer LR, et al: The acquired immunodeficiency syndrome in intravenous drug abusers and patients with a sexual risk: Clinical and postmortem comparisons. Hum Pathol 1987; 18:1109–1114
2. Wormser GP, Krupp LB, Hanrahan JP, et al: Acquired immunodeficiency syndrome in male prisoners. Ann Intern Med 1983; 98:297–303
3. Niedt GW, Schinella RA: Acquired immunodeficiency syndrome. Clinicopathologic study of 56 autopsies. Arch Pathol Lab Med 1985; 109:727–734
4. Tapper ML, Rotterdam HZ, Lerner CW, et al: Adrenal necrosis in the acquired immunodefi-

ciency syndrome. Ann Intern Med 1984; 100:239–241

5. Krigel RL, Friedman-Kien AE: Kaposi's sarcoma in AIDS. In: DeVita JR, Hellman S, Rosenberg SA, eds; AIDS: Etiology, Diagnosis, Treatment, and Prevention. pp 185–211, Philadelphia, JB Lippincott Co. 1985

6. Longo DL: Kaposi's sarcoma and other neoplasms. pp 96–98, in Fauci AS, moderator, In: Acquired immunodeficiency syndrome: epidemiologic, clinical, immunologic, and therapeutic considerations. Ann Intern Med 1984; 100:92–106

7. Guarda LA, Luna MA, Smith JL, et al: Acquired immune deficiency syndrome: Post mortem findings. Am J Clin Pathol 1984; 81:549–557

8. Knowles DM, Chamulak GA, Subar M, et al: Lymphoid neoplasia associated with the acquired immunodeficiency syndrome. Ann Intern Med 1988; 108:744–753

9. Reichert CM, O'Leary TJ, Levens DL, et al: Autopsy pathology in the acquired immune deficiency syndrome. Am J Pathol 1983; 112:357–382

10. Hui AN, Koss MN, Meyer PR: Necropsy findings in acquired immunodeficiency syndrome: A comparison of premortem diagnoses with postmortem findings. Hum Pathol 1984; 15:670–676

11. Welch K, Finkbeiner W, Alpers CE, et al: Autopsy findings in the acquired immune deficiency syndrome. JAMA 1984; 252:1152–1159

12. Moskowitz L, Hensley GT, Chan JC, et al: Immediate causes of death in acquired immunodeficiency syndrome. Arch Pathol Lab Med 1985; 109:735–738

13. Zeigler JL, Beckstead JA, Volberding PA, et al: Non-Hodgkin's lymphoma in 90 homosexual men: Relation to generalized lymphadenopathy and the acquired immunodeficiency syndrome (AIDS). N Engl J Med 1984; 311:565–570

14. Levine AM, Meyer PR, Begandy MK, et al: Development of B-cell lymphoma in homosexual men. Ann Intern Med 1984; 100:7–13

15. Wong B, Gold JWM, Brown AE, et al: Central nervous system toxoplasmosis in homosexual men and parenteral drug abusers. Ann Intern Med 1984; 100:36–42

16. Weber WR, Askin FB, Dehner LP: Lung biopsy in *Pneumocystis carinii* pneumonia: A histopathologic study of typical and atypical features. Am J Clin Pathol 1977; 67:11–19

17. Schinella RA, Clancey CA, Fazzini E, et al: *Pneumocystis carinii* as a cause of pulmonary fibrosis. Chest (in press).

18. Heyman MR, Rasmussen P: *Pneumocystis carinii* involvement of the bone marrow in acquired immunodeficiency syndrome. Am J Clin Pathol 1987; 87:780–783

19. Grimes MM, LaPook JD, Bar MH, et al: Disseminated *Pneumocystis carinii* infection in a patient with acquired immunodeficiency syndrome. Hum Pathol 1987; 18:307–308

20. Schinella RA, Breda SD, Hammerschlag PE: Otic infection due to *Pneumocystis carinii* in an appar-

ently healthy man with antibody to the human immunodeficiency virus. Ann Intern Med 1987; 106:399–400

21. Coulman CU, Greene I, Archibald RWR: Cutaneous pneumocystosis. Ann Intern Med 1987; 106:396–398

22. Naidich DP, Garay SM, Leitman BS, et al: Radiographic manifestations of pulmonary disease in the acquired immunodeficiency syndrome (AIDS). Semin Roentgenol 1987; 22:14–30

23. Goodman PC, Daley C, Minagi H: Spontaneous pneumothorax in AIDS patients with *Pneumocystis carinii* pneumonia. Am J Radiol 1986; 147:29–31

24. Katzenstein A-L A, Askin FB: Surgical Pathology of Non-neoplastic Lung Disease. Philadelphia W.B. Saunders, 1982, pp 67–69

25. Churg A, Golden J, Fliegel S, et al: Bronchopulmonary dysplasia in the adult. Am Rev Respir Dis 1983; 127:117–120

26. Greene JB, Sidhu GS, Lewin S, et al: *Mycobacterium avium-intracellulare*: A cause of life-threatening infection in homosexuals and drug abusers. Ann Intern Med 1982; 97:539–546

27. Pitchenik AE, Fischl MA, Dickinson GM, et al: Opportunistic infections and Kaposi's sarcoma among Haitians: Evidence of a new acquired immunodeficiency state. Ann Intern Med 1983; 98:277–284

28. Tarshis MS: The *Mycobacteria* in Gradwohl's clinical laboratory methods and diagnosis. Frankel S, Reitman S, Sonnenwirth AC (Eds), 7th Edition 1970; St. Louis, MO, C.V. Mosby Co. p. 1234

29. Barnes PF, Arevalo C: Six cases of *Mycobacterium tuberculosis* bacteremia. J Infect Dis 1987; 156:377–379

30. Viera J, Frank E, Spira TJ, et al: Acquired immune deficiency in Haitians: Opportunistic infections in previously healthy Haitian immigrants. N Engl J Med 1983; 308:125–129

31. Eng RHK, Bishburg E, Smith SM, et al: Bacteremia and fungemia in patients with acquired immune deficiency syndrome. Am J Clin Pathol 1986; 86:105–107

32. Sharer LR, Cho E-S, Epstein LG: Multinucleated giant cells and HTLV-III in AIDS Encephalopathy. Hum Pathol 1985; 16:760

33. Ewing EP, Chandler FW, Spira TJ, et al: Primary lymph node pathology in AIDS and AIDS-related lymphadenopathy. Arch Pathol Lab Med 1985; 109:977–981

34. Popovic M, Sarngadharan MG, Read E, et al: Detection, isolation, and continuous production of cytopathic retroviruses (HTLV-III) from patients with AIDS and pre-AIDS. Science 1984; 224:497–500

35. Anderson DW, Virmani R, Reilly J, et al: High prevalence of myocarditis in the acquired immune deficiency syndrome (AIDS). Lab Invest 1987; 56:1A

36. Roldan EO, Moskowitz L, Hensley GT: Pathology of the heart in acquired immunodeficiency syndrome. Arch Pathol Lab Med 1987; 111:943–946

16

Acquired Immunodeficiency Syndrome (AIDS) and the Laboratory Worker: A Survey

Stephen A. Geller

SINCE THE TIME OF ITS RECOGNITION, in 1981,[1,2] the acquired immunodeficiency syndrome (AIDS) has increasingly occupied the attention of both the scientific and lay communities. The spectre of AIDS as a major public health threat has contributed to extraordinary advances in the understanding of the nature of viruses, particularly retroviruses, and their modes of infectivity.[3,4] At the same time, knowledge about the nature of AIDS remains, for most of the population, fragmented and inaccurate, even among hospital personnel.[5]

The requirements for dealing with AIDS patients, on a societal as well as a medical plane, have caused re-examination of ethical[6-9] as well as therapeutic and diagnostic concepts. The number of AIDS patients in the United States is expected to exceed the 250,000 level by the beginning of the next decade,[10] and the economic implications are only beginning to be appreciated.[11-14] The full impact of AIDS on the medical community has not yet been felt. In urban medical centers as many as 25% of the admissions may be for AIDS, contributing significantly to the psychological burden for hospital personnel.[9]

The need for prudent behavior on the part of hospital staff members was suggested relatively early in the course of the recognition of AIDS[6] and the recommendations, at that time, included specific precautions for laboratory workers. Despite professional[15-18] and lay literature and educational activities indicating that the AIDS virus is not easily transmitted, considerable fears remain in the hospital setting where a majority of employees, both professional and paraprofessional, may still manifest considerable anxiety about working in a milieu with AIDS patients.[5] Indeed, pathologists interviewed immediately after a recent College of American Pathologists (CAP)-sponsored seminar, devoted to potential hazards of the autopsy, had an "obvious lack of eagerness to examine AIDS victims."[15]

We surveyed pathologists in order to determine prevalent views about AIDS, in preparation for a presentation, about the risks posed by AIDS, to laboratory personnel at a Spring 1987 CAP-seminar. This paper reports the results of that survey.

MATERIALS AND METHODS

A survey, concentrating on questions of particular interest to laboratory workers, was mailed to "Director, Department of Pathology" at 425 hospitals, including at least one hospital in each state, during January 1987. Hospitals were selected in the largest cities in each state, and, where possible, university, private, federal, and local governmental institutions were included. Respondents were asked to identify the size of their hospital and the region of the country in which it was located. Respondents were asked to include their name and address if they wanted a copy of the results sent to them, and were invited to submit relevant laboratory or hospital regulations, as well as any additional comments they might deem appropriate. A stamped, preaddressed return envelope was included along with an introductory letter discussing the purpose of the survey. The survey was divided into 18 questions, some of which consisted of more than one part.

For the purpose of this study, respondents were asked to consider AIDS, AIDS-related complex (ARC), and serologic evidence of infection with human immunodeficiency virus (HIV; HTLV-III) as synonymous. The specific questions are in Table 1.

RESULTS

There were 221 responses (52%), although not every respondent answered each question. Indeed, only one of the more than 40 potential questions was answered by all respondents. Two hundred twenty indicated their hospital size: 111 (51%) were from 300 bed or smaller hospitals; 60 (27%) were from hospitals of 300–600 bed size; 31 (14%) were from hospitals of 600–1000 bed size; and 18 (8%) were from institutions greater than 1000 beds in size. Of the 217 who indicated their hospital location, 25% were in the Northeast, 16% in the South, 16% in the Central zone, 13% in the Midwest, 6% in the Northwest, 8% in the Southwest, and 16% in the West. One hundred seventy-seven (80%) listed their name and address. Responses are shown in Table 1.

The data were analyzed to determine if specific trends could be discerned. Representative findings are shown in Table 2 where there is, in most instances, clearly a pattern of increasing positivity or negativity, depending on the question, and somewhat proportional to hospital size. A similar pattern, in terms of geographic location, could not be appreciated.

DISCUSSION

Analysis of the data shows a number of expected trends. The larger hospital laboratories are more likely to have developed specific procedures for dealing with AIDS, and, concommitantly, are less likely to demonstrate excessive concern in terms of this "epidemic" (Table 2).

For example, only 69% of smaller hospitals, with fewer than 300 beds, had a specific institutional policy for AIDS, and only 65% of the laboratories in this setting had a specific laboratory policy. In comparison, 88% of the more than 600 bed hospitals, and 82% of their laboratories, had developed specific policies. The medium-sized, 300–600 bed, hospitals were intermediate in this regard. Similarly, 68% of the under 300 bed hospitals and 68% of the 300–600 bed hospitals had special ways of identifying specimens. Eighty-six percent of the larger hospitals had such procedures.

The largest hospitals, in contrast, were less likely to have policies excluding personnel from working with AIDS patients or handling their specimens. None of the 18 hospitals greater than 1,000 bed size permit any personnel to refrain from AIDS contact, and only 4% of the 49 larger-than-600 bed hospitals responding excluded personnel from AIDS-related responsibilities. However, 13% of the small, and 12% of the intermediate, hospitals did exclude some employees from working with AIDS patients or their specimens. The two conditions cited most often as potentially exclusionary were pregnancy and immunodeficiency; 19% of the

TABLE I
Survey Questions and Responses

	Yes		No		Don't Know		Total
	#	(%)*	#	(%)	#	(%)	#
1. Is there a specific hospital policy for dealing with AIDS?	164	(75)	46	(21)	9	(3)	219
1a. If YES, does it include specifics about the handling of specimens?	133	(89)	12	(8)	4	(3)	149
2. Is there a specific laboratory policy concerning the handling of AIDS specimens? Please enclose a copy if available.	153	(71)	60	(28)	2	(1)	215
3. Are AIDS specimens handled using the same safety practices recommended for Hepatitis specimens?	207	(94)	12	(5)	1	(1)	220
3a. If NO, is AIDS Handled MORE or LESS cautiously?							
4. Do you have special ways of identifying specimens (blood, urine, feces, CSF, tissues, etc) submitted to the laboratory from AIDS patients?	158	(72)	58	(27)	2	(1)	218
4a. If YES, are your requisition forms specially marked?	123	(76)	37	(23)	2	(1)	162
4b. Are the specimen containers specially marked?	157	(95)	9	(5)	0	(0)	166
4c. Are these practices regularly followed?	135	(82)	20	(12)	9	(5)	164
4d. If YES, how often?							
5. Are any of your employees specifically excluded from handling AIDS patients or specimens from AIDS patients?	24	(11)	194	(88)	2	(1)	220
5a. If YES, please indicate exclusions.							
5b. Specifically, are pregnant employees excluded from working with AIDS patients or materials?	27	(19)	111	(77)	6	(4)	144
6. Are employees who may come in contact with blood, body fluids, or tissues from AIDS patients required to wear gloves when activities involve skin contact?	169	(78)	43	(20)	4	(2)	216
7. Are human serum samples which are used as controls or reagents for AIDS testing labeled with a warning statement concerning possible infectivity?	106	(66)	34	(21)	21	(13)	160
8. Are specimens (blood, urine, feces, CSF, tissues, etc.) disposed of in some manner other than that used for Hepatitis B?	23	(11)	193	(88)	3	(1)	219
8a. If YES, are specially labeled disposal containers used?	22	(63)	12	(34)	1	(3)	35
8b. Are wastes incinerated in a special manner?	21	(34)	35	(51)	5	(8)	61
8c. If YES, please describe:							
9. Are laboratory spills decontaminated in a special manner when the spill is from an AIDS patient?	90	(42)	124	(57)	2	(1)	216
10. Are AIDS specimens evaluated using the same instruments (SMAC, Coulter, Astra, etc.) as all other specimens?	201	(93)	1	(1)	15	(7)	216
10a. If YES, are the instruments subjected to special disinfecting procedures?	17	(9)	158	(86)	8	(4)	183
10b. If NO, are the specimens evaluated with manual methods?	3	(8)	24	(69)	8	(23)	35
11. Are "frozen sections" prepared from tissues removed from AIDS patients?	166	(79)	36	(17)	8	(4)	210
11a. If YES, are the cryostats subjected to special disinfecting procedures?	93	(59)	62	(39)	3	(2)	157
12. Are autopsies performed on AIDS patients?	188	(89)	19	(9)	4	(2)	211

3a. If NO, is AIDS Handled MORE or LESS cautiously?

	#	(%)
More	17	(89)
Less	2	(11)

4d. If YES, how often?

	#	(%)
25%	5	(4)
50%	33	(25)
75%	65	(49)
100%	30	(22)

TABLE I
Survey Questions and Responses— *Continued*

	Yes		No		Don't Know		Total
	#	(%)*	#	(%)	#	(%)	#
12a. If YES, do you use a special "isolation" room?	21	(11)	167	(87)	3	(2)	191
12b. Do you restrict non-essential personnel (clinicians, students, nurses, etc.) from entering the autopsy room?	157	(83)	30	(16)	3	(2)	190
12c. Do you use Hepatitis B procedures (masks, eye protection, prolonged fixation, etc.)?	179	(95)	7	(4)	2	(1)	188
12d. Do you use Jacob-Creutzfeldt procedures (masks, eye protection, NaOCl-soaked protective sheets, NaOH disinfection, etc.)?	63	(34)	117	(64)	3	(2)	183
12e. Do you use an electric saw (Stryker) for cranial dissection?	125	(71)	44	(25)	8	(4)	177
13. Have educational materials and seminars about AIDS been provided for the hospital employees?	195	(89)	10	(5)	13	(6)	218
13a. Has AIDS-education been provided especially for laboratory employees?	175	(85)	30	(14)	2	(1)	207
14. Are employees who have AIDS or ARC allowed to continue working?	99	(53)	3	(2)	84	(45)	186
14a. If NO, have you been subjected to grievance procedures?	0	(0)	9	(53)	8	(47)	17
14b. If YES, have you had morale/discipline problems with other employees?	13	(14)	50	(55)	28	(31)	91
15. Is testing for HIV (HTLV-3) antibody a required part of the preemployment examination?	3	(1)	197	(92)	13	(6)	213
16. Are serum samples from laboratory workers collected and stored for possible HIV (HTLV-3) testing as part of an on-going surveillance program?	8	(4)	196	(91)	12	(6)	216
17. If an employee refuses to work with AIDS patients or specimens, even after appropriate education and/or counseling, is dismissal likely?	85	(40)	48	(23)	79	(37)	212
18. Are you aware of any pathologist, technologist, or autopsy-room technician who has developed AIDS, ARC, or antibody to HIV (HTLV-3), other than those in one of the recognized high-risk groups?	0	(0)	216	(98)	5	(2)	221

*Percentages rounded to nearest whole number.

144 respondents to this question exclude pregnant patients. Five indicated that an employee who was an immune suppressed individual would be excused. Other indications included contagiousness of an employee, dermatitis, and other breaks in the integrity of skin. In five responses, it was noted that employees had the option of working with AIDS.

At least 11% of the responding hospitals do not perform autopsies on AIDS patients. Where an "isolation" facility is used for autopsy, it is most likely to be in a large hospital. The significance of this is not clear, since only the larger hospitals are likely to have the potential for devoting specific space for autopsies thought to be hazardous. In medical centers that have this type of facility, it is most likely used for hepatitis, as well as AIDS cases.

It is of some interest to note that only question 18 was answered by every respondent (Tables 1 and 2). Although anecdotal, it may still be of value to note that there is, thus far, no pathologist, technologist, or autopsy technician known to have developed AIDS, despite the fact that autopsies were performed on AIDS patients, in our largest cities, before the potential infectivity of this condition was recognized. This nonscienti-

TABLE II
Correlation of Hospital Size and Responses. Selected Questions

	Hospital Size (beds)	Number Responding	% Yes*	# No	% Don't Know
1. Is there a specific hospital policy for dealing with AIDS?	<300	111	69	25	6
	300–600	59	75	24	2
	600–1000	31	87	13	0
	>1000	18	89	6	6
2. Is there a specific laboratory policy concerning the handling of AIDS specimens?	<300	106	65	34	1
	300–600	59	73	27	0
	600–1000	31	81	16	3
	>1000	18	83	17	0
4. Do you have special ways of identifying specimens submitted to the laboratory from AIDS patients?	<300	109	68	31	1
	300–600	60	68	30	2
	600–1000	31	84	16	0
	>1000	18	89	11	0
5. Are any of your employees specifically excluded from handling AIDS patients or specimens from AIDS patients?	<300	110	13	85	2
	300–600	60	12	88	0
	600–1000	31	6	94	0
	>1000	18	0	100	0
12. Are autopsies performed on AIDS patients?	<300	105	86	11	3
	300–600	57	89	9	2
	600–1000	31	94	6	0
	>1000	18	100	0	0
12a. If autopsies are performed on AIDS patients, do you use a special "isolation" room?	<300	90	7	92	1
	300–600	54	9	89	2
	600–1000	29	17	79	3
	>1000	18	28	72	0

TABLE II
Correlation of Hospital Size and Responses. Selected Questions—*Continued*

	Hospital Size (beds)	Number Responding	% Yes*	# No	% Don't Know
13. Has AIDS-education been provided especially for laboratory employees?	<300	111	87	7	6
	300–600	59	92	3	5
	600–1000	30	93	7	0
	>1000	18	94	6	0
14. Are employees who have AIDS or ARC allowed to continue working?	<300	89	48	1	51
	300–600	50	52	4	44
	600–1000	30	70	0	30
	>1000	17	53	0	47

fic observation is supported by the recent literature dealing with the potential risk to health workers by contact with HIV-infected individuals.

Lifson and co-workers[16] demonstrated that virtually all of the 922 health workers reported to the Centers for Disease Control (CDC) as having AIDS belonged to recognized high-risk groups. Specific occupational exposures could not be identified for implication as the source of AIDS virus in any of the health care workers with AIDS, and they concluded that the risk of transmission of the causative virus in the occupational setting is low. Their work is confirmed by Henderson,[17] Moss,[18] and their respective coworkers who studied a total of 632 health care workers who had high exposure to AIDS patients. Included among this group were 179 who had percutaneous or mucous membrane exposures to blood or body fluids from infected individuals. None of these had serologic evidence of infection with the AIDS retrovirus, although there are isolated reports of seroconversion following needlestick[20-23] or after prolonged cutaneous exposure to a patient with AIDS.[24] Three recent incidents involving skin or mucous membrane exposure of female health-care workers to blood from HIV-infected individuals resulted in seroconversions.[25] Two of these women had skin areas whose integrity was interrupted as potential sites of contamination, and the third had mucous membrane exposure. No other risk factor could be identified in this group, although previous needle-stick exposure could not be excluded. Two of the women developed minor illnesses within 2 months of exposure, but none of them have developed AIDS as of the time of this writing.

A study of dentists and their assistants, most of whom were exposed to AIDS patients, failed to demonstrate serologic evidence of infection in any of the 255 individuals evaluated.[26] The reports cited above include more than 1,000 documented skin or mucous membrane exposures, and there have, thus far, been less than 15 instances of seroconversion. It has been emphasized that

AIDS is not a significant occupational risk[23,27] and "no health care worker in the world has contracted AIDS from a patient".[28]

How is the virus inactivated? HIV can be recovered from an aqueous environment for as long as a week, at room temperature, and for more than three days in a dried state at room temperature,[29] but is completely inactivated by heat, alcohols, formaldehyde solution, glutaraldehyde, 0.5% sodium hypochlorite (1:10 dilution of household "bleach"), phenols, and other chemicals.[29-31]

What are the recommended procedures for laboratory workers who may have contact with AIDS patients or specimens from those patients? The CDC has listed procedures to follow,[32] based on the Biosafety Level (BSL) 2 standards and special practices, equipment, and facilities as described in the CDC-NIH biosafety manual.[33] The summary statement emphasizes that "these are the same practices recommended for all clinical specimens".[32] Almost 20 of our survey respondents noted that they approach AIDS cases as they do hepatitis cases. This is clearly the single most prudent philosophy to follow. As we have discussed, the risk of seroconversion after percutaneous exposure is almost nonexistent,[20-23] and there is, thus far, no risk of acquiring AIDS by occupational exposure.[28] In contrast, the risk of hepatitis B infection, after needle-stick, may be as high as 30%.[34]

Two of the 221 respondents noted that their hospitals had not yet had a case of known AIDS. A small number noted that they had not yet been asked to perform an autopsy or a frozen section consultation on an AIDS patient; two of these specifically recorded that they would do so if requested. Only one respondent indicated that he would not perform an autopsy on an AIDS patient. Two others indicated that they would not perform an autopsy if the diagnosis was already confirmed, and three indicated that they only performed "limited" autopsies. It should, by now, be well recog-

nized, especially by pathologists, that many "confirmed" diagnoses are incorrect.[35-39] We believe that failure to perform an autopsy on any patient who dies in the hospital is a violation of our finest traditions of scientific inquiry and of the principles of true "quality assurance" for the practice of medicine. Further, there are no facts to support the failure to perform any diagnostic procedure in terms of degree of risk of these patients.

Geberding[7] has convincingly demonstrated that all possible strategies for implementing infection-control procedures in dealing with HIV-infected patients in the hospital setting will fail, for scientific, logistical, economic, and ethical reasons. She also clearly notes that "existing guidelines for reducing exposure to blood and body fluids will protect workers who care for patients with this pathogen." This statement is equally true for the laboratory.

Hensley,[40] in response to our survey, noted that it is the policy of the Broward County, Florida, Medical Examiner's Office to perform autopsies on all known victims of AIDS. In addition, they are engaged in a project, jointly with the CDC, to study sera for the presence of HIV-antibody on all persons undergoing autopsy at that facility. Results to date reveal that only about 15% of HIV-infected persons were diagnosed as AIDS or ARC during life. Hensley emphasizes that, if special precautions were taken only on those known to be HIV-antibody positive, 85% of the risk of transmission would be ignored.

Seventy-two percent of respondents identified their AIDS-patients' specimens in a special way, usually with a warning label. We, and others,[41] believe that this practice is incorrect, and potentially dangerous. Every form of patient contact must be considered to be a potential source of infection by HIV, hepatitis, and other pathogenic organisms.

We have not commented on all aspects of this survey, including some of the personnel issues queried. Forty-five percent of the respondents to question 14 did not know their institutional policy about continuing employment by workers who have AIDS or ARC. Thirty-one percent of those answering question 14b did not know about morale or discipline problems among employees working with AIDS individuals. This may be, in large part, because this problem is not yet prevalent in many cities. There is no doubt that many hospitals will soon be faced with these kinds of problems. It is likely that existing laws that pertain to handicapped and disabled persons will be used for the protection of AIDS patients.[42] Recommendations for developing guidelines have been made.[43]

Educational efforts need to be expanded, and concepts revised in the face of current knowledge. Pathologists and other laboratory workers are appropriately regarded as the bridge between the art and the science of medicine and must continue to accumulate and act upon available knowledge. In the case of AIDS, this can contribute to more appropriate practices in the hospital setting, and will help to control the elements of fear that may interfere with rational and humane practices and the maintainance of the highest levels of medical practice.

ACKNOWLEDGMENTS

Jeanne Shirley, MT, ASCP, and W. Stephen Nichols, M.D. provided useful suggestions in the preparation of the survey. David P. Geller developed the printed form used in the survey. Randy Garrett and Brenda Bell assured the timely distribution of the survey. Claire Berman assisted immeasurably in the evaluation of the data.

REFERENCES

1. Centers for Disease Control. *Pneumocystis* pneumonia — Los Angeles. MMWR 1981; 30:250 – 252
2. Centers for Disease Control. Kaposi's sarcoma and *Pneumocystis* pneumonia among homosexual men — New York City and California. MMWR 1981; 30:305 – 308
3. Gallo RC: The first human retrovirus. Sci Amer 1986; 255:88 – 98
4. Gallo RC: The AIDS virus. Sci Amer 1987; 256:46 – 56
5. Valenti WM, Anarella JP: Survey of hospital personnel on the understanding of the acquired immunodeficiency syndrome. Am J Infect Control 1986; 14:60 – 63
6. Levine C: AIDS: Public health and civil liberties. Hastings Cent Rep 1986; Dec (suppl):1 – 36
7. Geberding JL: Recommended infection-control policies for patients with human immunodeficiency virus infection. N Engl J Med 1986; 315:1562 – 1564
8. Bayer R, Levine C, Wolf SM: HIV antibody screening. An ethical framework for evaluating proposed programs. JAMA 1986; 256:1768 – 1674
9. Wachter RM: The impact of the acquired immunodeficiency syndrome on medical residency training. N Engl J Med 1986; 314:177 – 180
10. Eckholm E: AIDS, an unknown disease before 1981, grows into a worldwide scourge. NY Times, April 16, 1987, p 11
11. Hardy AM, Rauch K, Echenberg D, et al: The economic impact of the first 10,000 cases of acquired immunodeficiency syndrome in the United States. JAMA 1986; 255:209 – 211
12. Opinion. Who pays for AIDS? Nature 1986; 321:548
13. Scitovsky AA, Cline M, Lee PR: Medical care costs of patients with AIDS in San Francisco. JAMA 1986; 256:3103 – 3106
14. Seage GR, Landers S, Barry A, et al: Medical care costs of AIDS in Massachusetts. JAMA 1986: 256:3107 – 3109
15. Sande MA: Transmission of AIDS. The case against casual contagion. N Engl J Med 1986; 314:380 – 382
16. Lifson AR, Castro KG, McCray E, Jaffe HW: National surveillance of AIDS in health care workers. JAMA 1986; 256:3231 – 3234
17. Henderson DK, Saah AJ, Zak BJ, et al: Risk of nosocomial infection with human T-cell lymphotropic virus type III/lymphadenopathy-associated virus in a large cohort of intensively exposed health care workers. Ann Intern Med 1986; 104:644 – 647
18. Moss A, Osmond D, Bacchetti P, et al: Risk of seroconversion for acquired immunodeficiency syndrome (AIDS) in San Francisco health workers. J Occup Med 1986; 28:821 – 824
19. Goudreau R: Experts say doctors burying clues to understanding AIDS. Orlando Sentinel, Sept 29, 1986, pp. A1, A8
20. Anonymous: Needlestick transmission of HTLV-III from a patient infected in Africa. Lancet 1984; 2:1376 – 1377
21. Weiss SH, Saxinger C, Rechtman D, et al: HTLV-III infection among health care workers. JAMA 1985; 254:2089 – 2093
22. Stricoff RL, Morse DL: HTLV-III/LAV seroconversion following a deep intramuscular needlestick injury. N Engl J Med 1986; 314:1115
23. McCray E, and the Cooperative Needlestick Surveillance Group: Occupational risk of the acquired immunodeficiency syndrome among health care workers. N Engl J Med 1986; 314:1127 – 1132

24. Grint P, McEvoy M: Two associated cases of the acquired immune deficiency syndrome (AIDS). Communicable Dis Rep 1985; 42:4

25. Centers for Disease Control. Update: Human immunodeficiency virus infections in health-care workers exposed to blood of infected patients. MMWR 1987; 36:285–289

26. Flynn NM, Pollet SM, Van Horne JR, et al: Absence of HIV antibody among dental professionals exposed to infected patients. West J Med 1987; 146:439–442

27. Decker MD, Schaffner W: Risk of AIDS to health care workers. JAMA 1986; 256:3264–3265

28. Geddes AM: Risk of AIDS to health care workers. Br Med J 1986; 292:711–712

29. Resnick L, Veren K, Salahuddin Z, et al: Stability and inactivation of HTLV-III/LAV under clinical and laboratory environments. JAMA 1985; 255:1887–1891

30. Spire B, Barre-Sinoussi F, Montagnier L, Chermann, JC: Inactivation of lymphadenopathy associated virus by chemical disinfectants. Lancet 1984; 2:899–901

31. Martin LS, McDougal JS, Laskoski SL: Disinfection and inactivation of the human T lymphotropic virus type III/lymphadenopathy-associated virus. J Infect Dis 1985; 152:400–403

32. Centers for Disease Control: Human T-lymphotropic virus type III/lymphadenopathy associated virus: Agent summary statement. MMWR 1986; 35:540–549

33. Richardson JH, Barkley WE: Biosafety in microbiological and biomedical laboratories. Washington, DC: US Department of Health and Human Services, Public Health Service. HHS Publication no. (CDC) 86-8395, 1986; pp 11–13

34. Crossley K: Acquired immunodeficiency syndrome: Recommendations to prevent transmission for hospitals and health care workers. Minn Med 1986; 69:211–213

35. Goldman L, Sayson R, Robbins S, et al: The value of the autopsy in three medical eras. N Engl J Med 1983; 308:1000–1005

36. Zarling EJ, Sexton H, Milnor P: Failure to diagnose acute myocardial infarction. JAMA 1983; 250:1177–1181

37. Scottolini AG, Weinstein SR: The autopsy in clinical quality control. JAMA 1983; 250:1192–1194

38. Kircher T, Nelson J, Burdo H: The autopsy as a measure of accuracy of the death certificate. N Engl J Med 1985; 313:1263–1269

39. Bedell SE, Fulton EJ: Unexpected findings and complications at autopsy after cardiopulmonary resuscitation (CPR). Arch Intern Med 1986; 146:1725–1728

40. Hensley GT: Personal communication, 1987

41. Lipsky BA, McDonald LL, Vracko R, Tenover FC: Letter. Clin Microbiol Newsletter, February, 1987; p 15

42. Klein CA: AIDS and employment issues. Nurse Pract 1986; 11:87–90

43. Dong A: Health care employees with AIDS—set policies before problems arise. Dimens Health Serv 1986; 63:43

17

Defining and Implementing a National AIDS Prevention Strategy

Stephen C. Joseph

NO OTHER PUBLIC HEALTH CRISIS in recent history has challenged us on so many fronts and on such a scale as the AIDS epidemic. In New York City alone, as of June 1988, over 15,000 people have been diagnosed with AIDS since 1981, 23% of the national total. More than 7,800 have died. AIDS is the current leading cause of death in New York City among men aged 25–44 and women aged 25–34.[1]

In the first three months of 1988, the number of AIDS cases reported among IV drug abusers in New York City surpassed the number of cases among gay men in quarter-by-quarter analysis. While the numbers of both groups are increasing, the proportion of AIDS cases attributable to IV drug abuse is also increasing.[2]

Currently, upwards of 200,000 people in New York City are estimated to be infected with the human immunodeficiency virus (HIV), including some 50,000 gay and bisexual men, 120,000 intravenous drug abusers, and 23,000 to 36,000 women and heterosexual men without a history of IV drug abuse. The IV drug abuser is the primary source of the rise in HIV infection in women and children in New York City. Eighty percent of the 1,733 women with AIDS in New York City have been IV drug abusers or sex partners of IV drug abusers.

Most of the 325 children diagnosed with AIDS in New York City were infected from their mothers, 80% of whom were IV drug abusers or the sex partners of IV drug abusers. Between 300 and 800 HIV-infected children are estimated to be born in New York City each year.

The connection between AIDS, drugs, and poverty in New York City means that the epidemic is hitting minority communities especially hard. Thirty-one percent of the city's AIDS cases are among blacks; 23% are among Hispanics. Eighty-six percent of male IV drug abusers with AIDS, and 90% of the mothers of children with AIDS, are black or Hispanic.

Initially, AIDS was believed to be a disease of homosexual men and IV drug abusers. Subsequently, attention has turned to what was believed to be a "hidden epidemic": huge numbers of infected heterosexuals whose symptoms have not yet been observed. Further epidemiologic investigation and early results of serological surveys have shown, however, that HIV infection in heterosexuals is primarily linked to exposure to IV drug abusers or bisexual men. We have little current evidence for secondary or tertiary spread among heterosexuals, in contrast, for example, to the situation in Africa. This current interpretation of the data, however, does not negate the fact that there is a large pool of infected people in New York City, and that such a large pool does increase the probabilities of HIV spread through heterosexual sex. At particular risk are sex partners of IV drug abusers, who are mostly female and minority group members.

According to our best current projections, more than 43,000 people will have developed full-blown AIDS in New York City by the end of 1991; 32,000 will have died. More AIDS cases will have been diagnosed in New York City in the single year of 1991 than have shown up from 1981 through 1986.

Among men, close to 37,000 cumulative AIDS cases are projected for 1991, compared with 6,000 for women. By 1991, women will have accounted for 13% of the total cases, compared with 10 percent presently. Gay and bisexual men will represent 24,000 cases in 1991, 56% of the total. Among IV drug abusers, 14,500 cumulative cases are projected, 34% of the total.[3]

These projections are based on the assumption that the rates of the last 6 months will continue as a constant over the next 4 years. They reflect only cases already counted using the current standard case definition. Cases of AIDS-related illness can be estimated by multiplying adult incident cases of AIDS by ten, and pediatric cases by three.

The import of these projections is clear: The impact of AIDS on our citizens, our hospitals, and our cities will be beyond that of any modern public health crisis.

AIDS already poses serious and complex challenges to New York City: Understanding the causes and patterns of infection; controlling the spread of HIV; protecting individuals and families from AIDS-related discrimination and harassment; and providing those who are sick from the disease with appropriate levels of medical care and social service support. Irrespective of development of a vaccine or effective treatment, increasing resources will be needed for intensive prevention, health, and social service interventions.

To date, more AIDS patients have been hospitalized in New York City than we thought we would see until 1990. On any given day, more than 1,500 people with AIDS or AIDS-related illnesses occupy New York City hospital beds, including over 500 in municipal hospitals. With less than one-fourth of New York City's medical and surgical beds, the municipal hospital system, the Health and Hospitals Corporation (HHC), now provides care for 37% of the City's hospitalized AIDS patients. HHC's HIV-related patient census is expected to rise by at least 20% annually, including a disproportionately high share of substance abusers: three-quarters of the patients with AIDS at HHC hospitals contracted the virus from IV drug abuse, including direct IV drug abuse, sexual contact with an IV drug abuser, or being born to an IV drug abuser or their sex partner.

HHC programs for the increasing numbers of people with AIDS include AIDS-related assessment, a full continuity of inpatient and outpatient medical care, and extended care services. The interdisciplinary health care team is the core of inpatient services for persons with AIDS, providing continuity of care in HHC hospitals that see the largest number of people with AIDS. Bellevue Hospital, which has the largest average daily census of AIDS patients in the HHC system, has established a designated AIDS unit. The AIDS Long Term Care Program at Coler and Goldwater Hospitals remains the only significant source of institutionalized long-term care services to persons with AIDS in New York City, and one of only two such settings in the nation. An issue particular to people with AIDS in a long-term care facility is their need for substance abuse treatment while in the facility.

A community-based clinic, operated at the Community Health Project in coordination with Bellevue, provides a thorough physical and psychosocial assessment to members of risk groups who have AIDS-related illness. The City will open additional AIDS assessment centers in other areas of the City shortly, focusing on drug treatment and women's health services. Close to 800 patients are currently enrolled in a City-funded azidothymidine (AZT) treatment program at HHC facilities.

Half of the City's reported cases of AIDS in children have been treated at HHC facilities; 7% of HHC AIDS patients are children. A significant number of these children are orphans, abandoned, or lack family support structures and must remain in the hospital. They are difficult to place in foster care because of the stigma of AIDS. To help encourage their normal development and offer them routine medical monitoring, New York City has opened the nation's first pediatric day care program for children with AIDS.

New York City provides emergency shelter, and assists in housing-related matters, as well as AIDS-related problems with family and children's services, through the Human Resources Administration (HRA). A pilot AIDS Family Case Management Unit will tailor services to the income, housing, home care, and counseling needs of families where one or more persons has AIDS. A special social service unit assists persons with AIDS in all hospitals. HRA also runs an AIDS Helpline for information on public assistance, food stamps, and home care for persons with AIDS or AIDS-related conditions. Every month New York City provides housing, home care, and hospice services to about 1,000 people who are not in need of inpatient care. New York City has opened one of the first foster care programs for children with AIDS, and will establish a day nursery for children up to the age of five.

The Department of Mental Health is developing outpatient clinics and day-treatment services for persons with AIDS, as well as for families and friends affected by the AIDS crisis. The AIDS Discrimination Unit of the New York City Human Rights Commission is handling an increasing number of complaints of AIDS-related discrimination; last year, the Unit received 314 complaints, up from three complaints in 1983.

Against this background of response, and as the epidemic spreads, a number of critical public health policy issues have emerged.

We must increase massive public health education risk-reduction efforts. The New York City Department of Health has a multifaceted prevention and risk-reduction strategy that directs education at the general public, health and social service providers, and community groups, and targets outreach to people engaged in high-risk behavior.

The first in a series of explicit, hard-hitting, multimedia advertising campaigns promotes the use of condoms among heterosexuals as a means of preventing the transmission of AIDS. This campaign is extremely bold, incorporating many harsh facts that the media have chosen to ignore. It directly addresses the "safer sex with condoms" issue. Attention-getting and controversial, the campaign's arresting message is summed up by the tagline: "AIDS, if you think you can't get it, you're dead wrong." We have launched a second campaign directed at IV drug abusers, and a third campaign encouraging abstinence among adolescents.

We are also increasing outreach to people practicing high-risk behavior. Public health educators take their message of prevention into neighborhoods where IV drug abuse is concentrated to reach IV drug abusers and their sex partners, and we work with many city-wide and local organizations to reach those at risk through IV drug abuse.

Approximately half of the roughly 100,000 people who move through the New York City Correctional system each year are current or former IV drug abusers; 50–60% of these people are estimated to be HIV-positive. A joint program between the Departments of Health and Correction educates jail inmates about AIDS and distributes condoms to those at highest risk of infection, to slow transmission inside and outside of jail. Prison Health Services offer City jail inmates risk-reduction counseling and voluntary, confidential testing for HIV antibodies as part of our ongoing AIDS education and prevention program.

A public health education program targets the "sex industry" to reach people before they take part in unsafe sex. Public health educators distribute educational literature and condoms at sex clubs, massage parlors, and other places where patrons seek multiple sex encounters or unsafe sex.

We must rapidly and extensively increase voluntary, confidential risk-reduction counseling and HIV antibody testing. These measures help people to assess their risk for HIV infection, understand their HIV antibody status, and incorporate that knowledge into their behavior. Because testing requires counselors trained to help people understand the results and reduce the risk of transmitting the virus, compulsory testing for any groups is likely to be counterproductive. In New York City, our policy is that anyone should be able to know his or her antibody status, provided the test results are confidential, testing is voluntary, and counseling is available before and after testing.[4]

Testing in New York City is available through free, anonymous test sites; through any licensed physician; and at Health Department Sexually Transmitted Disease Clinics. Anonymous HIV testing sites are open in all five boroughs; the HIV screening capacity of our laboratories will more than double. Counselors in our contact notification program urge people who are HIV-infected to notify their contacts, and directly and actively assist them to do this when asked. We will shortly begin to offer contact notification services to AIDS and ARC patients of private physicians.

Physicians in New York City must accept a much larger responsibility in helping to contain the spread of HIV infection. Thus far, fewer than 3,000 of the more than 25,000 New York City physicians have sent blood specimens of at least one of their patients to our lab for testing. Every physician in New York must actively consider if patients are at risk of AIDS infection, must discuss risk-avoiding behavior as part of routine medical care of all patients, and must offer counseling and, where appropriate, testing to patients at risk.

As we call for counseling and testing of more people, and as more people seek information about their health status, the demand for counseling and testing has rapidly exceeded service supply. We need increased support to make voluntary, confidential counseling, testing sites, and opportunities more widely available. Expanded testing requires investments in money and trained personnel; the lack of trained counselors is now the critical constraint to the rapid expansion of testing nationwide.

We must increase efforts to break the connection between AIDS and substance abuse. AIDS prevention efforts must be linked to drug treatment programs and public health education programs to reach this difficult population. The future of the epidemic in New York and elsewhere in the nation lies here.

We are revising a proposal for a research project with the State Health Commissioner to study the effect of the availability of clean needles to a small, carefully selected and monitored group of IV drug addicts—a population that otherwise does not have much contact with a medical system. The data from such a research project will help us decide if laws in New York City prohibiting the possession of injection equipment without prescription need to be changed to help stem the spread of infection.

We must expand our knowledge base. The projections of the future course of AIDS mean that we must increase our surveillance and research. We must continue to investigate the nature of HIV and its transmission. as well as to assess how well risk-reduction messages change behavior.

We must eliminate the false dichotomy between civil liberties and public health. Our opposition to mandatory antibody testing does not sacrifice public health in the name of civil liberties or individual privacy. Public health officials have been virtually unanimous in agreeing that control measures such as mandatory testing would be an inefficient use of resources, and would drive people away from our public health system. HIV-infected people already face devastating discrimination in housing, employment, and insurance. They would not cooperate with our education, counseling, and testing if they feared measures that could lead to additional discrimination or quarantine.

Finally, we must increase coordinated planning, programming, and funding at the federal, state, and local levels. An Interagency Task Force coordinates the City's AIDS programs and services. This group recently delivered its first "Report to the Mayor," describing the range of programs thus far in response to the epidemic.[5]

Controlling the AIDS crisis requires the cooperation of the entire public and private sector. The City has initiated contracts with community organizations such as the Association for Drug Abuse, Prevention, and Treatment to reach drug abusers and their sex partners, as well as other contracts to groups for reaching Hispanics, blacks, and young homosexuals.

City agencies take part in the AIDS Service Delivery Consortium with state agencies, voluntary hospitals, and community-based organizations to develop a comprehensive strategy for managing the AIDS epidemic in the city. The Consortium will receive approximately $10 million in grant funds over a four-year period from the U.S. Public Health Service and the Robert Wood Johnson Foundation for improving and expanding services to persons with AIDS in New York City.

Spending for AIDS treatment, testing, counseling, education, and other programs in New York City in fiscal 1988 will be over $385 million, of which $98 million is City funds. This is up from $250 million, $75 million of which is City tax levy, in Fiscal 1987. In 1989, we project continuing increases in City funding for AIDS programs,

as well as a significant rise in AIDS funding for New York City from federal sources.

Even this will not be enough to keep up with the unrelenting progress of the epidemic. We have been fortunate in New York City to have the constant and vigorous support of the Mayor for our policy and program initiatives, including the more controversial ones. Analogous leadership has not been demonstrated at the federal level. A significant federal commitment is long overdue.

We need nothing less than a bold, effective, and comprehensive national prevention strategy. It must be directed at barring the spread of the virus among heterosexuals, as well as reducing the toll among homosexual men, IV drug abusers, and their sex partners and children.

Proposals by the national leadership for mandatory testing of small groups of people will do little to control the spread of infection among the majority of Americans who are at risk. Equally as unfortunate, they may divert our attention from where the real battles against AIDS ought to be fought.

Defining and implementing a national prevention strategy is already within our reach. It includes three major elements:

1. *A massive national public health education program.* This must consist of an "outer shell" of information to the general public, and an "inner shell" of targeted education for people practicing high-risk behavior. People *can* protect themselves against getting, and giving, AIDS—but we must discuss AIDS issues honestly, explicitly, and repeatedly.

2. *Rapid expansion of voluntary, confidential counseling and HIV antibody testing into every public and private clinical facility,* including physicians' offices, hospital outpatient departments, sexually transmitted disease clinics, family planning and abortion clinics, and publicly-funded anonymous test sites. Counseling and voluntary testing *do*

help people adopt risk-avoiding behavior. Along with education, these are our best current weapons against AIDS.

3. *Major efforts to curtail AIDS transmission via IV drug abuse.* There will be no slowing the spread of the AIDS virus or preventing its seepage into the heterosexual community without a meaningful war on drugs. Efforts must range from interdiction at the international level, to law enforcement at all levels, to more education programs, increased and liberalized methadone maintenance, and rapid and massive detoxification programs, plus availability of clean needle exchange. AIDS prevention efforts should include wide availability of needles and syringes in states where prescriptions are not needed to buy or distribute them.

A national prevention strategy demands a "moon-shot," war-footing approach to federal resource commitment, guided by aggressive, articulate, and visible leadership from the highest levels of the federal administration. With the exception of the outstanding example of Surgeon General Koop, that leadership has so far been lacking.

Our time is running out. If we do not institute a vigorous and comprehensive national prevention program within the next 18–24 months, we will fall behind in the epidemic among heterosexuals as we have with gay men and IV drug abusers. On the other hand, seizing the opportunity today would save large numbers of lives and substantially reduce the enormous burdens and costs that will be associated with the epidemic extending into the mid-1990s.

The time has come to center the national debate upon adoption of a national prevention strategy that works. Those of us in a position to influence policy must advance such a strategy against this mounting health problem in New York City and across the country.

REFERENCES

1. New York City AIDS surveillance data, New York City Department of Health, 1988
2. New York City AIDS surveillance data, New York City Department of Health, 1988
3. Office of Epidemiology, Surveillance, and Statistics, New York City Department of Health, 1988
4. HIV Counseling and Testing Policy, New York City Department of Health, March, 1987
5. AIDS IN NEW YORK CITY, Report to the Mayor from the Interagency Task Force on AIDS, April, 1987

Index